Human disease for dentistry

Human disease for dentistry

Farida Fortune

Professor of Oral Medicine
St Bartholomew's and
The London School of Medicine and Dentistry
London, UK

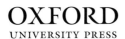
OXFORD
UNIVERSITY PRESS

OXFORD

UNIVERSITY PRESS

Great Clarendon Street, Oxford OX2 6DP

Oxford University Press is a department of the University of Oxford.
It furthers the University's objective of excellence in research, scholarship,
and education by publishing worldwide in

Oxford New York

Auckland Bangkok Buenos Aires Cape Town Chennai
Dar es Salaam Delhi Hong Kong Istanbul Karachi Kolkata
Kuala Lumpur Madrid Melbourne Mexico City Mumbai Nairobi
São Paulo Shanghai Taipei Tokyo Toronto

Oxford is a registered trade mark of Oxford University Press
in the UK and in certain other countries

Published in the United States
by Oxford University Press Inc., New York

A catalogue record for this title is available from the British Library

ISBN 0 19 263163 2 (pbk)

10 9 8 7 6 5 4 3 2 1

Typeset by Newgen Imaging Systems (P) Ltd., Chennai, India
Printed in Italy
on acid-free paper by
Legoprint S.p.A.

Contents

1 Patient assessment and surgical care

PATIENT ASSESSMENT

Patient assessment should be carried out on all patients before any procedure in the dental setting, whether in the general dental surgery under local anaesthetic, conscious sedation, or on premises licensed for use of general anaesthesia.

The assessment of the dental patient is very important. The purpose of the patient assessment is to:

- Establish rapport and effective lines of communication with the patient.
- Allay fear and anxiety.
- Obtain a current and past medical and dental history.
- Note current medication, responses to local or other anaesthetic agents, and allergies.
- Undertake an appropriate examination when necessary.
- Order special investigations or refer the patient for a specialist opinion before proceeding with treatment, if appropriate.
- Address issues of informed consent.
- Assess the risk of procedure for a particular patient at a point in time.

The ASA (American Society of Anesthesiologists) Physical Status Classification (Box 1.1) provides a useful tool in routine outpatient and inpatient dental care in the assessment of all patients. It helps to assess the risk of an untoward incident occurring during a patient treatment visit.

BOX 1.1 The ASA Physical Status Classification

I. Healthy patient

II. Patient with mild, controlled, functionally non-limiting systemic disease. Examples are well-controlled diabetes, hypertension, and epilepsy. A pregnant woman also falls into this category.

III. Patient with severe or poorly controlled systemic disease that is functionally limiting. Examples are poorly controlled diabetes, hypertension, epilepsy, and angina.

IV. Patient with severe systemic disease that is a constant threat to life. Examples are recent a cardiac event or surgery. These patients are usually inpatients who tend only to need emergency dental treatment.

V. Moribund patient not expected to survive 24 h with or without surgery.

PREOPERATIVE ASSESSMENT

Dental surgeons working in a hospital environment or special centres may have to assess patients preoperatively. The aim of the assessment is to detect, and treat if necessary, any risk factors before an anaesthetic or sedation procedure. The dental and medical history and examination of the patient are very important and should be carried out for all patients. History sheets given to patients can have limitations, unless preliminary information is checked and acted upon by the dentist.

The history

The dental surgeon should do a systems review checking the cardiovascular, respiratory, gastrointestinal, urogenital, and central nervous system. Important points to note are:

- Cardiac symptoms of pain, palpitations, or loss of consciousness.
- Shortness of breath at rest, sitting, standing, or lying, or on exertion.
- Congenital or other cardiac valvular defects, rheumatic fever, hypertension, or operations.
- Chest diseases including tuberculosis, asthma, and bronchitis.
- History of diabetes mellitus.
- History of gastrointestinal disease.
- Medication, including contraception and hormone replacement therapy (HRT), and allergies.
- Personal or family history of abnormal bleeding or bruising.
- Deep vein thrombosis or pulmonary emboli.
- Blood disorders or anaemia.
- Jaundice.
- Hepatitis status.
- Kidney or bladder problems.
- History of diseases affecting the nervous system.
- History of fits or faints.
- History of psychiatric disorders including depression.
- Previous operations or serious illness.
- Social history including addictions, e.g. alcohol, drugs, and tobacco.

The examination

The examination should include the following:

- Careful examination of the head and neck area.
- Neck mobility.
- Vital signs including pulse, blood pressure, and respiratory rate.
- Signs of heart failure.
- Sites for venous access.
- Oral access.
- Dental charting including prosthesis and presence of crown and bridgework.

Investigations

- Plain chest X-ray.
- Resting electrocardiogram (ECG).
- Full blood count and renal function (urea and electrolytes).
- Liver function tests (LFTs).
- Sickledex test if required.
- Random blood glucose.
- Dipstick test of the urine.
- Blood gases for ASA status II and III only.
- Lung function tests for ASA status II and III only.
- Haemostasis including international normalized ratio (INR), prothrombin time (PT), and partial thromboplastin time (PTT).
- Pregnancy test if required.

Dentists should be mindful of the NICE guidelines on preoperative tests: *The Use of Routine Preoperative Tests for Elective Surgery* (June 2003, for review June 2007).

CONSENT

Consent is the explanation given to the patient by the dentist before carrying out a procedure with the patient's agreement. Consent is based on the principle that each human being controls his/her own life and therefore has a right to determine what happens to their health and well-being. Treatment without consent is a crime unless in the best interest of the patient, e.g. in an emergency.

The Human Rights Act 1998 came into force in October 2000. Patients are protected by the European Convention on Human Rights (Box 1.2).

If a dentist carries out treatment without providing essential information about all aspects of the treatment carried out, this breeches the respect for private life and freedom of expression, including the right to receive and impart information. The explanation should take into account the patient's age, physical and mental state of health, intellect, beliefs, and culture.

Consent may be explicit, i.e. verbal or written, and may also be implied. Explicit consent applies to a treatment that has been explained to the patient. The patient should understand the information, formulate a decision based on the information provided, and give written or verbal consent. Implicit consent applies to treatment carried out when a patient by their action or behaviour

---

BOX 1.2 Articles of the European Convention on Human Rights relevant to consent

Article 3: prohibition of torture and inhuman and degrading treatment and punishment.
Article 8: right to respect for family life.
Article 9: freedom of thought, conscience, and religion.
Article 10: freedom of expression, which includes the right to receive and impart information.

and acting on general information does not object to a treatment. Examples are sitting in the chair and opening the mouth for local anaesthetic.

Legal constraints are pertinent. All dentists must familiarize themselves with the issues surrounding consent.

There are four parts to informed consent: sufficient explanation and information about treatment, the opportunity to ask questions, capacity, and its voluntary nature.

Sufficient explanation and information about treatment

The information should be given in language that is easily understood by the patient. The information should be of such a nature that the patient is informed fully and fairly leading them to be able to make an informed decision before agreeing to treatment. If any documents are involved they should be in plain, easily understood English.

All known risks should be communicated. This may be difficult, but should cover all significant risks and small risks with significant consequences. However, there is no requirement in English law that all risks, side-effects, and complications must be explained. Guidance may be obtained from The Senate of Surgery document published in 1998 entitled 'The surgeon's duty of care: guidance for surgeons on legal and ethical issues'. It states that a surgeon should:

. . . inform adult patients aged 16 and above of the nature of their condition, along with the type, purpose, prognosis, common side effects and significant risk of any proposed surgical treatments. Where appropriate, alternative treatment options (including non-surgical) should also be explained together with the consequences of no treatment. This information should be provided in the detail required by a reasonable person in the circumstances of the patient to make a relevant and informed judgment. . . .

The following bodies have given rulings relevant to views on 'sufficient information':

- The House of Lords ruled: Information given is a matter of medical opinion.
- The Law Lords ruled: Patients should be informed of substantial risk of grave consequences and be put in a position to make a balanced judgement.
- The Court of Appeal ruled recently: A doctor should normally inform a patient of significant risks which might affect the judgement of a reasonable patient.

The legal standard used when deciding if sufficient information was given to a patient is the same as when deciding if a dentist has been negligent in treating a patient. The 'Bolam test' is applied, i.e. if the treatment given conformed to a responsible body of medical opinion held by practitioners skilled in that field. Care should be taken in applying this principle, as the Court has been shown to be capable of being critical of a 'responsible body' of medical opinion.

The opportunity to ask questions

The dentist must give the patient an opportunity to ask questions, and must answer all queries. The dentist should be careful to disclose all the risks relevant to the patient's treatment in an understandable way.

Capacity

This is a legal term. It is the ability to comprehend, retain information, and weigh up the pros and cons of a suggested treatment:

- Anyone under the age of 18 (age of consent) but above 16 may give consent. They do not have the capacity to refuse consent.
- A minor under the age of 16 years may give consent if they understand both the nature of the treatment as well as the risks and possible complications. They are said to be 'Gillick competent'. The minor does not have the capacity to refuse treatment, although parents or the legal guardian cannot override the refusal to treatment which has to be determined by the Court.
- Parents or a legal guardian may give consent on behalf of a minor under the age of 16 and not Gillick competent.
- In those who are under capacity (mental, intellectual, or unconscious) and not a minor, consent except in an emergency has to be obtained from the Court.

Voluntary nature of consent

Sufficient information must be given to enable the patient to give consent freely and without duress. Any coercion will invalidate consent. The dentist providing the treatment should seek consent: the Department of Health Reference Guide to Consent for Examination and Treatment published in March 2001 states '. . . seeking consent may be delegated to another health professional, as long as that professional is suitably trained and qualified. . . . Inappropriate delegation . . . may mean 'consent' obtained is not valid.'

INTEROPERATIVE ASSESSMENT

It is important to monitor the vital signs during the procedure. Whether patients are being treated under local anaesthesia, sedation, or general anaesthesia constant vigilance to the state of the patient's well-being is required:

- Be vigilant and recognize early any signs of complications.
- Monitor vital signs such as blood pressure, pulse, and breathing.
- Monitor swallowing and check for gagging.
- Monitor the patient's level of consciousness.
- Check any intravenous lines or tubes if present.
- Maintain the patient's comfort with good local anaesthesia.
- Good positioning of the dental chair is essential.
- Monitor and constantly check any equipment being used.

POSTOPERATIVE ASSESSMENT

Recovery from a dental procedure can be a traumatic experience for patients. Dental procedures done under general anaesthetic or sedation may increase postoperative morbidity. Recovery entails the ability of the body's biochemical and physiological homeostatic mechanisms to return the patient to normal. Each unit should have a procedure to be able to assess that the patient can safely return to their home environment.

The protocols for postoperative discharge must be able to assess early recovery of vital signs which should be stable throughout, and whether the patient is fit to be discharged home. Several scoring methods are available. Both the Steward score and the modified Aldrete scoring system below have been adapted from Alexander Goodwin's 'Assessment for recovery in day stay' (Bath United Hospital, Bath, UK):

The Steward score

This method may be appropriate for patients having inhalation sedation. It is simple to administer in a dental practice environment. The Steward score assesses consciousness, the airway, and movement. The patient requires a score of 6 points before they can be discharged (Table 1.1).

Modified Aldrete scoring system

This assesses activity, respiration, circulation, consciousness, and oxygen saturation and may be considered when setting protocols to evaluate patients who have undergone intravenous sedation (Table 1.2). Nine or more points are required for recovery to be confirmed.

Table 1.1 The Steward score

Status	Score
Consciousness:	
Fully awake	2
Responding to stimuli	1
Not responding to stimuli	0
Airway:	
Coughing on command or crying	2
Maintaining a good airway	1
Airway needs maintenance	0
Movement:	
Moving limbs purposefully	2
Non-purposeful movement	1
Not moving	0

Table 1.2 The Modified Aldrete scoring system

Activity	Score
Movement—able to move, voluntarily or on command:	
Four extremities	2
Two extremities	1
No extremities	0
Respiration:	
Able to breathe deeply and cough freely	2
Dyspnoea, shallow, or limited breathing	1
Apnoea	0
Circulation:	
Blood pressure within 20 mmHg of preoperative level	2
Blood pressure within 20–50 mmHg of preoperative level	1
Blood pressure ±50 mmHg of preoperative level	0
Consciousness:	
Fully awake	2
Arousable on calling	1
Unresponsive	0
Oxygen saturation:	
Saturation >92%	2
Needs oxygen to maintain saturation >90%	1
Saturation <90% with oxygen	0

Before sending a patient home the patient must make their own assessment of their confidence to be discharged. If they do not feel well enough to go home, irrespective of the vital signs and scoring systems, their wishes should be respected.

Before discharge home make sure the vital signs have been stable for at least 1 h. The patient must be able to:

- orientate themselves in person, place, and time
- keep oral fluids down
- walk without assistance
- pass urine.

The patient must not have:

- pyrexia
- any nausea and vomiting
- excessive pain
- any active bleeding
- headache
- blurred vision.

NEGLIGENCE

Negligence has the following legal definition in English law:

Negligence is the omission to do something which a reasonable man, guided upon those considerations which ordinarily regulate the conduct of human affairs, would do, or doing something which a prudent and reasonable man would not do.

Medical or dental negligence is:

The failure to treat and care for a patient with a reasonable degree of skill and care. The standard of a dentist's care is measured against that of his or her peers. To prove that the dentist is negligent one must show that in making that mistake the dentist provided a standard of care that was unacceptable by the standards of the dental profession.

Causation must also be proved. This is the link between the alleged act of negligence and the damage or injury suffered. For negligence to occur there must be:

- A duty of care owed to the patient.
- A breach of duty of care.
- Causation in that breach caused damage.

Duty of care

When a patient is given treatment by a dentist it is implicit that the dentist has the skill conferred by his or her qualification and will exercise reasonable care commensurate with his or her peers in executing the treatment.

Breach of duty of care

Mr Justice McNair, presiding on the case of Bolam versus Friern Hospital Management Committee (1957), ruled that the doctor is not guilty 'if he has acted in accordance with a practice accepted as proper by a responsible body of medical men skilled in that particular art'.

'The Bolam test' is used when deciding whether or not a dentist has been negligent, i.e. the standard of dental practice is decided by dental opinion.

The 1998 case of Bolito versus City and Hackney Health Authority returned power to the Court to decide the standard of care. The judge ruled that if the responsible body of medical opinion could not withstand logical analysis, the action could be deemed negligent.

Causation and damage and/or injury

This refers to damage or injury caused directly due to the occurrence of a negligent act by the dentist. If the damage or injury may have been caused irrespective of the negligent act, no causation can be proved. Box 1.3 lists the factors affecting claims of negligence.

BOX 1.3 Factors affecting claims of negligence

- Limitation: an adult has 3 years from the date of the alleged negligence to bring a claim. This does not apply to children under 18 or those suffering incapacity.
- Contributory negligence: the patient has contributed to damage and/or injury suffered by ignoring guidance given by the dentist.
- Consent to a procedure does not preclude a dentist from acting negligently.

TRAUMA

Head injury

Head injury is a major cause of death in young adults, with more than 5000 deaths each year in the UK.

Head injury may result from direct or indirect impact. Direct injury may be caused by impact with a sharp object from a fall or a sharp object thrown at the head. Indirect injury occurs when the traumatic episode causes violent movement of the cranial contents. An example of indirect injury is a contra-coup injury, when the site of the impact is distant from the head. The consequent movement causes the brain to impact against the enclosed cranial cavity. The skull is more commonly lacerated than fractured during a traumatic episode.

Definitions

- Concussion: Transient disturbance of neurological function following head injury.
- Extradural haematoma: Collection of blood between the dura and the skull. The cause is usually a skull fracture such as trauma to the parieto-temporal region or to the middle cerebral artery.
- Intradural haematoma: Collection of blood or bleeding into the subdural space or within the brain itself.
- Sudural haematoma: Collection of blood between the brain and dura. Causes include age-related brain shrinkage, alcohol-related brain and vessel shrinkage, and tearing of blood vessels secondary to acceleration–deceleration injury.
- Subarachnoid haemorrhage: Collection of blood in the subarachnoid space. It is caused by the rupture of an arteriovenous malformation of the circle of Willis into the subarachnoid space. It is the commonest abnormality seen on MRI or CT scan following head injury.

Clinical features

Clinical features of head injury are:

- Dependent on the type of injury, the location of the injury, and time and changes in mental state since the injury.

- Extradural haematomas cause transient loss of consciousness, followed by an interval of lucidity. Thereafter the patient's unconsciousness persists.
- Subdural haematomas develop a persistent headache with neurological signs.
- Subarachnoid haemorrhages develop a headache and neurological problems.

The Hunt–Hess classification (Table 1.3) is used to grade subarachnoid haemorrhage. The Glasgow Coma Scale (Table 1.4) is used to assess the patient's neurological state over a period of time. A score of 14–15 indicates minor trauma to the head, 9–13 indicates moderate to severe trauma to the head, and a score of less than 8 indicates severe trauma to the head.

Table 1.3 Hunt–Hess classification of subarachnoid haemorrhage

Grade	Clinical problem
1	Mild headache and minor nuchal rigidity
2	Cranial nerve palsy, nuchal rigidity, severe headache
3	Lethargy, mild focal deficit, confusion
4	Stupor, hemiparesis, early decerebrate rigidity
5	Deep coma, decerebrate rigidity, moribund

Table 1.4 The Glasgow Coma Scale

Response	Clinical sign	Score
Eyes open	Spontaneously	4
	To speech	3
	To pain	2
	Eyes never open	1
Best verbal response	Orientated	5
	Confused	4
	Inappropriate words	3
	Incomprehensible sounds	2
	No verbal response	1
Best motor response	Obeys commands	6
	Localizes pain	5
	Withdrawal	4
	Flexion to pain	3
	Extension to pain	2
	No motor response	1

Investigations

Investigations include X-rays, computed tomography (CT) scan, and/or magnetic resonance imaging (MRI). Haematology should include blood sugar, full blood count (FBC), urea and electrolytes (U and Es), clotting screen, and blood alcohol level and drug screen.

Treatment

- ABC: the management of the Airway, Breathing, and Circulation supercedes all other treatment.
- If head injury is suspected to be severe an early neurological opinion should be sought.
- The aim is to prevent hypoxia and hypotension, but should this occur then treatment should be vigorous.
- Monitor intracranial pressure as this gives an idea of cerebral perfusion and thus cerebral ischaemia.
- Cerebral perfusion pressure = mean arterial pressure − intracranial pressure (ICP).
- An ICP of ≥15 mmHg may be caused by cerebral oedema or haemorrhage. This may be treated by mannitol infusion. In severe cases surgical decompression may be necessary.
- The role of steroids and prophylactic antibiotics is still controversial.

Facial laceration

Trauma to the face may cause severe psychological distress irrespective of the degree of the injury. Such injuries tend to bleed profusely and can be very frightening, especially for children. Injuries may affect the facial contours and aesthetics. Damage to the eyes, ears, nose, parotid glands, and facial nerve may have devastating consequences. Regional local anaesthesia should be used when repairing facial laceration to prevent distorting effects secondary to the volume effect of local anaesthesia.

Eyebrow injury

Eyebrow injury is usually caused by lacerations and bleeds profusely. For the best cosmetic results clean the opposing ends of the laceration but do not shave the eyebrows before repairing the laceration.

Lip injury or lacerations

The deep tissue such as the muscle must be repaired first before the surface skin. The vermillion border should be carefully opposed. Even minor discrepancies will have a major aesthetic impact.

Ear injury

The blood supply may be easily compromised during injury as well as during repair. The ear cartilage is avascular. The main problems are haematoma and necrosis of tissue. The use of splints may reduce the formation of haematoma.

Nose injury

The nasal blood supply is precarious, with the nasal cartilage being avascular. Adrenaline-free local anaesthetic should be used. As for the ear, the repair should be performed in layers.

Facial fractures

Bony fractures of the face are common. Trauma to teeth is a common consequence of facial injury. Risk factors for facial fractures are:

- Road traffic accidents associated with driver fatigue and alcohol or other substance abuse.
- Alcohol consumption *per se*.
- Male under the age of 25.
- Assaults inside the home are associated with female injuries.
- Assaults outside the home are associated with male injuries.
- Falls in the elderly and inebriated.

The British Association of Oral and Maxillofacial Surgeons (BAOMS) national facial injury survey indicates that:

- 500 000 facial injuries occur per year in the UK.
- A quarter of these are associated with alcohol consumption.
- A quarter are due to assaults.
- Although road traffic accidents accounted for only 5% of facial injuries 40% of these were serious.

Orbital fracture

The orbital floor is very thin. Severe trauma to the orbit is likely to fracture the floor rather than any other part of the orbit. In a blow-out fracture the orbital contents may be dislodged into the maxillary sinus. Damage to the eye itself may be caused by:

- corneal abrasion or tears
- orbital emphysema
- hyphema (blood in the anterior chamber)
- vitreous haemorrhage.

The functional impairment should be assessed by a surgical ophthalmologist.

Nasal bone fracture

Fracture of the nasal bone occurs commonly and results from direct trauma to the nose. The deformity may be significant with swelling, crepitus, and nasal discharge of blood being prominent. Septal haematomas also occur. The nasal bone may also be mobile.

Assessment of the fracture is usually clinical. Epistaxis if not self-limiting should be arrested with a nasal pack and the fracture should be reduced and specialist referral made.

Zygomatic fracture
This type of injury is frequently sustained by a direct blow in sport or a fight. The most obvious abnormality is flattening of the face on the side of fracture, with depression or step deformity. Other clinical features are:

- injury to the maxillary branch of the fifth cranial nerve (infraorbital branch)
- subconjunctival haemorrhage
- diplopia may be present
- change in level of the eye
- restricted eye movements
- the mouth may be lacerated or opening restricted.

X-ray or CT will image the fracture. Surgical treatment is indicated for displaced fractures.

Mandibular fracture
Mandibular fractures are common and may occur in the body or the ramus of the mandible during a traumatic incident. The most obvious clinical sign is malocclusion and mandibular displacement. Pain, tenderness, swelling, and deformity are common features. X-rays, both lateral and antero-posterior views, are required. Surgical fixation is usually indicated.

Maxillary fracture
Maxillary fracture is usually secondary to direct trauma. Clinical signs are:

- pain
- swelling
- rhinorrhoea
- malocclusion of the teeth
- mobility of the middle third of the face.

Classification of fractures
Facial fractures are classified as LeFort I, II, or III according to Table 1.5. CT scan and MRI can show the extent of the fracture to a degree which is not possible with plain X-rays.

Management of facial fractures
After emergency management of maintaining the airway, breathing, and circulation, the aim should be for primary repair: this will give the best cosmetic results. Deal with bleeding from lacerations, epistaxis, and rhinorrhoea. If rhinorrhoea is present prophylactic antibiotics are required to prevent meningitis.

Table 1.5   Classification of facial fractures

Le Fort I	Fracture of the maxilla only involving the nasal fossa. The fracture detaches the maxillary alveolus and palate
Le Fort II	Fracture of the maxilla, nasal bones, and medial orbits. It is a pyramidal fracture through the nasal bones medially and the maxillary sinus wall laterally
Le Fort III	Fracture of the maxilla, nasal bones, zygoma, ethmoids, vomer, and cranial base. The fracture through the orbit and fronto-zygomatic suture detaches the facial skeleton from the base of the skull

The oral-maxillo-facial surgeon should be involved early in patient assessment and treatment. The principles are:

- reduction of fractures
- stable internal fixation
- aim for early mobilization of the jaw.

Shock

Shock is an acute disturbance of the circulation resulting in inefficient or deficient delivery of the metabolic requirments of the tissues. There is a disproportion between the circulating blood volume and the size of the vascular tissues. The net result is gross circulatory failure and tissue hypoxia. There are four types of shock: hypovolaemic, cardiogenic, septic, and distributive.

Hypovolaemic shock

Hypovolaemic shock is caused by a large reduction in blood volume. It is the commonest type of shock. Causes of hypovolaemic shock are:

- Haemorrhage from severe wounds, perinatal bleeding, dissecting aortic aneurysm.
- Dehydration in paediatric patients from continued diarrhoea and vomiting.
- Intestinal loss from gut in obstruction, pancreatitis, and ascites.
- Severe burns.

The preload is decreased and the afterload increase, whereas myocardial contractility remains normal.

Cardiogenic shock

In cardiogenic shock the heart fails to act as a pump, with the result that insufficient blood is delivered to the organs. It usually occurs after myocardial infarction, secondary to loss of myocardial function. Other causes include:

- Myocarditis, pericardial infusion with tamponade.
- Drug toxicity, especially cocaine and chemotherapeutic agents.
- Pulmonary embolism.

The preload and afterload are increased and myocardial contractlity is decreased.

Septic shock

Septic shock occurs secondary to sepsis and scepticaemia or toxaemia. Gram-negative organisms are the main organisms associated with the scepticaemia. Initially both the preload and the afterload are decreased and myocardial contractility increases. In the late stages the preload and afterload are increased and myocardial contractility decreases.

Distributive shock

Distributive shock results from a severe decrease in the vascular tone. This results in vasodilatation and peripheral pooling of blood. The causes are:

- Head injury.
- Anaphylactic shock.
- Drugs, including barbiturates.
- Spinal cord injury.
- Late stages of septicaemia.

The preload and afterload are increased and myocardial contractility is increased.

Clinical features of shock

General features of shock are:

- tachycardia
- weak thready pulse
- hypotension
- tachypnoea
- cold peripheries
- peripheral cyanosis
- confusion.

Other specific features are related to the underlying cause:

- chest pain
- haemorrhage
- fever
- vomiting and diarrhoea
- dyspnoea
- dehydration.

Stages of shock

Shock can be subdivided into three stages:

- Stage I: Compensated shock
  - The low CO_2 is insufficient for the metabolic needs.
  - In the early stages the patient is anxious and restless with tachycardia and tacypnoea.
  - In the later stages the skin becomes cold and clammy and the pulse becomes weak and thready.
  - The systolic blood pressure drops although the diastolic blood pressure remains the same.
- Stage II: Decompensated shock
  - The patient remains warm because of decreased O_2 demand.
  - The pulse is weak and thready and the rate falls.
  - Blood pressure begins to fall.
  - Breathing becomes slow and shallow.
  - Confusion is secondary to cerebral hypoxia.
  - Oliguria.
- Stage III: Irreversible
  - The myocardium, central nervous system, and respiration are depressed.
  - There is massive vasodilatation with peripheral pooling.
  - Major organ failure occurs, including the kidneys.
  - The patient will die without major organ support.

Treatment of shock

- Keep the patient nil by mouth, with all fluids given intravenously.
- Maintain the airway and breathing.
- Use high-flow oxygen and artificial ventilation.
- Maintain the circulation.
- Control any haemorrhage.
- Elevate the feet to increase venous return.
- Control the ambient temperature.
- Treat underlying specific problem.

Box 1.4 Mortality rates

In the UK there are 37 000 cases of septic shock per year with mortality rates of 40%. There is a 70% to 100% mortality rate for cardiogenic shock: 45% to 50% of patients die within 1 h. There is a 50% mortality for distributive shock.

2 Cardiovascular system

Understanding the cardiovascular system is particularly relevant to dentistry: cardiovascular disease is the most frequent cause of death, and the increasing number of elderly people in the population are particularly liable to disorders of the cardiovascular system.

EXAMINATION OF THE CARDIOVASCULAR SYSTEM

Examination of the cardiovascular system should cover the following in particular:

- general appearance
- hands
- arterial pulse
- arterial blood pressure
- venous pulse
- jugulo-venous pressure
- the chest and heart
- peripheral oedema.

General appearance

The characteristic features of many diseases in which the cardiovascular system is involved may be apparent:

- shortness of breath
- cyanosis
- clubbing
- pallor
- malar flush
- oedema of the ankles or sacrum.

Signs indicating particular cardiovascular diseases may also be apparent:

- Malar flush may be associated with mitral stenosis.
- Marfanoid habitus may be associated with aortic incompetence.
- Down syndrome may be associated with atrial septal defect.

The hands

- Note the **colour of the hands**: pale or white hands indicate poor perfusion; blue peripheries may indicate peripheral and/or central cyanosis.

- Assess the **temperature of the hands**: warm hands usually indicate good perfusion; cold hands may indicate peripheral vascular disease or low cardiac output.
- Look for **clubbing** (see Box 2.1): clubbing is a curvature of the nails in two directions.
- Look for **splinter haemorrhages**: these are common in bacterial endocarditis. Quinke's sign is the alternate blanching and flushing seen in severe aortic incompetence.

The arterial pulse and cardiac rate

Revise your anatomy, paying attention to the **radial, carotid, brachial**, and **femoral pulses**. In an emergency you should be able to palpate for all of these with no difficulty.

The **radial artery** is the most conventional to choose for palpation of the pulse. It is also the most accessible in the fully clothed patient. The **carotid artery** gives the best indication of arterial wave form. The **brachial artery** may give an idea of the wave form and is used for palpation and auscultation when measuring the blood pressure. The arterial wave forms and volumes are shown in Table 2.1.

The **cardiac rate** varies greatly. The physiological limit is wide: between 80 and 90 beats/min is considered normal but in athletes the rate may be as

---

BOX 2.1 Causes of clubbing

- Cardiac disorders: cyanotic congenital heart disease, bacterial endocarditis, left to right shunts.
- Respiratory disorders: suppurative lung disease, i.e. bronchiectasis, empyema, lung abscess, cystic fibrosis, carcinoma of the bronchus, idiopathic fibrosing alveolitis, asbestosis and pleural mesothelioma.
- Others: Crohn's disease, cirrhosis of the liver, tropical diseases, idiopathic or familial clubbing.

Table 2.1 Arterial waveforms and volumes

Normal	Better felt at brachial/carotid
Small volume	Mitral stenosis, shock, pericardial effusion
Large volume	Hyperdynamic, e.g. anaemia, thyrotoxicosis
Collapsing	Aortic incompetence
Plateau	Aortic stenosis
Alternative	Alternate strong–weak beats, e.g. left ventricular failure
Paradoxus	Volume decreases on inspiration, e.g. constrictive pericarditis

low as 50–60 beats/min. **Brachycardia** is a rate of less than 60 beats/min and **tachycardia** is a rate of more than 100 beats/min.

An appropriate artery should be used to assess the **rate, rhythm, volume,** and **character** of the pulse as well as the state of the arterial wall. Remember that exercise and anxiety will affect the pulse rate.

On palpation the **cardiac rhythm** is usually regular. An irregular pulse may be due to sinus arrhythmia (increases on inspiration, and on expiration decreases (slows down)), which is a normal feature in the young. An irregularly irregular pulse is commonly caused by atrial fibrillation (AF), or ectopics.

The state of the arterial wall can be an important sign: in Mönckeberg's sclerosis the artery feels like lead piping; in elderly patients the arterial wall is more easily palpable but gives little information as it becomes stiff.

Measurement of blood pressure

Blood pressure measurement is often performed badly. The patient must be comfortable and relaxed when the measurement is attempted. The systolic blood pressure may vary by 50 mmHg in an anxious patient who subsequently relaxes.

Equipment
The mercury manometer is the simplest apparatus:

- Make sure the glass manometer is clean and there are no air bubbles in the mercury column.
- Check the valve and rubber bulb for air leaks.
- The cuff should be long enough to encompass the arm adequately. Make sure the correct cuff width is used—10 cm for an adult, 15 cm for an obese adult, and 5 cm for a child.
- Check the stitching around the inflatable rubber pad, so that when the pressure is raised it does not herniate from below the cloth.

When recording the blood pressure, specify:

- The limb used—this is usually the right arm, held horizontally.
- The position of the patient, whether the patient is standing or lying down.
- The variation in respiration (if significant, e.g. in severe asthma).

Practical procedure
- Palpate for the brachial artery in the antecubital fossa.
- Inflate the cuff until the pulsation disappears and continue to over 200 mmHg.
- Deflate the cuff when the pulsation is first felt; this gives an indication of systolic pressure. This helps to eliminate any falsely low reading caused by the auscultatory gap (see below).
- Place the diaphragm over the brachial artery.
- Inflate the cuff until the mercury rises higher than the systolic pressure previously found by palpation (remember this is unpleasant for the patient): release

the valve slowly and steadily, listening carefully. The **Karotkoff sounds** begin as soft muffled thuds.

- The systolic blood pressure is the level at which the sounds are first heard (Phase 1).
- The sound becomes louder until the pitch is sustained (Phases 2 and 3) (the 2nd and 3rd Karotkoff sounds).
- As the pressure continues to fall the sounds become softer (Phase IV) (the 4th Karotkoff sound), and then disappear (Phase V) (the 5th Karotkoff sound).
- Record the first and fifth Karotkoff sounds.

Occasionally the sounds disappear soon after the systolic pressure has been recorded and reappear well above the diastolic pressure. This is called the **auscultatory gap**.

The venous pulse and jugulo-venous pressure

Inspection of the **jugular venous pulse** is important. The internal and external jugular communicate with the right atrium and so give an indication of right atrial pressure.

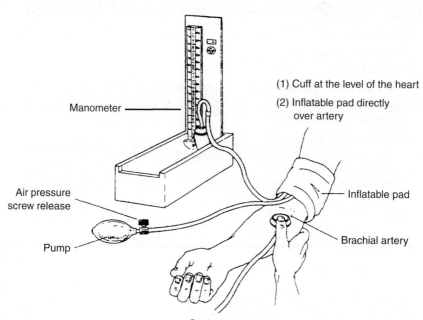

Manometer

(1) Cuff at the level of the heart
(2) Inflatable pad directly over artery

Air pressure screw release

Inflatable pad

Pump

Brachial artery

Stethoscope—diaphragm placed over artery

The patient should lie comfortably at an angle of 40° so that the sternocleidomastoid is relaxed. Look for pulsation in the neck veins (rarely visible in health). Take care to distinguish venous from arterial pulsation.

The **jugulo-venous pressure**:

- has an upper level
- may be detected by expiration, or pressure over the right upper abdomen (hepato-jugular reflex)
- is non-palpable
- falls on inspiration
- is biphasic.

Peripheral oedema

Test for dependent oedema over the ankles and sacrum, which may be a sign of right heart failure. Non-pitting oedema may be caused by lymphatic obstruction.

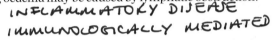
INFLAMMATORY DISEASE
IMMUNOLOGICALLY MEDIATED

RHEUMATIC FEVER

Rheumatic fever is a multisystem disease which occurs after a streptococcal infection. It occurs mainly in 5–15 year age group. Table 2.2 shows the geographical incidence of rheumatic fever.

BOX 2.2 Summary points on dental patients with cardiovascular disease

Dental patients with cardiovascular disease may be compromised by:

- An inability to tolerate prolonged dental procedures.
- Limited mobility.
- An inability to lie flat during treatment (due to breathlessness).
- Drug interactions.
- Excessive bleeding because of current therapy, e.g. aspirin, warfarin.
- The need for antibiotic prophylaxis in patients at risk.
- Anxiety, which may precipitate angina in predisposed individuals. This may require emergency treatment because of a cardiovascular event during routine treatment, the inability to tolerate a general anaesthetic, or the inability to tolerate some local anaesthetics.

Table 2.2 Geographical incidence of rheumatic fever

Country	Incidence per 100 000 population	Patient age (years)
UK	0.2	5–15
USA	9	5–15
Eastern Europe	12	1–15
Iran	60–100	0–20
Middle East	26	5–14

Aetiology

Group A and B haemolytic streptococci cause rheumatic fever in 0.3–3% of children with injection of the pharynx. There is a latent period 2–6 weeks before the onset of rheumatic fever. Patients from low socioeconomic groups who live in overcrowded conditions and are HLA-DR4 positive are prone to infection.

Rheumatic fever occurs after repeated oropharyngeal streptococcal infections causing an exaggerated B-lymphocyte antibody response. The streptococcal antigens cross-react with the host's connective tissue. The bacterial sugar (cell wall *n*-acetylgycosamine) component shares antigenic homology with glycoprotein found in the connective tissue of human heart valves.

The pathological process is a **vasculitis** affecting the connective tissue. **Aschoff's body** is the pathological lesion and consists of an aggregate of large cells with polymorphs and basophils around an avascular fibrinoid core. The cardiac lesion is characterized by a **pancarditis** with the endocardium being the most severely involved.

Chronic rheumatic fever may develop in 50% of patients with acute rheumatic fever.

Clinical features

The diagnosis is made on clinical grounds using the **Duckett-Jones** criteria (Table 2.3). The presence of two major and one minor criteria indicates a high probability of rheumatic fever. This is greatly strengthened by evidence of preceding streptococcal infection.

Carditis

Carditis occurs in 40–50% of patients and lasts between 3 and 6 months. Cardiac involvement is the most important manifestation of the disease, occurs about 2 weeks after polyarthritis and involves all the cardiac tissue. It is a **pancarditis**. There is a 1% mortality in patients with carditis.

Table 2.3 The Duckett–Jones criteria

Major criteria	Carditis
	Polyarthritis
	Erythema margination
	Subcutaneous nodules
	Chorea
Minor criteria	Fever
	Arthralgia
	Previous rheumatic fever
	Raised acute phase proteins ECR, CRP, ferritin
	Prolonged P–R interval on ECG

CHRONIC R.F. => Ribrous scarring / calcification
=> stenosis + regurgitation

The clinical features vary:

- Patients may be asymptomatic: asymptomatic cases are usually only recognized after the presentation of other clinical signs or cardiomegaly on the chest X-ray.
- Patients may present with congestive cardiac failure.
- Patients usually present with increasing breathlessness, palpitations, which may be intermittent, and/or chest pain.
- Mortality in patients with carditis is associated with the development of congestive cardiac failure.

Myocarditis involves the myocardium. All of the myocardium may be involved but the clinical consequences are usually due to left and right ventricular involvement. Patients present with left ventricular failure which may lead to right ventricular failure and subsequent congestive cardiac failure.

In **endocarditis** the mitral valve is the most commonly affected. The valvulitis which involves nodules on the mitral and aortic valves results in murmurs, which may change. The Carey Coombs murmur, a soft diastolic murmur, is associated with mitral valve involvement. Mitral valve disease may occur alone or in association with the aortic valve failure. When mitral and aortic valve disease occur together the disease is associated with a high mortality rate.

Mitral valve involvement results in **pericarditis** which is caused by inflammation of the cardiac pericardium. A pericardial rub is due to fluid in the pericardial space.

Polyarthritis
Polyarthritis occurs in 80–90% of patients. It is the initial clinical manifestation after the streptococcal sore throat. The arthritis is migratory and lasts for 4–6 weeks. It affects the large joints such as the knee, ankle, elbow, hip, and shoulder. The onset of pain is sudden and is associated with one or more joints, lasts for a week, and is accompanied by swelling.

Chorea
Chorea occurs in 10% of patients. Sydenham's chorea, also called St Vitus' dance, may occur 4 to 6 months after the other clinical signs. Sydenham's chorea consists of emotional liability and involuntary movements of the face and limbs. It disappears during sleep. It is caused by involvement of the central nervous system. The chorea may reappear during sleep or pregnancy.

Subcutaneous nodules
These are rare. They are small (up to 0.5 cm), non-tender, mobile, and firm and occur over bony prominences.

Erythema nodosum

Erythema nodosum are larger than subcutaneous nodules. They occur over the shins. The lesions appear as deep red nodules which are painful and tender on palpation.

Erythema margination

Erythema margination occurs in 65% of patients. It is associated with carditis. It has a serpinginious edge with a fading centre. The rash is painless and non-pruritic and spreads over the trunk and limbs.

Treatment

Treatment consists of bed rest and supportive therapy.

Bed rest

Bed rest is important in the acute phase until the temperature, acute phase proteins (ESR, CRP), and white cell count return to normal.

Drugs

Aspirin is given in doses of 60–100 mg/kg/day to give a therapeutic level 25–30 mg/dl. It should be continued until the acute phase proteins return to normal. Corticosteroids are used in patients with severe carditis. Diazepam is used to control the choreiform movements.

Complications

Fifty per cent of patients develop chronic rheumatic fever. Thirty per cent of patients with carditis during the initial attack will develop abnormal cardiac valves.

BOX 2.3 Summary points on dental patients with a history of rheumatic fever

- Thirty per cent of patients with a history of rheumatic fever may have valvular disease.
- The patient may be on antistreptococcal prophylaxis, e.g. penicillin.
- The patient may have a vascular prosthesis putting them into a high-risk category.
- The patient may be taking oral anticoagulants.
- The patient may be taking cardiac drugs, e.g. digoxin, angiotensin-converting enzyme inhibitors, diuretics, or beta-blockers.
- The patient may have chronic heart failure, making supine dentistry difficult.
- All patients should have a careful cardiac assessment.
- Dental treatment should be carefully planned and carried out by competent trained staff.
- Always consult the patient's physician.

Penicillin is the drug of choice as a prophylactic to prevent chronic rheumatic fever developing. It can be given either as a monthly intramuscular injection of benzathine penicillin or as oral phenoxymethyl penicillin, 250 mg twice a day (b.d.).

Long-term consequences of rheumatic fever

The long term consequences of rheumatic fever are particularly important to dental practice. Patients with chronic valvular heart disease need antibiotic prophylaxis. The mitral valve is affected in 80–90% of cases. The other valves are affected in the order aortic, then tricuspid, then pulmonary.

INFECTIVE ENDOCARDITIS

Infective endocarditis is caused by a microbial infection of the endocardium, including the cardiac valves (prosthetic or native).

Epidemiology

There has been an increase in the incidence of bacterial endocarditis despite the widespread use of antibiotics. The reasons for this are:

- an ageing population;
- increased survival after complicated cardiac procedures;
- increased intravenous drug abuse.

There has been a decrease in incidence in underdeveloped countries due to:

- insufficient facilities for the treatment of congenital heart disease;
- insufficient medical treatment of rheumatic fever.

Table 2.4 summarizes the geographical incidence of bacterial endocarditis and Table 2.5 shows the prevalence of infective endocarditis in underlying cardiac disease.

Pathogenesis

Pathogenesis of bacterial endocarditis involves the following stages:

- The endothelium is damaged by pre-existing disease.
- Micro-organisms from the gastrointestinal tract, the skin, the genitourinary, and the respiratory tract cause a bacteraemia.

Table 2.4 Geographical incidence of bacterial endocarditis

Country/Area	Incidence per 100 000
UK	6–7
USA	18
Eastern Europe	20
Middle East	20

Table 2.5 The prevalence of infective endocarditis in underlying cardiac disease

Underlying disease	Prevalence of infective endocarditis
Rheumatic heart disease	24%
Congenital cardiac abnormalities	25%
Other cardiac abnormalities	20%
Native valves with no pre-existing cardiac disease	31%

Table 2.6 Organisms which cause infective endocarditis in different patient groups

Patient group	Organism
Young and middle aged	*Streptococcus viridans*
Elderly	*Streptococcus viridans*
	Streptococcus faecalis
Drug addicts	*Streptococcus, Haemophilus*
Patients with prosthetic valves	Post-surgical early *Staphylococcus epidermidis*
	Post-surgical late *Streptococcus viridans*
Surgical cases	*Staphylococcus epidermidis*
Immunosuppressed patients	Candida, aspergillas
Farming communities (farm holidays)	*Coxiella burnetti*

- Sixty per cent of cases are caused by the *Streptococcus viridans* group.
- The streptococci produce carbohydrates which stick to the endocardium and consequently the valves.
- Direct implantation of bacteria on the endocardium causes rapid destruction and obliteration of a previously normal valve.
- Only 50% of patients with infective endocarditis have a history of cardiac disease.

The following organisms cause infective endocarditis:

- Streptococcal bacteria (viridans and enterococci): 65%.
- Staphylococcal bacteria: 10–30%.
- Anaerobic bacteria (Gram-negative bacilli): 0–5%.
- Other organisms (fungi, *Chlamydia*, rickettsia): 0–1%.

Table 2.6 shows which organisms cause infective endocarditis in different patient groups and Box 2.4 details the infection of abnormal valve lesions.

Clinical features

Infective endocarditis is a clinical syndrome consisting of cardiac disease, infection, embolism, and immunological phenomena which develop slowly

BOX 2.4 Abnormal valve lesions which become infected

- Any lesion with a regurgitant stream and a large pressure drop across a small orifice: mitral regurgitation, aortic regurgitation, small ventricular septal defect, mitral valve with prolapse and regurgitation.
- Prosthetic valve endocarditis.
- Valve-bearing conduits.
- Atrial septal defect (ASD) and stenotic mitral valve are low-risk lesions.

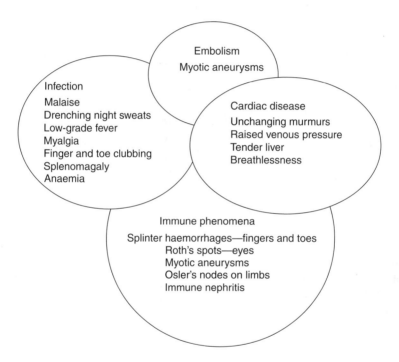

(see Figure). It is impotant to maintain a high index of suspicion. Dentists should always examine the hands as part of the dental examination (clubbing and splinter haemorrhages). A dipstick test of the urine may pick up microscopic haematuria and proteinuria.

Investigations

- Urine: microscopic haematuria and proteinuria.
- Blood cultures: four sets of cultures should be taken within the first 2 h.
- Echocardiogram: a 2D echo gives a good definition of the valves.
- Chest X-ray.
- ECG.

> **BOX 2.5** Dental management in a patient at risk of endocarditis
> - Take care with all dental procedures associated with a significant bacteraemia.
> - Careful treatment planning is required to minimize the number of treatment sessions.
> - When using local analgesia prophylaxis is given 1 h before treatment.
> - Give 3 g oral amoxil*: if this is contraindicated use 600 mg oral clindamycin.
> - Check hospital policy and the British National Formulary (BNF) for regimes under general anaesthetic.
> - Check hospital policy and the BNF for regimes associated with 'high risk' patients.
> - Specialist procedures, e.g. endodontics and orthodontics, should be discussed with a cardiologist and microbiologist.
> *In USA and Europe 2 g of amoxil is used.

Treatment

Treatment should involve multidisciplinary management by a cardiac surgeon, cardiologist, and microbiologist. The dental surgeon's opinion should be sought if the organisms are thought to have arisen from oral pathology.

Prevention

Since 60% of the organisms causing endocarditis may originate in the oral cavity, the role of the dentist is very important. A history of congenital heart disease, rheumatic fever, or previous endocarditis should result in careful treatment planning in conjunction with the patient's physician. Antiobiotic prophylaxis must be given for the following dental procedures known to be associated with a significant bacteraemia:

- Oral surgery: any invasive procedures.
- Periodontology: periodontal surgery, deep scaling.
- Orthodontics: extractions, subgingival points.
- Conservation: endodontics, deep scaling, extractions.

Box 2.5 summarizes the dental management of a patient at risk of infective endocarditis.

HYPERTENSION

Blood pressure naturally rises gradually with age and the definition of hypertension is difficult and depends on epidemiological studies.

Isolated systolic hypertension may be defined as:

- At 20 years of age a systolic pressure over 140 mmHg with a diastolic pressure of less than 90 mmHg.
- At 50 years of age a systolic pressure over 159 mmHg with a diastolic pressure of less than 95 mmHg.

Before initiating treatment both systolic and diastolic pressures must be considered.

There are several reasons for the problems with the definition of hypertension:

- It depends on epidemiology (Framington study).
- Blood pressure measurements are not consistent.
- Blood pressure measurements fall over time (acclimatization).
- The degree of awareness varies—women are more likely to have their blood pressure measured than men.

Ninety to ninety-five per cent of cases are **primary or essential hypertension**, with no known cause. Five per cent of cases are due to **secondary hypertension**. A number of causes of secondary hypertension have been identified:

- Coarctation of the aorta.
- Endocrine causes: acromegaly, Conn's syndrome, Cushing's syndrome, hyperthyroidism, phaeochromocytoma.
- Iatrogenic causes: steroids, oral contraceptives, non-steroidal anti-inflammatory drugs (NSAIDs), coffee.

Epidemiology

This is the number of new cases of hypertension diagnosed per year; with hypertension this is age dependent. Table 2.7 shows the incidence of hypertension.

The following risk factors are associated with hypertension:

- Age—risk increases with age.
- Alcohol.
- Drugs (NSAIDs, oral contraceptives, steroids, sympathomimetics).
- Family history—there is a polygenic influence. The major gene has not yet been characterized.
- Obesity—particularly centripedal obesity.
- Stress.
- Blacks and Asians have an increased morbidity.
- Migration—blood pressure rises with migration, e.g. rural to urban areas.

Clinical features

Most patients are asymptomatic. The most common symptom experienced is a throbbing sensation. There may be specific symptoms related to hypertensive

Table 2.7 Incidence of hypertension

Age in years	% of cases
20–40	1–2
40–60	2–4
60–80	4–8

complications such as chest pain secondary to coronary artery disease, breathlessness due to heart failure, or symptoms of cerebrovascular disease.

Most patients have no physical signs other than the recorded high blood pressure. There may be signs of the underlying cause, especially in the young, and signs of the complications of hypertension.

After the patient has been examined and a full history has been taken, check for the following:

- Associated diseases.
- Side-effects of medication.
- Drug interaction with dental prescriptions.
- Labile and difficult to control blood pressure.
- Clinical consequences of the sustained increase in hypertension in cardiac, vascular, and renal systems.

Problems arising from sustained hypertension

Sustained hypertension can give rise to the following problems or complications:

- cerebrovascular accident
- coronary artery disease
- heart failure
- dissecting aneurysm
- renal disease
- ocular disease.

BOX 2.6 Effect of drugs on the dental management of hypertensive patients

It is essential to take a full medical and drug history in patients who have hypertension. All drugs used have side-effects, many with important dental implications:

- **Diuretics:** thiazides may increase blood sugar and are associated with lichen planus. They have a hypotensive effect.
- **Beta-blockers: these** enhance the hypertensive effect when used in combination with general anaesthetics and NSAIDs and antagonize the hypertension effect when used in combination with local dental anaesthetics and adrenaline. Note the increased risk of lidocaine and bupivicaine toxicity.
- **Ace inhibitors** enhance the hypertensive effect with general anaesthetics, local dental anaesthetics, and corticosteroids. Note the increased risk of renal failure with NSAIDs: absorption of tetracycline is reduced.
- **Calcium antagonists:** verapamil increases the hypotensive effect of general anaesthetics. Verapamil and diltiazem increase the plasma concentration of midazolam. Calcium antagonists are associated with gingival hyperplasia.

Treatment

The following classes of drugs are used in the treatment of hypertension:

- diuretics
- beta-blockers
- angiotensin-converting enzyme (ACE) inhibitors.
- calcium antagonists.

HEART FAILURE

Heart failure is a clinical syndrome due to cardiac dysfunction—the failure of the heart to pump blood effectively. There are some situations in which a patient may present to a dental surgeon:

- Acute heart failure may occur in the dental chair, secondary to the patient suffering a myocardial infarction.
- Patients with chronic heart failure or cor pulmonale (right heart failure secondary to lung disease) may present to the dentist for routine oral care.

    Several clinical syndromes exist:

- Acute heart failure which is usually secondary to acute left ventricular failure.
- Cor pulmonale (associated with chronic lung disease secondary to left heart failure).
- Cardiogenic shock which is usually secondary to myocardial infarction clinically.

Heart failure is characterized by low systemic blood pressure, poor peripheral perfusion, oliguria, and anuria.

Epidemiology

In the UK 1–2% of the general population are hypertensive. The number of new cases of heart failure per year varies. The figures increase with age and after myocardial infarct (see Table 2.8).

Clinical features

Acute heart failure

Acute heart failure is a medical emergency. It occurs during or shortly after a myocardial infarct.

Table 2.8 Incidence of heart failure

Age in years	Incidence per 100 000
55	1
55–64	3–5
65–74	5–10
75–84	10–12

BOX 2.7 Clinical features of acute heart failure

Symptoms

- Severe breathlessness at rest.
- *Amno agnii*–a feeling of impending doom.

Signs

- The patient is acutely unwell.
- Severe breathlessness.
- Tachypnoea.
- Tachycardia.
- Gallop rhythm.
- Hypotension.
- Pulmonary crepitation.
- Cold clammy skin with dilated pupils.

Investigations

The following investigations are useful:

- chest X-ray
- ECG
- echocardiogram
- stress test—either an exercise ECG or a thallium scan.

Treatment

In a dental surgery emergency measures would entail:

- Reassuring the patient.
- Stop all treatment and call for help.
- Sit the patient upright.
- Administer oxygen: 6 l/min.
- Administer diamorphine 2.5–5 mg (only under supervision in a hospital setting).
- Insert an intravenous line.
- Administer frusemide (furosemide) 80 mg intravenously (only under supervision in a hospital setting).
- Monitor ECG if available.
- Monitor output.

Chronic heart failure

Chronic heart failure may be the reason for an elderly patient presenting with breathlessness on exertion or being unable to tolerate lying flat in the dental chair during routine dental treatment.

BOX 2.8 Clinical features of chronic heart failure

Symptoms

- Breathlessness.
- Tiredness.
- Peripheral oedema.
- Cough and wheeze (inspiratory and expiratory).
- Nocturia.
- Nausea and anorexia.

Signs

- Tachycardia.
- Displaced apex beat.
- Peripheral oedema.
- Raised jugulo-venous pressure.
- Hepatomegaly.
- Tachypnoea.
- Cold extremities.

BOX 2.9 Dental management of patients with chronic heart failure

- Develop a good relationship with the patient and provide a well-thought-out treatment plan.
- Encourage patients to take prescribed medication, e.g. diuretics, which are often neglected if the patient has a dental appointment.
- Carry out the procedure with the patient in a comfortable position and not lying flat. Watch out for drug interactions—patients may be taking diuretics, ACE inhibitors, anti-arrhythmia drugs, and anticoagulants.
- Underlying pulmonary disease may affect treatment.

Treatment
- Health education.
- Diuretics.
- ACE inhibitors are disease modifying and appear to increase survival time by 50–60%.

ISCHAEMIC HEART DISEASE (CORONARY HEART DISEASE)

Ischaemic heart disease is disease of the coronary arteries due to atheroma and is the most important cause of early death in the West. The clinical syndromes associated with ischaemic heart disease are **angina pectoris, myocardial infarction**, and **sudden death**.

Pathology

The basic pathology is atherosclerosis of the coronary arteries. This consists of focal proliferation of collagen inside the intima. This results in decreased flow and progressive patchy stenosis of the arterial vessel walls.

The following risk factors have been identified for the development of ischaemic heart disease:

- age
- sex
- family history
- high serum lipids
- high blood pressure
- smoking
- obesity
- lack of exercise
- psychosocial factors
- systemic disease, e.g. diabetes.

Angina pectoris

Angina pectoris is pain caused by reversible ischaemia of the coronary arteries. The angina may be stable or unstable. **Stable angina** is chest pain which is characterized by central chest pain or pain radiating down the left arm or to the angle of jaw. The pain is precipitated by exercise and relieved by rest. **Unstable angina** is chest pain which occurs with increasing intensity. It becomes more frequent over a period of time. Unstable angina is caused either by small emboli, which impact distally, or obstruction caused by intermittent occlusion of the coronary arteries.

Myocardial infarction

The pain in myocardial infarction is caused by irreversible ischaemia of the coronary arteries. It is caused by obstruction of the lumen of one or more coronary arteries. Myocardial infarction is potentially fatal and in the UK it accounts for 250 000 deaths each year. Over 33% of all deaths occur within the first 2 h of an attack. Anticoagulants and defibrillators reduce mortality by 10–20%.

Clinical features

Eighty to ninety per cent of patients experience **pain**. Features of the pain are:

- It may or may not be precipitated by a history of angina.
- It lasts longer than angina pain and is typically resistant to treatment.
- It can be described as tight crushing pain which may radiate into either the arm or jaw. The pain lasts for 10–20 min.
- It may be confused with epigastric problems, such as gastro-oesophageal reflux or peptic ulceration.

> **BOX 2.10** Non-cardiac causes of chest pain which may affect a patient in the dental chair
>
> - Skin—herpes zoster.
> - Anxiety and hyperventilation.
> - Muscle and costochondral pain—Tietze's syndrome, chest wall tenderness.
> - Musculoskeletal disorders.
> - Epigastric causes, indigestion, heartburn, peptic ulceration.
> - Acute pancreatitis.
> - Dissecting aneurysm.
> - Pleuritic pain.
> - Pulmonary embolism.
> - Pneumonia.

The diagnosis of chest pain is important as early administration of thrombolytic therapy of 300 mg aspirin by the dentist to a patient in his or her care may decrease the mortality.

Other clinical features myocardial infarction are:

- Signs due to vagal stimulation: vomiting.
- Signs due to sympathetic stimulation: pallor, sweating.
- Tachycardia.
- Signs due to hypoxia: hypotension, poor peripheral perfusion, third heart sound, raised jugulo-venous pressure, narrow pulse pressure.

Investigations

An ECG is likely to confirm the diagnosis. However, a normal ECG does not exclude the diagnosis. Look for ST segment elevation or changes consistent with left bundle branch block. Tropinin T, a myocardial fibrillar protein, is specific and is a rapid aid to diagnosis. Assessment of cardiac enzymes is done: peripheral blood should be taken back to assess levels of creative kinase (CK), aspartate aminotransferase (AST), and lactate dehydrogenase (LDH). Daily serial levels are requested.

Acute management

The priority is to ensure early access to defibrillation and thrombolytic therapy:

- **Thrombolysis**: use of thrombolytics can reduce hospital mortality by 25–50%.
- **Aspirin**: should be administered by the dentist who should inform the ambulance team and the physician.
- **Streptokinase (SK)** and **tissue plasminogen activator (tPA)** (Alteplase) are both used. SK is cheaper than tPA. In the UK, SK is the first-line thrombolytic agent. It is infused intravenously over 1 h. It is antigenic and may cause serious allergic reactions.

> **BOX 2.11** Acute management of myocardial infarction in the
> dental surgery (pre-admission to hospital)
>
> - Reassure the patient and stop the dental treatment.
> - Administer oxygen
> - Administer 300 mg of aspirin
> - Phone the ambulance direct
> - Pain relief is also very important as anxiety increases the release of adrenaline and
>   noradrenaline. (Diamorphine 2.5–5 mg is good for pain relief but is not available
>   in dental surgeries.)
> - Give nitrous oxide and oxygen
> - The dentist should accompany the patient to hospital. Most ambulances are
>   equipped with semi-automatic advisory defibrillators.

> **BOX 2.12** Dental management of the patient with ischaemic
> heart disease
>
> - The patient may have a tendency to bleed because of anticoagulants, e.g. warfarin
>   or aspirin.
> - The patient may have bradycardia because of beta-blockers and delayed recovery
>   after vasovagal episodes.
> - There is no evidence that adrenaline in local analgesics is cardiotoxic except in
>   patients who have an abnormal cardiac rhythm, which may be exacerbated with
>   intravascular injection.
> - The patient may have a pacemaker.
> - The patient may be breathless when laid flat.
> - Do not delay emergency treatment. Pain increases stimulation of catecholamines.
> - No antibiotic prophylaxis is required after coronary artery bypass or angioplasty.
> - Routine treatment depends on cardiac status: 3 weeks after angioplasty; 6 weeks
>   to 3 months after infarction; no delay after pacemaker implantation.
> - Keep up to date with practical skills to manage severe angina and skills for
>   cardiopulmonary resuscitation.

CONGENITAL HEART DISEASE

Congenital heart disease affects 1% of live births. It is the commonest cause
of childhood heart disease in the developed world. It can be either idiopathic or
caused by viral infection of the mother during pregnancy (e.g. by rubella or
cytomegalovirus).

Types of defect

Acyanotic valvular defects

Acyanotic defects are those valve lesions which are not associated with
cyanosis: ventricular septal defect (VSD), atrial septal defect (ASD), patent
ductus arteriosus (PDA), and coarctation of the aorta:

- **Ventricular septal defect** is the commonest congenital defect. It results in
  a defect between the two ventricles. The size of the defect may vary from a

pinhole to 2–3 cm. The flow of blood through the defect is from left to right. Where the jet of blood hits the endocardium thickening occurs and the thickened endocardium becomes a site for endocarditis. In large defects some of the blood is then recirculated through the lungs causing pulmonary hypertension with consequent reversal of shunt from right to left through the defect. It is the right to left shunt that causes the development of cyanosis.

- **Arial septal defect** is located near the foramen ovale. It is associated with Down syndrome. This defect has little effect on cardiac function and therefore has an acyonotic presentation. Survival is good but in large uncorrected lesions right ventricular failure may develop. The risk of bacterial endocarditis is lower than in VSD.
- **Patent ductus arteriosus** is an opening between the aorta and pulmonary artery. The opening normally closes during the third month of life. The shunt is from left to right. Bacterial endocarditis occurs occasionally. There can be complications due to right ventricular failure.
- **Coarctation of the aorta** is caused by narrowing of the aorta beyond the origin of the subclavian veins. The head and neck are unaffected. It results in restricted blood supply to the lower body. Clinically the radial and brachial pulses are strong and the femoral pulse weak (this gives rise to radiofemoral delay if the radial and femoral pulses are palpated simultaneously). Complications include bacterial endocarditis and left ventricular failure.

Cyanotic valvular defects

Tetralogy of Fallot, which has an unknown aetiology, consists of four defects: ventricular septal defect, pulmonary vein stenosis, straddling of the interventricular septum by the aorta into which blood flows from both ventricles, and compensatory right ventricular failure.

There are a number of clinical features:

- the most apparent feature is severe central cyanosis
- shortness of breath
- cerebral anoxia with consequent fainting
- children tend to squat to prevent dyspnoea

BOX 2.13 Dental relevance of congenital heart disease

- Risk of infective endocarditis.
- Dental treatment needs careful treatment planning to reduce sepsis.
- Associated congenital cardiac lesions may occur in Down and Turner syndrome or occasionally cleft palate.
- In right-to-left shunts rarely cerebral abscesses have been reported to have resulted from dental sepsis.
- All patients with structural defects are at risk of endocarditis.
- Patients at risk are: ostium secundum ASD, mitral valve prolapse without mitral regurgitation, 6 months post-surgery for PDA, ASD, VSD repair.

- poor growth
- clubbing
- heart failure
- polycythaemia
- endocarditis (less common).

STENOSIS = valve does not open
REGULERGITATION = valve does not close.

VALVULAR HEART DISEASE

Left heart valvular disease

Mitral stenosis

Aetiology

There is thickening of the valve leaflets with calcification and closure of the commissures. Degenerative mitral stenosis is associated with age-related calcification. Rheumatic heart disease, which is endemic in developing world, can also cause mitral stenosis.

Clinical features

Symptoms:

- Diagnosis is often difficult.
- The commonest symptoms are those of increasing breathlessness and fatigue.
- There may be recurrent chest infections.
- Haemoptysis.

Signs:

- Malar flush.
- Atrial fibrillation.
- Loud first sound, opening snap and mid diastolic murmur (use the bell of the stethoscope with the patient in the left lateral position).
- Pulmonary oedema.

Investigations

- Chest X-ray
- Echocardiography—a 2D echo will show leaflet thickening and the lack of movement.
- Haemodynamic studies will give an idea of the pressures and valve area involved.

Management

- Endocarditis prophylaxis should be given to all patients.
- Medical treatment is required for atrial fibrillation and anticoagulation is necessary.
- Surgical treatment: percutaneous mitral commissurotomy (PMC), mitral valve replacement.

Complications

Complications of mitral stenosis include heart failure, atrial fibrillation, mural thrombus, and infective endocarditis.

Mitral regurgitation

Aetiology

In the UK 2–5% of the population have mitral valve prolapse which can have the following causes:

- Rheumatic heart disease (in developing countries).
- Degenerative heart disease (in the West).
- Ischaemic heart disease resulting in acute or chronic rupture of the chordae tendinae or papillary muscle.
- Infective endocarditis.
- Congestive and hypertrophic cardiomyopathy.
- Rarely, autoimmune disease and endomyocardial fibrosis.

Clinical features

Symptoms:

- Mitral regurgitation may be asymptomatic for years.
- The commonest symptoms are breathlessness and fatigue.

Signs:

- Loud pansystolic murmur (unless caused by ischaemic heart disease) at the apex.
- Left ventricular failure.

Investigations

- Chest X-ray shows a large atrium and ventricle.
- ECG may show left atrial overload.
- Echocardiography confirms the diagnosis by continuous wave or colour Doppler.
- Trans-oesophageal imaging and left ventricular angiography allow assessment of severity.

Management

- Medical management: ACE inhibitors decrease the volume load in chronic disease; ACE inhibitors and diuretics are used for heart failure; anticoagulants if atrial fibrillation is present.
- Surgical management: indicated for severe acute disease, chronic disease and symptoms, and asymptomatic patients with left ventricular dysfunction.

Aortic stenosis

Aortic stenosis is stenosis of the aortic valve resulting in obstruction to the left ventricular outflow.

Aetiology

Causes of aortic stenosis include:

- A congenital bicuspid valve.
- Degenerative calcification: this causes sclerosis with little obstruction in 25% of the elderly but 2% will have stenotic valve disease.
- Rheumatic heart disease.

Clinical features

Symptoms:

- This condition may be asymptomatic for long periods.
- The onset of symptoms indicates severe obstruction: angina, breathlessness, dizziness, sudden death.

Signs:

- harsh ejection systolic murmur
- loud second sound
- slow-rising small-volume pulse.

Investigations

Echocardiography is used to visualize and quantify the severity of the defect. Coronary angiography is performed in all patients preoperatively.

Management

All patients need endocarditis prophylaxis. For **asymptomatic patients** there should be regular review, with patients being told to present with the onset of symptoms. Patients should avoid active competitive sports. **Symptomatic patients** should be offered valve replacement.

Aortic regurgitation

Aortic regurgitation results from valve dysfunction, or incompetence or dilatation of the aortic root.

Aetiology

Causes of aortic regurgitation include rheumatic heart disease, hypertension, aortic dissection, Marfan's syndrome, bacterial endocarditis, and syphilis.

Clinical features

Symptoms:

- breathlessness
- angina
- palpitations
- fever in endocarditis
- severe chest pain in aortic dissection.

Signs:

- Collapsing pulse with wide pulse pressure.
- High-pitched ejection diastolic murmur.
- Corrigan's sign is a visible carotid pulsation in the neck.
- Quinke's pulse is a visible pulsation in the nail beds.
- In acute cases there is rapid breathing and pulse.

Investigations
Chest X-ray shows cardiomegaly and echocardiography is diagnostic.

Management
Surgery is the only effective treatment. ACE inhibitors can be used for afterload reduction.

Right heart valvular disease

Tricuspid stenosis
The most common cause of tricuspid stenosis is rheumatic heart disease.

Clinical features
- Tiredness and fatigue.
- Oedema of the legs.
- Giant 'a' waves at the neck caused by the atrium contracting against the stenosed valve.

Investigations
Use chest X-ray and echocardiography.

Management
Management is by the use of diuretics and surgical valve replacement.

Tricuspid regurgitation
Tricuspid regurgitation is due to right ventricular enlargement which has been caused by rheumatic heart disease, congenital heart disease, or endocarditis resulting from intravenous drug abuse.

Clinical features
- Giant 'v' waves in the jugular venous pulse.
- Tiredness and fatigue.
- Leg oedema.
- Ascites, and jaundice from hepatic congestion.

Management
Management is by the use of diuretics, Ace inhibitors, and surgical valve replacement.

Anticoagulation in patients with valvular disease

All mechanical prostheses require anticoagulation and lifelong treatment is necessary for patients with prosthetic valves:

- Warfarin is the anticoagulant of choice and is monitored through anticoagulant clinics using the international normalized ratio (INR).
- The INR is kept between 2.5 and 4.0.
- The Starr–Edwards caged ball and the Bjork–Shiley disc valves need an INR of between 3.0 and 4.5.
- Bioprosthetic valves are only anticoagulated for 3 months after placement and an INR of 2.5–3.5 is aimed for.
- Patients with atrial fibrillation need anticoagulation.
- Warfarin is changed to heparin in pregnancy and in patients requiring surgery.

Prophylactic antibiotics in valvular heart disease

Prophylactic antibiotics are used to prevent the development of infective endocarditis. The causes of endocarditis are:

- Dental procedures (the most common cause).
- Endoscopy.
- Intravenous drug abuse causing right-sided lesions.
- Cutaneous infections (rarely): the causative organisms are: streptococci, staphylococci, and Gram-negative bacilli, fungi, and rickettsial organisms (rarely).

DISTURBANCES OF HEART RHYTHM

Atrial fibrillation (AF)

Atrial fibrillation is the most common cardiac rhythm disorder. It is thus a major risk factor for thromboembolism and stroke, and is *the* most important risk factor for stroke in the elderly.

Atrial fibrillation is the loss of normal sinus rhythm as a result of numerous re-entrant electrical impulses within the atria. This leads to asynchronous electrical activity in the conducting system and atrial systolic function is lost. The contractions or 'fibrillations', at a rate 400–600 per minute, are conducted in an irregular pattern through the atrioventricular (AV) node. This leads to an irregular rapid ventricular response resulting in decreased volume and stasis.

Aetiology
There are both cardiac and non-cardiac causes of AF.

Cardiac causes of AF
Most patients have underlying cardiovascular disease, including coronary artery disease, especially after myocardial infarction. Uncomplicated coronary

artery disease is not commonly associated with AF. Other cardiac cause include:

- valvular heart disease
- hypertension
- post-cardiothoracic surgery
- cardiomyopathy hypertrophic, restrictive or dilated
- congenital heart disease
- constrictive pericarditis.

Non-cardiac causes

- Alcohol intake, especially in young people who binge drink.
- Thyrotoxicosis.
- Diabetes.
- Chronic obstructive lung disease.
- Infection or any fever.
- Pulmonary embolism.

Clinical features

AF is classified as acute if it is present for less than 48 h and chronic if it is present for more than 48 h. The main symptom is palpitations. The pulse is irregularly irregular, but this may be difficult to recognize if the pulse is slow. The cardiac apex beat is faster than the radial pulse. Patients may develop systemic emboli causing stroke, causing renal failure, or limb ischaemia. Other clinical features will depend on the underlying cause.

Investigations

The ECG shows irregularity in the QRST complex and absent P waves. Echocardiography is also useful.

Treatment

Treatment aims to control the heart rhythm and rate. Control of the rhythm will help decrease the risk of stroke:

Acute AF

Acute AF may be self-limiting following acute myocardial infarction or alcohol. Anticoagulate and consider cardioversion:

- Paroxysmal AF: cardioversion and antithrombotic therapy.
- Persistent AF: anticoagulation, cardioversion, anti-arrhythmic treatment.
- Permanent AF: drugs for heart rate control, antithrombotic therapy, cardioversion in resistant cases.

Chronic AF

- Paroxysmal AF: this is self-terminating.
- Persistent AF: responds to pharmacological or electrical cardioversion.
- Permanent AF: resistant cardioversion.

Medication

Drugs are used for cardioversion and to try and maintain sinus rhythm. The following drugs are suitable for long-term use:

- Class Ic drugs flecainide and propafenone are contraindicated in AF due to ventricular impairment and ischaemic heart disease.
- The class Ic drugs flecainide and propafenone are more effective than the class III drug amiodarone.
- Beta-blockers must only be instituted by a specialist physician in patients with heart failure.
- Digoxin is effective; overdose causes dysrhythmias, nausea, and vomiting.

Cardioversion

Electrical DC cardioversion has a higher success rate than any drug currently available. Care should be taken as the risk of thromboembolism is increased at the time of cardioversion. Electrical cadioversion is given under general anaesthetic. The patient is anticoagulated for 3 weeks before cardioversion. A DC shock is given over the chest wall overlying the heart (precordium). Anticoagulation is continued for 4 weeks after the procedure.

In acute cases where no prior anticoagulation has been given heparin should be administered, cardioversion performed, and oral anticoagulation continued for 4 weeks. In patients who present with their first episode of acute AF (of less than 48 h) cardioversion without anticoagulation is safe.

Antithrombolic therapy

The main complication of antithrombolic therapy is a thromboembolic stroke. There are three categories of risk for developing a stroke:

- **High-risk patients** (annual risk of cerebrovascular accident (CVA) 8–12%): these patients have suffered a previous transient ischaemic attack (TIA) or CVA. They are older than 65 years and have one or more of the clinical risk factors of diabetes, hypertension, valve disease, heart failure, thyroid disease, and impaired left ventricular function.
- **Moderate-risk patients** (annual risk of CVA 4%): these patients have the same clinical risk factors as high-risk patients but are less than 65 years old.
- **Low-risk patients** (annual risk of CVA 1%): no history of embolism, hypertension, or diabetes.

Treatment

Treatment depends on risk assessment. For high-risk use warfarin and maintain the INR between 2.0 and 3.0. For moderate-risk patients give warfarin or aspirin and for low-risk patients give aspirin 75–300 mg daily. Echocardiography may prove helpful in establishing whether underlying cardiac problems exist.

Supraventricular tachycardia

In supraventricular tachycardia (SVT) the heart beats at a fast rate of 150–260 beats per minute. SVT is benign but can produce severe symptoms; Wolff–Parkinson–White (WPW) syndrome, however, can be life-threatening. WPW syndrome consists of increased atrial rate and an electrical connection (accessory pathway) directly from the atria to the ventricle and in addition to the AV node, resulting in very rapid conduction into the ventricles by two pathways.

Clinical features

There is an abrupt onset of tachycardia with no obvious precipitating cause. Cases often present at A&E. There is polyuria. The haemodynamics are usually stable.

Investigations

The ECG shows narrow-complex tachycardia. Long-term ECG monitoring is useful.

Management

Acute management is to stop the tachycardia with vagal manoeuvres—exert firm pressure on the carotid for 5 s or a Valsalva manoeuvre with the patient squatting or supine and breathing against a closed glottis for 15 s. If this is unsuccessful use a rapid injection of incremental doses of 3–12 mg of adenosine bolus which is usually effective. In resistant cases a slow intravenous bolus of verapamil, 5 mg followed by another 5 mg will terminate the tachycardia.

Long-term management depends on the patient. No treatment is necessary for infrequent attacks with minimal symptoms. For frequent attacks consider anti-arrhythmic medication or radiofrequency (RF) ablation. Simple anti-arrhythmics (beta-blockers and verapamil) are safe. RF ablation should be before the use of amiodarone. WPW syndrome requires RF ablation.

Atrial flutter

Atrial flutter involves a regular macro re-entry circuit within the right atrium that drives the left atrium. The atrioventricular node cannot conduct as fast as the circus rate, resulting in a 2 : 1 or 3 : 1 block.

Investigation

The ECG is characteristic with a regular rate of 300 beats per minute. It has characteristic saw-tooth pattern. Any change in the baseline ECG suggests that the diagnosis is likely to be atrial fibrillation.

Management

Drug treatment is always the initial management, but may not be effective in cardioverting atrial flutter. Anti-coagulation should be considered in all patients. Electrical cardioversion is almost always successful in preventing recurrence but some patients may go on to develop atrial fibrillation. 'Ablate and pace' treatment involves ablation and implantation of a pacemaker: this is the first-line therapy for tachy–brady syndrome.

Ventricular arrhythmias

Ventricular arrhythmias are common and are usually benign. In patients with coronary artery disease there is an increased risk of cardiac mortality and cardiac arrest. Ventricular arrhythmias range from asymptomatic ventricular ectopic beats to sustained ventricular tachycardia and cardiac arrest.

Ventricular tachycardia

Ventricular tachycardia (VT) is asymptomatic or has the symptoms of coronary artery disease. ECG is the investigation of choice.

Diagnosis
The differential diagnosis of ventricular tachycardia includes supraventricular tachycardia (SVT) with bundle branch block and SVT with accessory pathway conduction.

Making the diagnosis may be difficult. It is important because drugs given to treat SVT may be harmful in patients with ventricular tachycardia and can lead to ventricular fibrillation. If the diagnosis is in doubt the patient should be treated for ventricular tachycardia.

Management
Management should tackle the underlying heart disease:

- In patients who are haemodynamically stable use anti-arrhythmic drugs or overdrive ventricular pacing.
- If patients are haemodynamically compromised DC cardioversion should be carried out. Once the patient is in sinus rhythm further investigations should be carried out to stop further attacks.

Mortality in patients with sustained ventricular tachycardia and coronary artery disease is 20% at 2 years.

Ventricular fibrillation

Ventricular fibrillation (VF) accounts for 5% of patients resuscitated from sudden cardiac arrest:

- Brugada's syndrome is inherited as an autosomal dominant trait. There is an abnormality of the cardiac sodium channel. It is associated with syncope or sudden death.
- Long-QT syndrome may be congenital or acquired. Congenital long-QT syndrome is familial and presents with syncope or sudden death. Acquired

long-QT syndrome is often associated with drugs or electrolyte abnormalities. It is characterized by *torsade de pointes* (self-terminating ventricular tachycardia).

• Wolff–Parkinson–White syndrome is a rare cause of ventricular fibrillation in normal hearts. Atrial fibrillation is rapidly conducted over the accessory pathway and can degenerate into ventricular fibrillation. There is usually a delta wave on the ECG after resuscitation.

CARDIOPULMONARY RESUSCITATION (CPR)

Cardiopulmonary resuscitation is the resuscitation of a collapsed patient facing imminent death from a reversible cause. Collapse can result from ventricular fibrillation or cardiac standstill, including asystole and pulseless electrical activity.

There are many reasons why a patient may require CPR:

• **In acute cases**: trauma, electrocution, cerebrovascular insult, haemorrhage, anaphylaxis, pulmonary embolism, severe hypoxia, severe hypovolaemia, tension pneumothorax, cardiac tamponade.
• **In children and young adults**: respiratory arrest, airway obstruction, drug overdose.

The chain of survival

These are the steps that optimize the likelihood of survival following cardiac arrest:

• Early access to specialist centre.
• Early cardiopulmonary resuscitation.
• Early defibrillation.
• Early advanced care.

BOX 2.14 The principles of effective resuscitation

• Decreasing the delay before therapy is initiated is vital for success.
• Call for help early in the sequence.
• Make contact with the victim as soon as possible.
• Use appropriate expertise and equipment.
• Remove any danger to the patient and rescuer.
• Assess the patient's clinical state.
• Give basic life support (BLS) to improve both cardiac and cerebral oxygenation until definitive treatment is available.
• Give advanced life support (ALS) to correct the underlying problem using defibrillation and intravenous cannulation.

> **BOX 2.15** Useful references on CPR for practical use
> - Guidelines 2000 for cardiopulmonary resuscitation and emergency cardiovascular care. An international consensus on science. *Resuscitation* 2000; **46**: 1–448.
> - Resuscitation Council (UK). *Cardiopulmonary Resuscitation. Guidance for Clinical Practice and Training in Primary Care*. London: Resuscitation Council, 2000.
> - Resuscitation Council (UK). *The Legal Status of Those Who Attempt Resuscitation*. London: Resuscitation Council, 2000.

Guidelines for CPR

These have been carefully formulated and agreed by The International Liaison Committee on Resuscitation (ILCOR) (March 2000) and combine US, European, Australian, Canadian, South African and Latin American protocols. The ILCOR agreed steps of apparently straightforward algorithms.

The new CPR guidelines for 'peri-arrest arrhythmias' also give treatment algorithms. They cover narrow- and broad-complex tachycardias, bradycardias, and atrial fibrillation. Resuscitation guidelines for pregnancy and neonates are also available.

The lay rescuer

The lay rescuer should:

- Check for responsiveness and breathing.
- Give **two breaths** to confirm that the patient is unresponsive.
- Checking for circulation now deliberately omits feeling for a carotid (or other) pulse. Palpation for major pulses is time-consuming and often inaccurate. This is replaced by **checking for unresponsiveness, flaccidity, and skin changes**.
- The **overall appearance of death is sufficient to justify full basic CPR** by a lay rescuer.
- The rate of **chest compression is 100 per minute** and **the ratio of compression to ventilation 15:2** regardless of how many rescuers are involved. A rapid rate and fewer interruptions of chest compression produce a significantly better coronary blood flow.
- A ventilation volume of 700–1000 ml is recommended, which is consistent with the amount that would ordinarily make the chest rise and fall in a normal manner.

The health professional

The health professional should make a rapid almost simultaneous assessment of responsiveness, pulse, and breathing especially. Unless a pulse is present defibrillation should be instituted with minimum delay. Expert help should be sought urgently.

Advanced life support

The emphasis of advanced life support is on immediate defibrillation for VF or pulseless VT. A health professional should give a precordial thump before defibrillation. Basic life support (BLS) should take only a minimal time before the application of the defibrillator/monitor.

Treatment pathways are divided in two:

- Diagnose VF or pulseless VT: this requires immediate defibrillation.
- Diagnose asystole and/or pulseless electrical activity.
- In VF or pulseless VT defibrillate with up to three consecutive shocks administered within 1 min. No BLS is needed during this phase.
- Check the pulse after a shock only if there is a rhythm suggesting cardiac output.
- The initial energy sequence for conventional defibrillators is 200 J, then 200 J, followed by 300 J.
- If defibrillation fails or a non-shockable rhythm is present airway support is required.
- Give chest compression at a rate of 100 per minute.
- Do not interrupt the procedure for pulse checks and defibrillation.
- Remember there is no need for synchrony or defibrillation with ventilation.

VASCULAR DISORDERS

Aortic aneurysm

Aneurysms are not uncommon; they are caused by abnormal widening of the aorta involving the intima and media. The defect is in the media. There are two

---

BOX 2.16 Pharmacological agents recommended during CPR

- **Adrenaline** 1 mg every 3 min. This improves cerebral and coronary blood flow. Vasopressin may be an acceptable alternative.
- **Amiodarone** is the first-line agent for shock-refractory VF/VT and is given initially as a 300 mg bolus. Lidocaine is an alternative to amiodarone.
- **Magnesium** is suggested for refractory VT/VF in patients who could be magnesium or potassium depleted. Bretylium is no longer recommended.
- **Atropine** in a single bolus of 3 mg is used for pulseless electrical activity or a rate of <60 per minute.
- A buffering agent, namely **sodium bicarbonate**, is used late in the management of cardiac arrest. Intravenous bicarbonate may have damaging effects on cardiac or cerebral tissue. Use only if there is pre-existing metabolic acidosis or very late in the arrest procedure when full blood gas analyses are available. It is not known if the use of a buffering agent improves the outcome.

types of aneurysm:

- Fusiform, due to diffuse dilatation of a segment of the aorta.
- Saccular, involving part of the circumference resulting in pocket-like protrusions with a mouth.

Aneurysms have various causes including: atherosclerosis, trauma, cystic medial necrosis secondary to Marfan syndrome or Ehlers–Danlos syndrome, syphilis, and candida.

Dissection of the aorta

Dissection of the aorta is the most important acute problem of the aorta. It is uncommon and is caused by a break in the intima allowing blood to enter the artery wall and cause further separation of the layers. Table 2.9 shows the sites of the aorta most often affected by dissection.

Clinical features

There are a number of clinical features which occur in dissection of the aorta:

- Deep-seated pain which may suddenly develop a severe stabbing quality.
- Pain is usually migratory starting at the site of origin of the dissection.
- Pain is frequently felt in the anterior chest but may migrate to the scapular region.

Other symptoms are site dependent:

- Dissection of the ascending aorta may have associated brady-arrhythmias.
- Carotid dissection may present with sudden neurological deficit.
- A third of patients develop aortic regurgitation.
- Hypotension. The blood pressure may be different in both arms.

Investigation and treatment

Investigation is by X-ray, ECG, transoesophageal echocardiography, or MRI scan.

Table 2.9 Sites of the aorta most often affected by dissection

Site	Per cent of cases
Ascending	65%
Descending	20%
Aortic arch	10%
Abdomen	5%

Treatment involves surgical correction with stent-graft placement. Medical treatment is required to stabilize the patient prior to the operation.

Arterial occlusion

Arterial occlusion results from sudden interruption of the blood flow, usually in a limb. It can be caused by thrombotic disease, arteriosclerosis obliterans, myeloproliferative disorders, intravascular coagulation, trauma, or embolism from the heart or aneurysms. Cardiac causes are left atrial enlargement and mural thrombi in the left ventricle secondary to myocardial infarction.

Clinical features

- Pain in the affected limb.
- Pallor, coldness, and numbness with the loss of skin sensation within an hour.
- Loss of pulses distal to the site of occlusion.
- Muscle contraction occurs after approximately 6 h.

Treatment

When the pulses are absent an immediate operative procedure is indicated. If the limb remains viable angioplasty may be indicated. The patient should be anticoagulated.

Buerger's disease (thromboangiitis obliterans)

This was first described by Buerger in 1908. It is a progressive occlusion of veins, arteries, and nerves and is not related to the development of atheroma. There is an intense inflammation in the vessels. It starts in the small arteries of the hands and feet and occurs in young males between 20 and 40 years old.

Clinical features

- Superficial thrombophlebitis which is nodular and migratory.
- The nodules are red and tender and 50% of patients have a Raynaud-like syndrome.
- Exercise-induced pain is localized to the instep and is relieved by rest.
- The feet appear intensely red.
- The foot pulses are absent; there are femoral and popliteal pulses.
- Eventually the pain becomes intense and still occurs at rest. There is severe ulceration.

Treatment

Cessation of smoking—most patients continue to smoke, leading inevitably to amputation.

Varicose veins

Varicosities occur in the superficial veins. They become dilated and convoluted secondary to incompetent valves, especially of the saphenous veins. Risk factors are:

- female sex
- familial history
- arteriovenous fistulae
- increase in abdominal pressure.

Clinical features
- Feeling of 'heaviness' in the legs.
- Cosmetic deformity.
- Leg discomfort increases towards the end of the day. Raising the legs will decrease discomfort.

Treatment
Wearing of compression stockings may be sufficient. In severe cases ligation and stripping may be indicated.

Deep vein thrombosis (DVT)

As the name suggests, this is thrombosis of the deep veins. There are a number of precipitating factors:

- Prolonged bed rest.
- After prolonged surgical procedures such as hip replacement.
- Related to carcinoma of the lung, pancreas, and small and large intestine.
- Direct pressure from any large mass in the pelvis, such as a tumour or pregnancy.
- Oral contraception.
- Hormone replacement therapy.
- Vascular thrombotic disease.
- The post-partum period.
- Intravascular coagulation.
- Trauma.
- Bacterial infection.

Clinical features
Clinical features are mainly non-specific and include swelling and oedema of the limb and the clinical features of the underlying problem. Pulmonary embolism is frequently the first indication of the presence of a deep vein thrombosis.

Investigations and treatment

Investigations are Doppler ultrasound and a Ventilation–Perfusion scan if pulmonary embolism is suspected.

Heparin is used to initiate treatment. Warfarin is given orally.

Dental relevance of DVT

The dentist should be aware of the interaction of warfarin with other medication. Patients with a DVT may have underlying problems which increase their dental risk assessment.

3 Gastrointestinal tract

The basic function of gastrointestinal tract is to convert food into a form in which it may be absorbed. Material unsuitable for absorption passes out as faeces about 24–36 h after ingestion.

COMPONENTS AND FUNCTIONS OF THE GASTROINTESTINAL TRACT

Mouth

The mouth is involved in the processes of mastication, sensation—touch, temperature, pressure, and taste—salivation, chewing, and swallowing.

Salivation

Salivation is under nervous control: parasympathetic stimulation results in a copious flow of saliva and sympathetic stimulation results in a small volume of viscid, 'sticky' saliva. There is no humoral control of salivation.

Functions of saliva

The main functions of saliva are mechanical—lubrication, aiding mastication, swallowing, and taste, and articulation in speech. Saliva contains the enzyme salivary amylase (ptyalin) which begins the digestion of starch (this is later stopped by acidity in stomach). Saliva also has an antimicrobial and general cleaning action as well as an important role in the prevention of caries.

Swallowing

Swallowing occurs in three stages:

- In the mouth, under voluntary control: contraction at the base of tongue forces the food bolus into the pharynx.
- In the pharynx swallowing becomes a reflex: openings to the larynx and trachea, nasopharynx and the back of the mouth are shut off. Respiration is inhibited. The bolus is passed into the oesophagus.
- When the bolus passes into the oesophagus there is receptive relaxation and peristaltic waves are initiated.

Cardiac sphincter

The cardiac sphincter is the valve between the distal end of the oesophagus and the stomach. It is normally closed but opens shortly after swallowing (vagal activity). After propelling the bolus into the stomach the peristaltic wave shuts it and prevents reflux.

Achalasia is failure of the cardiac sphincter to open on swallowing. Food accumulates in the oesophagus.

Stomach

The stomach produces four types of secretion:

- gastric juice (hydrochloric acid and enzymes)
- mucus
- intrinsic factor
- gastrin—involved in hormonal control of gastric juice.

Only water, alcohol, and aspirin are absorbed in the stomach.

Gastric juice

The secretion of gastric juice is stimulated by:

- Vagal activity—a reflex response to the presence of food in the mouth (cephalic phase).
- Gastrin from the gastric antrum in response to the presence of food and also released by vagal activity (gastric phase).
- Gastrin from the duodenum in response to the presence of chyme (intestinal phase).
- Distension of stomach also causes minor stimulation by intrinsic innervation.
- Histamine acting via the histamine H2 receptor stimulates gastric secretion.

Secretion of gastric juice is inhibited by:

- enterogastrone
- cholecystokin–pancreozymin (CCK-PZ)
- gastric inhibitory peptides (GIP).

The hormones CCK-PZ and enterogastrone are secreted by the duodenum.

The differential secretion of acid and enzymes is not fully understood. The gastric enzymes are different forms of the inactive precursor pepsinogen which are converted to active pepsin by the acid environment. Pepsin functions to break down proteins to form short-chain peptides. Pepsin also 'clots' milk.

Mucus

Mucus is a large molecular weight mucoprotein which forms a hydrated gel. Secretion of mucus is stimulated by:

- mucosal irritation—either mechanical or chemical,
- acid in the lumen of the stomach,
- both vagal and sympathetic stimulation.

Mucus functions to protect the gastric mucosa and lubricate the gastric surface. It contains bicarbonate which acts as a buffer near the mucosa.

Intrinsic factor

Intrinsic factor is a glycoprotein of molecular weight about 55 000. The secretion of intrinsic factor is controlled by the same factors which control the secretion of gastric acid.

Intrinsic factor is necessary for the absorption of vitamin B_{12} from the distal ileum. Intrinsic factor does not normally enter the portal bloodstream; if it does, antibodies to it may develop.

Gastrin

Gastrin is secreted from the gastric antrum. It is a polypeptide with 17 amino acids but occurs in a number of different forms. Secretion of gastrin is stimulated by:

- the presence of food in the gastric antrum and duodenum,
- vagal stimulation.

Gastrin increases gastric acid secretion, increases pepsin secretion, increases gastric antral motility, and enhances the growth of the gastric and duodenal mucosa.

Gastric motility

Gastric motility comprises receptive relaxation and peristalsis. This mixes the stomach contents with gastric juice, converts them to semi-liquid chyme, and propels the contents through the stomach and into the duodenum.

Gastric motility is stimulated by the vagus nerve, gastrin, and motilin, and is inhibited by sympathetic nerves, enterogastrone, and gastric inhibitory peptide (GIP).

Gastric disorders

The main gastric disorders are peptic ulceration, Zollinger–Ellison syndrome, carcinoma, the consequences of gastrectomy, and vomiting.

Pancreatic exocrine secretion

About 0.5–0.8 l of exocrine secretion are produced by the pancreas each day; the fluid is isotonic with plasma and is alkaline, having a pH of about 8.5. Pancreatic secretion is controlled by vagal stimulation which sensitizes the exocrine pancreas to the effects of secretin and pancreozymin. Secretin produces a secretion of mainly water and electrolytes. Pancreozymin (cholecystokinin–pancreozymin, CCK-PZ) produces a secretion which is rich in enzymes. Pancreatic enzymes are stored in zymogen granules, secreted together; and have a neutral to slightly alkaline optimum pH.

Proteases

The proteases break down proteins and peptides to amino acids; they are secreted as inactive precursors which are converted to the active forms by the action of enterokinase from the duodenum:

- Trypinsogens, converted to the active trypsins.
- Chymotrypsinogen, converted to the active chymotrypsin.
- Procarboxypeptidases, converted to the active carboxypeptidases.

Amylase

Pancreatic amylase breaks down starch and related polysaccharides to maltose.

Lipase

Pancreatic lipase breaks down long-chain fatty acids, diglycerides, monoglycerides, and glycerol. The enzymic activity is enhanced by bile salts. Ribonucleases and deoxyribonucleases break down nucleic acids to nucleotides.

Bile

The liver produces about 0.3–1.2 l of bile each day. Bile is secreted continuously by the hepatic parenchymal cells to be stored and concentrated in the gall-bladder. It is then released from the gall-bladder when required by the body. It is a fluid which is iso-osmotic with plasma and is slightly alkaline, having a pH of 7.3–7.7. Bile contains:

- Bile salts.
- Taurocholic acid.
- Glycocholic acid.
- Conjugated products of cholesterol with taurine or glycine (ratio 1:2 in humans); secreted as the sodium salts, they constitute about two-thirds of the total solids in bile. 90% is reabsorbed in the ileum and recirculated through the liver (enterohepatic circulation). Total pool = 2.4 g; daily synthesis = 0.2–0.4 g.

Bile has a role in fat digestion and absorption, activation of pancreatic lipase, increasing pancreatic exocrine secretion, and causing the release of enterokinase.

Cholesterol

The concentration of cholesterol in bile is 15–45 mmol/l; the plasma concentration is 3.5–6.5 mmol/l.

Phospholipids

Phospholipids are present in bile mainly as lecithin (about 7 g/l).

Bile pigments

The bile pigments bilirubin and biliverdin are excretory products with no physiological function. They give colour to the bile and are excreted conjugated as bilirubin diglucuronide.

Control of bile secretion

The main control of the hepatic secretion of bile is by bile salts. Gall-bladder contraction is controlled by CCK-PZ with the vagus having a mior role. CCK-PZ relaxes the gall-bladder sphincter as the gall-bladder contracts.

Small intestine

The small intestine secretes about 3 l/day of **intestinal juice** (succus entericus) from the intestinal glands in the crypts of Lieberkuhn. There are three types of secretory cells: **goblet cells** which secrete mucus, **argentaffin cells** which secrete hormones, and **paneth cells** which secrete enzymes.

Control of the secretion of intestinal juice

There is a low level of secretion for first hour or two after a meal which therafter rapidly increases. Secretion occurs along the whole length of the small intestine but is most obvious at upper end. The main control is the presence of chyme which both mechanically and chemically stimulates the mucosa. Vasoactive intestinal polypeptide (VIP) and secretin may also play a part controlling the secretion of intestinal juice.

Enzymes in intestinal juice

Intestinal juice contains:

- enterokinase (activates the trypsinogens of pancreatic juice)
- maltase
- invertase
- dipeptidase
- alkaline phosphatase.

Brunner glands

The Brunner glands are found only in the duodenum, mainly at the beginning. A small basal secretion becomes copious after the ingestion of a meal. The stimulus for secretion is mainly gastrin and secretin. The Brunner glands secrete mainly alkaline mucus which serves to protect the duodenal wall from the acid from the stomach.

Absorption in the small intestine

The presence of villi greatly increases the area available for absorption of glucose, amino acids, fats, vitamins, iron, bile salts, and water and electrolytes.

Movement of the small intestine

Segmentation allows mixing of the contents with secretions and exposure to absorptive surfaces. Movement are both pendular and peristaltic and serve to propel the contents along the small intestine. Movement is stimulated by:

- vagal activity
- motilin (a hormone secreted by the duodenal mucosa)
- CCK-PZ.

Movement is inhibited by sympathetic activity.

Disorders of the small intestine and associated structures
There are a number of disorders affecting the small intestine:

- duodenal ulceration
- pancreatitis
- gallstones
- adynamic ileus
- resection of parts of the small intestine
- portal obstruction
- jaundice, ascites, cirrhosis
- malabsorption syndrome
- intestinal obstruction.

Large intestine

The ileocaecal valve closes at the entrance of the large intestine. Rhythmic opening and closing starts a few minutes after a meal. The mechanism is uncertain and is probably under hormonal (gastrin) and nervous (vagus) control.

The large intestine secretes **mucus** from goblet cells. This is controlled locally by mechanical stimulation. The mucus lubricates the contents and neutralizes acids formed by bacterial action.

Movement
Movement is via segmentation and peristalsis as in the small intestine. There is also mass action contraction which moves the bulk of the contents from one region of the colon into the next.

Absorption
The large intestine absorbs 90% of the water entering caecum, sodium, potassium, chloride, glucose, and vitamins produced by bacterial action.

Disorders of the large intestine
There are a number of disorders affecting the large intestine:

- constipation
- megacolon (Hirschsprung's disease)
- diarrhoea—gastroenteritis, infectious disease, e.g. typhoid, cholera
- Crohn's disease

- ulcerative colitis
- diverticular disease
- colectomy and colostomy.

EATING DISORDERS

The mouth is part of the gastrointestinal tract, and the clinical features of diseases affecting the upper and lower gut are frequently manifested in the mouth. The mouth also plays an important part in the psychological framework of a person and as such is seen as an area of control of bodily function. Eating disorders may result from:

- Markedly restricted intake or vomiting and purging of food taken in.
- Constant and massive increase in dietary fat, protein, and carbohydrates seen in the morbidly obese patients.

Most cases of eating disorders are undiagnosed. In UK between 165 000 and 300 000 people have eating disorders associated with anorexia or bulimia. In 1980 6% of the population were obese; by 2001 the figure was 20%. The National Audit Office in 'Tackling Obesity' estimates the cost of obesity to be £3.6 billion by 2010.

Obesity

A person is said to be obese if they have a body mass index (BMI) of greater than 30. The BMI is calculated by dividing the weight in kg by the square of the individual's height (in m).

Health risks and associated problems
Truncal fat deposition incurs a greater risk of morbidity. The major risks arise from diabetes, cancer, gallstones, and social problems.

Diabetes
Obesity is associated with Type 2 diabetes. An obese person has a 40–90 times increased risk of diabetes.

Coronary artery disease
Seventy five to 80% of patients with coronary artery disease are obese.

Cancer
The World Health Organization (WHO) lists obesity as the second most common preventable cause of cancer. Carcinomas associated with obesity are:

- post-menopausal breast cancer
- kidney cancer
- oesophageal cancer.

Gallstones

The associated risk of gallstones is increased seven times in obese people. However, rapid weight loss of more than 3 kg a week predisposes to gallstones.

Social problems

There are a number of social problems encountered by obese people, especially:

- reduced mobility
- difficulty with personal hygiene
- loss of self-esteem
- increased depressive episodes
- discrimination in employment.

Treatment of obesity

The major focus in treatment of obesity should be on:

- Change in lifestyle, which should include a lifeplan which is focused on the patient as a person.
- Weight loss with a change in content and pattern of eating.
- Physiological changes resulting from increased exercise and dietary intake.
- Psychological support by increasing self-esteem and encouraging the patient to feel the need for change.

Anorexia nervosa

Aetiology

The aetiology of anorexia nervosa is unknown. The condition involves a psychological regression to childhood. The conflicts aroused in adolescence cannot be tolerated by the girl or her family, resulting in a retreat into childhood, arrested physical development, and hypothalamic dysfunction. There are a number of 'family theories', in which the patient's symptoms 'stabilize' the family. All conflict in the family then centres on the patient, resulting in the submergence of other conflicts.

The psychological characteristics of anorexia nervosa include:

- a tendency to perfectionism
- a setting of high standards
- social isolation and sexually naïvety
- loss of self-esteem.

Clinical features

The male to female ratio is 1 : 10 and the age onset is below 25 years. Patients conceal their eating disorder and are frequently extensively investigated for underlying disease. The main diagnostic factors for anorexia as given in the American Psychiatric Association Diagnostic and Statistical Manual, 1994 are shown in Box 3.1.

> **BOX 3.1** Diagnostic factors for anorexia taken from the American Psychiatric Association Diagnostic and Statistical Manual, 1994
>
> - Refusal to maintain weight at a minimal normal level for height and age, such that body weight is 15% below that expected for the individual's height and age.
> - An intense fear of gaining weight or of becoming fat.
> - A distorted notion of body shape and image, such that the individual continues to complain of feeling fat even at very low weights.
> - Amenorrhea in females of post-menarcheal age, or an equivalent endocrine disturbance in males.
> - The main problem appears to be the overwhelming fear of fatness, with a distorted body image. They are obsessed with talking about food and frequently, cook compulsively.
> - Patients continue to visualize themselves as fat or even obese even when they are below normal body weight for their age, height and sex.

Bulimia nervosa

Bulimia nervosa is associated with the obsessive drive to lose weight by binge eating and vomiting. The male to female ratio is 1 : 20 (however, there are an increasing number of males). The age of onset is around 17–18 years. Psychologically, bulimics tend to have more outgoing personalities than anorexics and are not socially isolated; they may or may not be sexually experienced.

Aetiology

The aetiology of bulimia nervosa is unknown; however, a complex mix of individual family and social factors is likely to be involved. Patients have problems with authority. This may result from interactions between the patient and their parents. The patient may be a perfectionist, or more frequently comes from a high-achieving, high-performance family. There may be a family history of eating disorder, depression, alcoholism, or drug abuse.

Clinical features

The diagnostic criteria for bulimia nervosa are: recurrent bingeing; feelings of lack of control; use of dieting, fasting, vomiting, and purging to control the weight; abnormal concern about shape and weight; and two or more binge episodes per week for at least 3 months.

Patients frequently conceal symptoms—both the bingeing and the vomiting. Calorie intake varies from 40–500 calories to over 3000 calories. Episodes may be intermittent.

The main diagnostic factors for bulimia as given in the American Psychiatric Association Diagnostic and Statistical Manual, 1994 are shown in Box 3.2.

> **BOX 3.2** Diagnostic factors for bulimia taken from the American Psychiatric Association Diagnostic and Statistical Manual, 1994
>
> - Eating in a discrete period of time an amount of food that is definitely larger than most people would eat.
> - A sense of lack of control over eating during the episode.
> - Recurrent, inappropriate, compensatory behaviours (such as self-induced vomiting, use of laxatives or diuretics, strict dieting and/or excessive exercise) in order to prevent weight gain.
> - The binge eating and compensatory behaviour occur on average at least twice a week for 3 months.
> - Self-evaluation is unduly influenced by body shape and weight.

Clinical signs
- Increase in rate of dental caries.
- Acid erosion palatally on the dentition.
- Frequent sore throat and hoarse voice.
- Swollen, painless enlarged parotids, especially in males, which become persistent.
- Metabolic disturbances such as hyperkalaemic alkalosis.

Treatment

Treatment may be necessary because of depression, or because of associated metabolic problems. Bulimia is easier to treat than anorexia. Most patients can be treated on an outpatient basis with individual or group psychotherapy. With treatment, 70% of patients cease bulimic behaviour completely.

There are a number of factors which indicate a poor prognosis in eating disorders:

- anxiety
- depression
- social isolation
- poor family/parental interrelationships
- bulimia resistant to treatment
- vomiting and purging
- prolonged illness
- persistent severe weight loss.

Clinical complications in eating disorders

Eating disorders can give rise to a number of clinical complications:

- Loss of fertility.
- Osteoporosis, especially spontaneous fractures or following minor trauma.
- Cardiac disease, especially hypokalaemia-induced arrhythmias.

- Renal failure.
- Sialosis of salivary glands.
- Ulceration or stomach rupture.
- Erosion of tooth enamel.

The mortality rate is very high at around 13–20% per annum. A greater proportion of those with anorexia die each year than those with bulimia. The main causes of death are starvation, cachexia, and suicide.

BOX 3.3 Dental relevance of common eating-related gastrointestinal problems

Difficulty in chewing

Difficulty in chewing is most commonly related to causes of dental origin. Non-dental causes include:

- Dry mouth.
- Sore ulcerated mouth.
- Burning mouth syndrome.
- Pain of non-dental origin, e.g. trigeminal neuralgia or glossopharyngeal neuralgia.
- Oropharyngeal infection—bacterial, fungal, or viral.

Odynophagia

Odynophagia means painful swallowing. Pain is experienced on swallowing the food bolus. There is usually no obstruction impeding the passage of the bolus. Infections such as oropharyngeal candidosis or Herpes simplex may be responsible.

Globus

Patients describe a lump in the throat. This is usually felt at the level of the larynx. Patients do not experience difficulty or pain on swallowing.

Regurgitation

Regurgitation of liquid food into the mouth usually presents as a bad taste or sore mouth or throat. It is usually related to posture or may be self-induced as part of an eating disorder.

Dysphagia

Dysphagia implies difficulty in swallowing. This may occur at the beginning of swallowing a normal sized bolus; repeated attempts are made with difficulty. This results in spluttering and coughing. The abnormality may be in the mouth or oropharynx. When the obstruction is further down in the oesophagus the initial stage of swallowing occurs, followed by a feeling of food being 'held up'. In these cases the location of the patient's dysphagia is an unreliable guide to the location of the blockage.

HIATUS HERNIA

A hiatus hernia occurs when the upper part of the stomach, which is joined to the oesophagus, moves up into the chest through the hole (called a hiatus) in the diaphragm. Hiatus hernia is a common condition which occurs in 10% of the population. Those most at risk are middle-aged or elderly women. Obesity increases the risk.

There are a number of different types of hiatus hernia:

- **Sliding hiatus hernia:** this is the most common type. It is frequently asymptomatic. The herniated portion of the stomach slides into and out of the chest cavity.
- **Fixed hiatus hernia:** the upper part of the stomach may be fixed in the chest. Patients may or may not be symptomatic.
- **Complicated hiatus hernia:** this is the most infrequent type. There is herniation of the entire stomach into the chest. Patients tend to be symptomatic and require surgery.

Clinical features

Hiatus hernia can have the following clinical features:

- Central epigastric pain.
- Burning pain which occurs after meals and on lying down. Pain may occur during the night and wake the patient.
- Reflux of fluid. Patients complain of a foul taste on waking.
- Other symptoms include a feeling of bloating, frequent belching, and dysphagia.

Complications of hiatus hernia can include:

- Reflux of acid into the oesophagus.
- Anaemia.
- Scarring causing stricture formation.
- Aspiration of stomach contents into the lungs.

Investigations and treatment

Hiatus hernia is best visualized with a barium swallow. Endoscopy may be used if the symptoms of pain are severe.

Lifestyle measures play an important role in treatment:

- Large meals should be avoided: small portions of food should be eaten every few hours.
- No food should be eaten in the 2–3 h before bedtime.
- Bending or stooping should be avoided.
- Obese patients should lose weight.
- To avoid night-time problems the head of the bed should be raised 20–30 cm from the floor.

If medication is required antacids are helpful. H2 antagonists or proton pump inhibitors can be used to decrease acid secretion.

Surgery may be necessary in patients with complicated hiatus hernia who develop complications.

GASTRO-OESOPHAGEAL REFLUX DISEASE (GORD)

Gastro-oesophageal reflux disease occurs in about 8 % of the population in the West. The causes are multifactorial and include:

- A malfunctioning lower oesophageal sphincter with defective relaxation of the sphincter and an abnormal basal tone.
- Abnormal motility of the lower oesophageal body, resulting in deficient or intermittent inefficiency of peristalsis.

Helicobacter pylori infection is **not** related to the pathogenesis of GORD.

Clinical features

Symptoms usually occur after a meal. Reflux is the main symptom but there may also be regurgitation, heartburn, nausea, bloating, and epigastric pain or discomfort.

Investigations and treatment

Endoscopy and barium swallow may be performed, but both investigations may be normal in GORD.

Proton pump inhibitors are the drugs of first choice in GORD. Antacids and H2 antagonists may also be useful. Surgery is only performed as a treatment of last resort.

OESOPHAGEAL VARICES

The portal vein takes blood from the stomach, spleen, and small and large intestine to the liver. It delivers blood to the liver at a rate of 1500 ml/min. Obstruction of flow in the portal vein will increase the portal venous pressure. A high portal pressure causes the development of portosystemic collaterals which dilate the veins proximal to the obstruction. The enlarged veins become tortuous, resulting in oesophageal varices.

Aetiology

In the UK alcohol consumption and viral infections resulting in cirrhosis are the main causes of portal hypertension. Once chronic liver disease such as cirrhosis develops, oesophageal varices arise in approximately a third of patients in the first 6 years. The risk of bleeding is high, with a third of patients having a major bleed within the first 18 months of identification of the varices. Bleeding from oesophageal varices is a life-threatening condition and accounts for approximately 10% of episodes of haematemesis from the upper GI tract.

Causes

- alcoholic liver disease
- viral hepatitis
- primary biliary cirrhosis
- veno-occlusive disease
- portal vein thrombosis
- Budd–Chiari syndrome.

Budd–Chiari syndrome is a condition caused by obstruction to hepatic venous outflow by diseases such as polycythemia rubra vera, myeloproliferative disorders, tumours, and pregnancy. The clinical features are abdominal pain, hepatomegaly, and ascites. The condition results in portal hypertension and varices.

Investigations

A number of investigations can be performed:

- Liver function tests.
- Prothrombin time.
- Full blood count as patients are often anaemic.
- Ultrasound of the upper abdomen.
- Endoscopy to visualize the extent of varices.

Treatment

In a stable patient consider an elective procedure to prevent varices and haematemesis, for example sclerotherapy, variceal banding ligation, or elective portocaval or splenorenal shunts. The administration of beta-blockers in patients with cirrhosis will reduce the portal pressure.

In an emergency in a patient with bleeding varices:

- Gain intravenous access, cross-match blood, and insert a CVP line.
- Check blood sugar.
- Transfuse colloid, then cross-matched whole blood.
- Endoscopy should be performed early to identify the bleeding site and stop bleeding.
- Sclerotherapy or band ligation may be tried.
- A combination of somatostatin or octreotide together with endoscopic therapy gives the best outcome.
- Continued bleeding is dealt with using a Sengstaken–Blakemore tube, inflating the balloon against the varicosity to staunch blood flow.
- Surgery.

DYSPHAGIA

Dysphagia is a persistent difficulty in swallowing. It has a large number of causes:

- **Oropharyngeal problems**: aphthous ulcers or glossitis, xerostomia secondary to drugs, anxiety, or Sjögren's syndrome, tonsillitis, pharyngitis secondary to cytomegalovirus (CMV), Epstein–Barr virus (EBV), herpes, or candidal infection, pharyngeal pouch secondary to diverticulum, retropharyngeal abscess, tonsillar mass.
- **Oesophageal problems**: foreign body causing an obstruction, diverticulum, oesophageal stricture secondary to reflux, oesophageal web in Plummer–Vinson syndrome in severe iron deficiency.
- **Neurogenic problems**: stroke, bulbar palsy, achalasia, myasthenia gravis, multiple sclerosis, Wilson's disease (hepatolenticular degeneration), botulism, lead poisoning, low levels of magnesium.
- **Extrinsic lesions compressing the oesophagus**: lymphadenopathy, tumours in the neck and mediastinum, retrosternal goitre, carcinoma of the bronchus, aortic aneurysm.

Clinical features

- Delay in or inability to swallow.
- Food sticking in the throat.
- Regurgitation of food—liquids first solids later.
- Difficulty swallowing solid foods and later liquids.
- Chest discomfort when swallowing.
- Coughing during or after swallowing.
- Weight loss because of swallowing difficulty.
- Recurrent episodes of pneumonia.

Investigations and treatment

Suitable investigations are barium swallow and fluoroscopy, endoscopy, and manometry. Treatment depends on the underlying cause.

Achalasia

Achalasia is a disorder of motility of the oesophagus. It occurs in both males and females at an incidence of 1 per 100 000 population per year.

Aetiology
The aetiology of achalasia is unknown. The principal abnormality is thought to be the degeneration of the neuronal bodies in the myenteric plexus. In South America, Chagas disease caused by *Trypanosoma cruzii* has a similar clinical picture.

Clinical features
- Dysphagia for fluids and solids occurs.
- Weight loss may indicate late-stage disease.
- Forty to 50% of patients complain of retrosternal chest pain.
- The main characteristic is failure of the lower oesophageal sphincter to relax on swallowing.
- The oesophageal body loses its ability to contract. Some non-peristaltic contractions may be present.
- Regurgitation of undigested solids during or shortly after a meal occurs in 80% of patients.
- Some patients induce regurgitation to relieve an uncomfortable feeling of retrosternal fullness.
- Fluid may be regurgitated into the pharynx.
- Nocturnal coughing may result from fluid regurgitation.
- Occasionally food or fluid is aspirated into the lungs.

Investigations and treatment
Investigations are barium swallow with fluoroscopy and manometry.

Possible treatments include botulinum toxin injections, medication with isosorbide dinitrate or nifedipine to increase vasodilatation, surgical treatment with endoscopy and pneumatic dilatation, or extramucosal oesophagomyotomy (Heller's operation).

OESOPHAGEAL CANCER

In the UK carcinoma of the oesophagus is a relatively uncommon, accounting for 4000 deaths per annum. It has a very poor prognosis. The 5-year survival rate is under 10%. The incidence of oesophageal cancer in a number of countries is shown in Table 3.1. The male to female ration of cases is 3 : 1.

Risk factors associated with oesophageal cancer
Adenocarcinoma occurs in the lower third of the oesophagus. Risk factors for **adenocarcinoma** are:

- Barrett's oesophagus—a condition affecting the lining of the lower oesophagus in which the normal healthy squamous cells are replaced by abnormal

Table 3.1 Incidence of oesophageal cancer

Country	Cases per 100 000 population
United Kingdom	7.5
South Africa and Iran	>35
Northern China	>139

columnar epithelium. Barrett's oesophagus is often due to gastro-oesophageal reflux.

- Cytotoxic drugs.
- Tobacco smoke.
- Alcohol.

Squamous cell carcinoma occurs in the upper two-thirds of the oesophagus. Risk factors for **squamous cell carcinoma** are:

- Smoking.
- Alcohol.
- Trauma—caustic stricture.
- Malnutrition and dietary deficiency, especially vitamins A, C, B_2, and molybdenum (molybdenum can reduce the production or counteract the actions of nitrosamines (see below)).
- Plummer–Vinson syndrome (also known as Brown–Patterson–Kelly syndrome): a disorder linked to severe, long-term iron deficiency anaemia, which causes swallowing difficulty due to web-like membranes of tissue growing in the throat.
- Achalasia.
- Human papilloma virus (HPV) infection.
- Consumption of nitrosamine-containing foods.

Clinical presentation

In almost all patients oesophageal cancer presents as difficulty in swallowing. Symptoms occur late since the lumen has to be less than 12 mm in diameter before dysphagia occurs. Dysphagia is initially to solids then to liquids. There may also be:

- End-stage saliva dysphagia.
- Enlarged cervical nodes—lymph node metastasis occurs early.
- Oesophageal pain.
- Haematemesis. The tumour may erode local structures, e.g. the aorta, and give massive haematemesis.
- Weight loss, malaise, and anorexia.

Investigation and treatment

Endoscopy and biopsy and barium swallow are used to establish the diagnosis. Ultrasound, chest X-ray, and CT scan of the abdomen are used to stage the tumour.

Treatment is aimed at palliation in malignant dysphagia, but survival is limited. Surgical resection requires a large margin of excision. Radiotherapy may be used—adenocarcinoma is less sensitive to radiotherapy than squamous cell carcinoma. Chemotherapy with cisplatinum is used as an adjunct to resection. Other modes of treatment include: combination therapy, dilatation endoscopy, endoprosthesis (stent), and endoscopic tumour ablation.

> **BOX 3.4** Dental relevance of oesophageal cancer
>
> - If a patient presents with difficulty swallowing take a careful history of the dysphagia.
> - Examination of the neck may reveal cervical lymphadenopathy, especially a Virchow's node on the left side in the anterior triangle between the two heads.
> - 40% of patients with tumours limited to the mucosa already have metastatic spread.

Table 3.2 Causes of upper gastrointestinal bleeding

Cause	Percentage of cases
Duodenal ulcer	30
Gastric ulcer	15
Gastric erosion	15
Oesophageal varices	12
Miscellaneous, e.g. oesophageal tumours or inflammation, vascular malformations	10
Undiagnosed causes	10
Mallory–Weiss tear	8

Prognosis

The overall median survival for a patient with oesophageal cancer is 1 year. The 5-year survival rate is 5%. There is a 5–10% mortality with oesophagectomy.

GASTROINTESTINAL HAEMORRHAGE

Bleeding can occur from any part of the gastrointestinal tract from the mouth to the anus. Gastrointestinal bleeding is a common medical/surgical emergency. Mortality associated with gastrointestinal bleeding is approximately 10% and is increased in the elderly.

Causes of upper gastrointestinal bleeding

Table 3.2 shows the main causes of **upper gastrointestinal bleeding**.
Causes of **lower gastrointestinal bleeding** include:

- haemorrhoids
- rectal and anal ulceration/tears/fissures
- inflammatory bowel disease
- polyps
- diverticular disease
- carcinoma of the colon/rectum
- angiodysplasia

BOX 3.5 Dental relevance of gastrointestinal bleeding

- Acute blood loss in young adults is usually a result of repeated retching which results in a Mallory–Weiss tear.
- Chronic blood loss from any part of the gastrointestinal tract may be occult.
- There may be no symptoms except malaise and tiredness.
- Patients, especially elderly men, may present with sore mouths, recurrent oral ulceration, or generalized pallor.
- A low Hb with a microcytic blood film and a low ferritin may be found on routine investigations.
- Elderly female patients may present with dysphagia, pallor, smooth sore tongue, or glossitis and angular cheilitis.
- Chronic blood loss may result in cardiac failure.
- Patients may have problems with general anaesthetic or intravenous sedation.

- arteriovenous malformation
- ischaemic colitis
- Meckell's diverticulum
- drugs, e.g. non-steroidal anti-inflammatory drugs (NSAIDs)
- trauma.

PEPTIC ULCERATION

Peptic ulceration results from a discrete break in either the duodenal or the gastric mucosa. In 1993–1994 peptic ulceration was the cause of death in 2778 people in England and Wales between the ages of 25 and 74 years.

Duodenal ulceration

Epidemiology and aetiology
Duodenal ulceration is a common condition occurring in 10% of the population. However, the incidence is declining developed countries. The male : female ratio is 1 : 1 and the peak incidence is between 40 and 55 years of age. Sixty-five to 70% of patients relapse 1 year after treatment.

   Factors associated with duodenal ulceration are:

- *Helicobacter pylori* infection.
- An increased rate of gastric emptying.
- Drugs which damage the mucosal lining, e.g. NSAIDs.
- Stress.

Clinical features
Do not make a diagnosis of duodenal ulceration on symptoms alone.
Clinical features include:

- Pain which wakes patient around 2 a.m.; it is situated in the epigastrium and is intermittent.

BOX 3.6 *Helicobacter pylori*

- *H. pylori* is an organism which lives in the mucous layer of the gastric mucosa.
- 20% of 20-year-olds test positive for *H. pylori*.
- 80% of 80-year-olds test positive for *H. pylori*.
- *H. pylori* infection can be detected by breath test and biopsy.
- *H. pylori* is more commonly associated with duodenal than gastric ulcers.

- Haemorrhage.
- Perforation.
- Pyloric stenosis.

Investigations

Endoscopy is the most reliable investigation: aphthous type ulceration is seen. Cells are taken for biopsy and culture. Also: barium meal—double contrast, breath test, and full blood count.

Benign gastric ulcer

Benign gastric ulcer results form a discrete break in the gastric mucosa. The most common site is the lesser curve. The size of these ulcers is variable.

Aetiology

Men are more often affected than women, and the condition is more common in the elderly. Incidence is increased in socioeconomic groups 4 and 5. Forty-five to 50% of patients relapse 1 year after treatment.

Clinical features

The clinical features are:

- Pain.
- Anaemia secondary to occult bleeding.
- Perforation.
- Benign gastric ulcer runs more a chronic course than duodenal ulcer.

Investigations

- Endoscopy: biopsy is most important to exclude gastric cancer.
- Barium meal.
- Full blood picture to exclude anaemia.

Treatment for peptic ulceration

Treatment is aimed at symptom relief, healing, and prevention of recurrence:

- Reduce alcohol intake.
- Stop smoking.

> **BOX 3.7** Dental relevance of peptic ulceration
> - Blood loss may result in iron deficiency anaemia with consequent sore mouth.
> - Oral features are sore mouth, glossitis, and angular cheilitis.
> - Long-standing anaemia may result in Plummer–Vinson syndrome.
> - Dysphagia may present problems with general anaesthetic.
> - H2 antagonist cimetidine blocks cytochrome P-450 resulting in an increased half-life for warfarin, phenytoin, metronidazole, and fluconazole.

- Eradicate *H. pylori* infection.
- Medication:
- Duodenal ulceration may be reduced by H2 antagonists. A 6-week course of cimetidine and ranitidine causes healing. H2 antagonists are ineffective at preventing gastric ulceration.
- Sucralfate, a mixture of aluminium hydroxide and sucrose.
- Bismuth.
- Antacids.
- Omeprazole, a hydrogen/potassium ATPase inhibitor.
- Misoprostol.
- Specific: cyclo-oxygenase 2 (COX-2) inhibitors: there is no justification for using simultaneous prescription of gastroprotective agents with COX-2 selective inhibitors.
- Where NSAID treatment needs to be continued in patients who have active peptic ulceration, a proton-pump inhibitor may be the concurrent treatment.
- Surgery: only used when there is haemorrhage, perforation, or for prevention of pyloric stenosis.

CARCINOMA OF THE STOMACH

Carcinoma of the stomach is the second most common cancer worldwide.

Aetiology

There are a number of premalignant conditions associated with stomach cancer:

- gastric adenomatous polyps
- chronic atrophic gastritis
- intestinal metaplasia
- gastric ulcer (benign)
- previous gastric surgery.

A number of causal factors for stomach cancer have been identified:

- *H. pylori* infection (gastric lymphoma and maltoma are particularly associated with *H. pylori* infection).

- Blood group A.
- There is a family history in approximately 10% cases: familial gastric cancer has been associated with E-cadherin mutation in New Zealand.
- Lead and zinc in drinking water.
- Diets high in starch and low in vitamin C.
- Cigarette smoking.
- Alcohol consumption (spirits).
- A diet containing pickled and smoked fish.

Epidemiology

The incidence increases with age (peak incidence occurs at 50–70 years of age). Stomach cancer is more common in males (male : female ratio 2 : 1) and varies with geographical location. Table 3.3 shows the variable geographical incidence of stomach cancer.

Clinical features

Symptoms are usually non-specific and patients present late. Symptoms may include:

- indigestion/dyspepsia
- anorexia and early satiety
- nausea and vomiting
- weight loss
- haematemesis
- melaena.

About 10–15% of patients present with signs of metatatic disease: supraclavicular node on the left side (Virchow's node), jaundice ascites, hepatomegaly, or abdominal mass.

Table 3.3 Geographical incidence of stomach cancer

Country/region	Incidence per 100 000 population
Japan	70
Southern Africa	60
Chile	30
Hungary	30
Iceland	30
USA	10
UK	5–10
Central Africa	0.01

Investigations

Diagnosis is made by endoscopy and cytology and biopsy. Once diagnosis is made the tumour should be staged by performing abdominal ultrasound, CT scan, or laparoscopy.

Management

Management of stomach cancer is primarily by radical surgical resection. Stomach cancer is relatively radioresistant. Chemotherapy is only used in patients with inoperable disease. A combination of mitomycin C, 5-fluorouracil and doxorubin is used but only 5% of patients go into complete remission.

Post curative surgical treatment, survival is 65–85% in Japan (early cancers may be as high as 90%) and 35–75% in the UK.

Screening

National mass population screening in Japan using endoscopy and X-rays has increased the detection of cancer. Twenty five per cent of all stomach cancers are detected this way. Patients with polyps, atrophic gastritis, and dysplasia or metaplasia should have annual screening.

CROHN'S DISEASE

Crohn's disease is a chronic inflammatory disorder which can affect any part of the gastrointestinal tract from the mouth to the anus.

Epidemiology

Crohn's disease occurs with a varying incidence worldwide: there are 2–4 cases per 100 000 population in Europe and the USA and 0.2–0.4 cases per 100 000 in Japan. It is very rare in developing countries. The peak age of incidence is 20–60 years. More women than men are affected.

Pathology

- Skin lesion.
- Aphthous ulceration
- Oral and mucosal involvement.
- Transmural inflammation, but predominantly submucosal.
- Inflammation infiltrate—lymphocytes, macrophages, and plasma cells.
- Histologically 50–70% of patients have non-caseating granulomas.

Aetiology

There may be genetic factors associated with the aetiology of Crohn's disease as 20% of patients have an affected family member. There is a higher incidence amongst identical compared with non-identical twins. Forty to 50% of patients with intestinal Crohn's have mutations in the *CARD15* (*NOD2*) gene on chromosome 16. Other factors include:

- Smoking—increases the relative risk by three to four times.
- Infective organisms. Several organisms have been postulated to be involved: *Mycobacterium paratuberculosis* is found in the gut of cattle and other ruminants, causing a disease called Johne's disease; measles.
- Diet—increased intake of refined sugar
- Immune mechanism.

Clinical features

Crohn's disease has a number of clinical features. Table 3.4 shows the percentage of patients having the various features.

Complications

A large number of complications and manifestations, both intestinal and extra-intestinal, are associated with Crohn's disease.
   Intestinal complications include:

- acute dilation, perforation, massive haemorrhage (all less common than in ulcerative colitis)
- strictures—leading to obstruction
- fistulas
- perianal disease
- ileocaecal disease
- blind-loop syndromes
- malabsorption.

   Some **extra-intestinal manifestation** of Crohn's disease are listed in Table 3.5.

Table 3.4 Crohn's disease: percentage of patients with various clinical features

Clinical feature	Per cent of patients
Diarrhoea	70–90
Abdominal pain	45–66
Anal lesions	50–80
Rectal bleeding	45
Weight loss	65–75
Fever	30–40
Fistula	8–10

Table 3.5 Some extra-intestinal manifestation of Crohn's disease

Manifestation	Incidence (%)
Related to disease activity:	
Aphthous ulceration	20
Erythema nodosum	5–10
Pyoderma gangrenosum	0.5
Acute arthritis (large joints affected, transient, non-destructive)	6–12
Eye complications: conjunctivitis, episcleritis, uveitis	3–10
Unrelated to disease activity:	
Sacro-ilitis (usually asymptomatic)	18
Ankylosing spondylitis (75% of patients are positive for HLA-B27. May progress following proctocolectomy)	2–6

Investigations

Iron and folate and B_{12} are low. Erythrocyte sedimentaton rate (ESR), C-reactive protein (CRP), and orosomucoids (alpha glycoproteins) may all be raised. Stool examination shows excess fat present if the small bowel is affected. Sigmoidoscopy, colonoscopy, and rectal biopsy should be performed to exclude large bowel involvement. Suitable imaging procedures include indium-labelled white cell scan, CT scan, and MRI scan.

Treatment

Diet plays an important part in treatment. Enteral feeding is widely used. Elemental diets (amino acids and glucose) are as effective a treatment as steroids. An increase in dietary fibre as part of a balanced diet is necessary, especially in children. Folate and B_{12} supplements may be necessary.

A wide range of drugs are used to treat Crohn's disease:

- Corticosteroids—in all forms. Budesonide 6 mg as maintenance is not associated with loss of bone density.
- Azathioprine is used in maintenance therapy.
- Oral cyclosporin.
- Infliximab (a tumour necrosis factor-alpha (TNF-α) blocker) is used in patients with fistulas and those unresponsive to other treatments.
- Sulfasalazine in active colonic disease.
- Mesalazine in active colonic disease.
- Metronidazole.

Seventy-five per cent of patients require at least one surgical procedure.

Prognosis

The risk of recurrent attacks is 70–85%. Patients have an increased risk of developing gastrointestinal carcinoma after 15 years.

> **BOX 3.8** Dental relevance of Crohn's disease
>
> - Oral Crohn's disease may affect most patients with gastrointestinal disease at some time during the lifetime course of the disease.
> - Children may present with oral Crohn's as the first clinical feature of systemic disease.
> - Patients may present with oral Crohn's as the sole manifestation.
> - Visible lesions include gingival infiltration, linear oral ulcers, cobblestone buccal mucosa, and swollen lips.
> - There may be facial reddening in areas where intraoral lesions have penetrated onto the facial surface.
> - Patients may have difficulty with oral hygiene because of oral soreness.
> - Regular hygienist appointments are necessary.
> - Some foods, preservatives and perfume additives tend to exacerbate oral lesions.
> - Oral lesions respond well to depot steroid infiltration with triamcinolone.
> - Extra-gut problems such as arthritis may interfere with the patient's mobility and dexterity.
> - Disease affecting the ileocaecal region may result in malabsorption of iron, B_{12}, and folate with consequent effects on the oral mucosa.

ULCERATIVE COLITIS

Ulcerative colitis is a chronic inflammatory disease which remits and relapses. It presents between the ages of 20 and 40 years. Incidence is 7–10 per 100 000 in the European population; 10–15 per 100 000 in the North American population. Whites are more affected than Blacks.

Aetiology

The aetiology of ulcerative colitis is unknown. It is an uncommon disease. There appears to be a genetic basis, there being a strong positive correlation with ankylosing spondylitis and HLA-B27. There is an association with coeliac disease in relatives. Smoking has a negative risk association. Once disease is established it may have an immunological basis.

Clinical features

Disease patterns can vary:

- Weight loss and malaise with intermittent diarrhoea.
- The disease classically starts at the anus and rectum and ascends the colon with time.
- There may be a single mild episode.
- There may be acute episodes of severe bloody diarrhoea. The acute form has high morbidity.
- Fever and abdominal distention may precede toxic megacolon and perforation.

A large range of clinical features may be present:

- Diarrhoea with mucous and blood.
- Abdominal pain.
- Erythema nodosum or pyoderma gangrenosum.
- Ulceration in the mouth, the rest of the gastrointestinal tract, and the skin.
- Mouth ulcers tend to be of the major type.
- Transient episcleritis and iritis.
- Deep vein thrombosis.
- Arthropathy.
- Sacroiliitis.
- Ankylosing spondylitis.
- Seronegative arthritis.
- Hepatobiliary disease—cirrhosis and sclerosing cholangitis.
- Amyloidosis.
- Development of carcinoma of the colon: 10% increase after 10 years.

Investigations

Investigations should look for anaemia, raised ESR, and leucocytosis during active disease. Barium enema shows loss of the haustral pattern with straightening and shortening of the large intestine. Also colonoscopy and sigmoidoscopy. Sigmoidoscopy appearance varies with disease type:

- In quiescent disease the surface mucosa appears granular.
- In active disease there is pus and blood and the mucosa looks red.
- In an acute episode of active disease there is pus and blood with ulceration and contact bleeding.

Treatment

- Symptomatic patients can be given codeine phosphate, sulfasalazine, or prednisolone, including suppositories for rectal symptoms.
- In active colitis pentasa 4 g daily and balsalazide 7.75 g daily may be used instead of steroids.
- Azathioprine used as steroids, which should be withdrawn after two relapses of disease activity in 1 year.

BOX 3.9 Dental relevance of ulcerative colitis

- Oral ulcers. These are large and persistent and resemble major aphthae. There may be single or bilateral lesions on the tongue.
- Nutritional problems may result in glossitis.
- Hepatic disease may cause problems with bleeding and drug metabolism.
- Ankylosing spondylitis may cause respiratory problems; this may affect oral access. Take care with the odontoid peg when reclining the patient in the dental chair.
- Ankylosing spondylitis may be associated with aortic incompetence. Patients may require antibiotic cover.

- Cyclosporin therapy should be instituted when CRP is greater than 45 mg/l.
- 5-Acetylsalicylic acid drugs reduce the risk of carcinoma in extensive colitis.
- High-protein diet and vitamin and iron supplements.
- Surgery is indicated for perforation, haemorrhage, severe complications, or repeated relapse.

Differential diagnosis of Crohn's disease and ulcerative colitis

The differential diagnosis between Crohn's disease and ulcerative colitis may be very difficult (Table 3.6). A third disease called indeterminate colitis may be diagnosed when the disease resembles ulcerative colitis and extends beyond the large intestine.

COELIAC DISEASE

Coeliac disease is also called gluten-sensitive enteropathy. It is a small-bowel enteropathy which is caused by sensitivity to gluten. It may be either early (classical) or late onset.

Table 3.6 Differential diagnosis of Crohn's disease and ulcerative colitis

	Ulcerative colitis	Crohn's disease
Clinical features:		
Bloody diarrhoea	Common	Less common
Abdominal mass	Rare	Common
Perianal disease	Less common	Common
Signs of malabsorption	None	Common (small bowel disease)
Radiological features:		
Rectal involvement	Invariable	Uncommon
Distribution	Continuous	Segmental, discontinuous
Mucosa	Fine ulceration, plasma cells, 'double contour'	'Cobblestones', 'rose thorn' ulcers
Strictures	Rare	Common
Fistulas	Very rare	May occur
Histological features:		
Distribution	Mucosal	Transmural
Cellular infiltrate	Neutrophils, plasma cells, eosinophils	Lymphocytes, plasma cells, macrophages
Glands	Mucin depletion, gland destruction, crypt destruction	Gland preservation
Special features	None	Granulomas, aphthous ulcers, histiocyte lined fissures

Epidemiology

Prevalence of coeliac disease in the UK is 1 in 1200. In North America it is 1 in 3000. Coeliacs have a 40 times increased risk for development of intestinal lymphomas and a 10 times increased risk for the development of oral tumours. Removal of gluten from the diet decreases the risks to normal after 5 years. Coeliac disease is associated with HLA-DR3, -DQ2, -DR5/DR7, and -DR4-DQ8.

Pathogenesis

Wheat contains endosperm proteins (white flour) which makes up 70% of the grain. The rest is outer husk (bran) and the wheat germ. White flour contains albumin, globulins, and gluten. The gluten is composed of gliadin and glutenins: the gliadin is toxic to the mucosa.

Coeliac disease is associated with autoimmune disease, e.g. thyroid, diabetes, chronic active hepatitis, Down syndrome, and dermatitis herpetiformis.

Clinical features

Coeliac disease may be asymptomatic and diagnosis is frequently delayed.
Common features are:

- In children: abdominal bloating, diarrhoea; failure to thrive, short stature; anaemia; anorexia; vomiting.
- In adults: anaemia; glossitis; clubbing of the fingers and toes.

Less common features are: osteoporosis, hypocalcaemia, psychiatric symptoms, depression, infertility, amenorrhoea or oligorrhoea, delayed puberty, male impotence.

Investigations

- Haematology and serology: anaemia (hypochromic, macrocytic); red cell folate (low); B_{12} may be low; iron levels low; antibodies to gliadin, reticulin, and endomysium; 10% of patients have IgA deficiency; albumin may be low; hypocalcaemia; hypomagnesaemia.
- Small intestine biopsy—three specimens are needed: mucosal atrophy which ranges from mild blunting to total absence of villi; crypt hyperplagia; infiltration of intraepithelial lymphocytes; lamina propria is infiltrated with plasma cells.
- Gluten challenge: to show histological evidence of gluten intolerance. This should never be carried out in children during growth spurts.
- Radiology: barium follow-through shows loss of jejunal feathery folds resulting in flocculation
- Hydrogen and ^{12}C breath test.
- Glucose tolerance test—flat with no increase or decrease in the blood concentration of glucose.

> **BOX 3.10** Dental relevance of coeliac disease
> - Anaemic patients present with glossitis.
> - Lack of iron, B_{12}, and folate contributes to oral symptoms.
> - Patients may have autoimmune diseases such as diabetes and hypothyroidism which increases the likelihood of intraoral candidosis.
> - Dermatitis herpetiformis may occur in the mouth.
> - Biopsy shows granular IgA at the basement membrane, at the apex of the Rete ridges.
> - Oral carcinomas have an increased incidence in patients with coeliac disease.

Treatment

Coeliacs should avoid foods containing wheat, rye, and barley. Corticosteriods are rarely used. Oats are considered safe by the UK and Finnish Coelic Societies but not all groups in the USA agree.

IRRITABLE BOWEL SYNDROME

A definition of irritable bowel syndrome has been agreed (Rome 11: a multi-national consensus document on functional gastrointestinal disorders. *Gut* 1999; Suppl.11):

- At least 12 weeks, which need not be consecutive, in the preceding 12 months of abdominal discomfort or pain that has two of the following features:
  - relieved with defecation, and/or
  - onset associated with a change in frequency of stool, and/or
  - onset associated with change in form (appearance) of stool.

However, this definition does not take into account common complaints of dietary triggers, bloating, or the need to defecate shortly after eating (gastrocolic reflex).

Aetiology

The aetiology of irritable bowel syndrome is unknown. Several mechanisms have been postulated including increased visceral sensitivity and psychosocial factors. More women than men present with features of irritable bowel syndrome.

Clinical features

Symptoms include bloating, which may be triggered by food or which may occur with increased frequency alternating with constipation. There is a change in the form of the stools.

There are usually no clinical signs; bloating may be observed.

Investigations and treatment

Intestinal pathology should be excluded and the patient strongly reassured. Treatment may consist of:

- Antispasmodic drugs such as mebeverine or alverine.
- Peppermint oil may help bloating.
- Dietary advice to remove dietary triggers.
- Amitriptyline may be helpful.

Differential diagnosis

There are a number of differential diagnoses:

- inflammatory bowel disease
- coeliac disease
- giardiasis
- hypolactasia
- depression or other psychiatric disease.

CARCINOMA OF THE COLON AND RECTUM

In the UK cancers of the colon and rectum are the second most common type of cancer and the second most common cause of death on the national cancer registry, with 19 000 ascribed deaths per year. There are 27 000 new cases every year. Western countries have both a high incidence and high prevalence.

Table 3.7 shows the sites of occurrence of cancers of the colon and rectum.

Aetiology

Environmental factors, especially a diet rich in refined carbohydrate, play a part in increasing the risk of developing carcinoma of the colon. A family history found in 15–20% of patients.

Table 3.7 Sites of colonic cancer

Site	Percentage of cases
Rectum	38%
Sigmoid colon	21%
Caecum	12%
Rectosigmoid	7%
Ascending, transverse, and descending colon	15% in total (5% each)
Anus, hepatic flexure	4% in total (2% each)

Predisposing factors include:

- Increasing age: most often seen in patients over 50 years of age.
- Hereditary familial adenomatous polyposis coli.
- Hereditary non-polyposis coli.
- Inflammatory bowel disease (risk increases with the length of time the disease has been present).

Intestinal polyps
Intestinal polyps may be:

- Neoplastic—familial polyposis coli (**point to remember for dentist**: associated with Gardener's syndrome—epidermoid cysts, osteomas, dentigerous cysts, lipomas).
- Hamartomatous: juvenile polyposis syndrome, Peutz–Jehger syndrome.
- Inflammatory: secondary to ulcerative colitis.
- Pseudo-polyposis: Cronkhite–Canada syndrome—generalized gastrointestinal polyposis with alopecia, pigmentation, and nail dystrophy.

Clinical features

- Non-specific symptoms such as weight loss and malaise.
- Specific features include emergency admissions with bowel obstruction or perforation.
- Alteration of bowel habit. This may be increasing constipation or alternating diarrhoea and constipation. An association with rectal bleeding should raise the index of suspicion.
- Rectal bleeding—bright red blood mixed with the stool indicates left colonic cancers. With right-sided cancers the blood tends to be darker.
- Tenesmus, a feeling of incomplete emptying of the bowels.
- Pain over the lower abdomen.
- Pallor from iron deficiency anaemia is usually associated with right-sided colonic cancer.
- Rectal examination and sigmoidoscopy may reveal a mass of blood in the stool.

Investigations and treatment

There are numerous investigatons to help with diagnosis:

- Faecal occult blood.
- Sigmoidoscopy and colonoscopy.
- Radiology—double-contrast barium enema is useful.
- Full blood count to look for anaemia.
- Liver function tests to see if there is any liver involvement or metastases.
- Look for an increase in carcino-embryonic antigen (CEA).

BOX 3.11 Dental relevance of carcinoma of the colon and rectum
- Patient presenting with unexpected weight loss, anaemia, secondary infection.
- Anaemia may cause glossitis, smooth tongue and ulceration, mucosal pallor.

Treatment depends on whether disease is local, metastatic, or synchronous (5% of patients):

- For **local disease**: surgical resection may be curative—for Dukes stage A tumours there is 90% 5-year survival, for Dukes stage B 75% 5-year survival. Pre-operative radiotherapy reduces the local recurrence rate. Post-operative radiotherapy is not effective.
- For **disease with metastases**: if symptomatic perform surgical resection and apply a stent (not in the rectum because of tenesmus); if asymptomatic chemotherapy is used but survival is less than 50% at 6 months.

PANCREATITIS

Acute pancreatitis

Acute pancreatitis causes sudden, severe abdominal pain necessitating acute admission to hospital. It is common, as indicated by an incidence of 10–20 per 100 000 population.

Aetiology
Numerous factors have been implicated in the aetiology of acute pancreatitis:

- Common factors: alcohol, gallstones, obstruction by carcinoma, parasites, and ampullary stenosis.
- Less common factors: infection, ischaemia, ERCP (endoscopic retrograde cholangiopancreatography), drugs, e.g. oestrogens, azathioprine, antibiotics.

Clinical features
Acute pancreatitis is characterized by:

- Pain and tenderness. The pain is severe and radiates into the back.
- Vomiting.
- Dehydration.
- Hypoxia causing confusion.
- Hypovolaemic shock.
- Jaundice (in 15% of patients).
- Grey–Turner/Cullen sign (uncommon, occurring in 5% of patients). This is discoloration of the flanks and periumbilical area.

Investigations
Serum lipase and serum amylase, which is usually three times the upper limit of normal. Neither amylase nor lipase are specific for acute pancreatitis. Plain

abdominal and chest X-ray, abdominal ultrasound, and CT scan in severe cases.

Treatment

The patient should be admitted to the acute unit and shock and hypoxia treated. Analgesics are important and opiates are usually required. Prophylactic antibiotics should be administered. Surgical intervention may be necessary in necrotizing pancreatitis. Parenteral feeding is also required.

Complications

There may be development of pseudocysts and fistulae after an acute episode. Patients with necrotizing pancreatitis usually develop diabetes mellitus.

Chronic pancreatitis

Chronic pancreatitis is a chronic disease affecting the pancreas; it is progressive and results in changes that are irreversible. The incidence is 1 per 100 000 population in the UK and the prevalence is 65 per 100 000 population. In South Africa the incidence is 40–70 per 100 000 population.

Aetiology

Alcohol consumption is the major cause. Tropical pancreatitis is seen in childhood. Both tropical pancreatitis and alcohol-induced pancreatitis are a chronic calcifying type of pancreatitis. Gallstones and tumours results in chronic obstructive pancreatitis.

Clinical features

There are initial episodes of acute symptoms and signs with severe pain and epigastric tenderness. This is followed later by symptoms of diabetes and pancreatic insufficiency, with decreasing pain.

Investigations

Plain abdominal X-ray, ultrasound, and CT scan of the abdomen. ERCP is the 'gold standard' investigation and demonstrates ductal problems associated with stenosis, abnormal anatomy, gallstones or bile duct stenosis. Biochemical tests are required for amylase and lipase, which may be raised during exacerbations, and faecal pancreatic elastase-1, which correlates with pancreatic function.

BOX 3.12 Dental implications of pancreatitis

- Patients may be addicted to opiates.
- Look for drug interactions.
- There may be alcohol abuse.
- Diabetes mellitus may be present.

Treatment

Alcohol intake should be stopped: alcohol is the main contributory factor to the development of chronic pancreatitis in the UK. Pain control is important, but care must be taken to monitor for addiction to opiates. The patient's nutritional status must be monitered and nutritional supplements added as required. Steatorrhoea should be treated with pancreatic enzymes, and diabetes mellitus should be treated. Surgical intervention is occasionally necessary.

4   The nervous system

The dental surgeon is frequently faced with patients presenting with complaints arising from the nervous system. The commonest is pain of dental origin. However, the nature of the pain may be vague and pain of non-dental origin may be present but be interpreted as dental pain, resulting in the unnecessary extraction of sound teeth.

The nervous system is composed of the **central** and **peripheral** nervous system with multifaceted functions including the collection and interpretation of sensory and motor information trafficking to and from the periphery, and the higher cerebral functions of reason, emotion, and intellectual function.

EXAMINATION OF THE NERVOUS SYSTEM

The purpose of taking a history and examining the nervous system is to be able to locate the lesion anatomically and understand the underlying pathological process. The history is very important and will result in the correct diagnosis in over 90% of cases. Make sure open questioning is used and the patient is allowed to give the history in their own time and words. Careful inquiry about the patient's age, occupation, and handedness is important—right-handedness assumes a dominant left hemisphere and left-handedness assumes a dominant left hemisphere.

Note the details of the primary and main symptom or sign:

- Date of the initial event.
- Nature of the primary event.
- Time taken for deficit to develop.
- Recurrence or persistence of the primary event.
- Provoking or relieving factors.
- Time for development of symptoms to peak and improve.
- Associated clinical symptoms and signs.

The systems review, as in any medical history, should be undertaken before starting the examination.

The examination should include:

- higher cerebral function
- cranial nerves
- motor systems
- tone

- power
- coordination
- reflexes
- sensation
- gait.

Examination of the higher cerebral functions

First note the state of consciousness:

- Alert?
- Confused?
- Comatose?
- Test the patient's intellectual skill.
- Is the patient orientated in time and place?

Then examine the memory:

- Ask the patient to recall their name and address, and repeat after 5 min.
- Assess concentration: serial subtraction of 7 from 100.
- Test general knowledge, e.g. current events.
- Note the patient's emotional state.

Next look at speech:

- Is there dysarthria (disorder of articulation)?
- Is there dysphasia?
- Is dysphasia receptive, i.e. failure to understand the spoken or written word, or expressive, i.e. unable to name objects verbally or in writing?
- Mixed dysphasias are common.
- Is there apraxia (inability to perform purposeful acts despite adequate power, coordination, and comprehension)?

Examination of the cranial nerves

Olfactory nerve (I)
Test the sense of smell, especially after head injury, when a tumour suspected, or when there is a loss of taste.

Optic nerve (II)
Check the visual acuity (with spectacles if worn) and check the visual fields (peripheral and central). The pupils respond to lesions of the visual pathway:

- With a parasympathetic oculomotor nerve (III) lesion the pupils are dilated.
- With a sympathetic lesion the pupils are constricted.
- A failure to react to light indicates optic or third nerve lesions.
- An Argyll Robertson pupil reacts to accommodation but not to light.

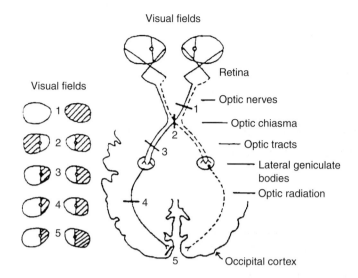

Perform ophthalmoscopy for:

- Abnormalities in the anterior or posterior chamber or lens.
- Swelling or pallor of the optic disc.
- Size and regularity of the retinal arteries and veins.
- The presence or absence of haemorrhages, exudates, or pigmentation.
- The presence of any other obvious lesions.

Third (III), fourth (IV), and sixth (VI) cranial nerves

Note that the trochlear nerve (IV) supplies the superior oblique The abducens nerve (VI) supplies the external ocular muscles and also carries parasympathetic fibres to the pupil.

Third nerve lesions cause:

- Ptosis (drooping of the upper eyelid).
- Fixation of the eye downwards and outwards.
- Fixation and dilation of the pupils.

Fourth nerve lesions result in an inability to turn the eye down and in (medially) and sixth nerve lesions result in an inability to turn the eye out (laterally).

The trigeminal nerve (V)

To test the sensory function of the trigeminal nerve use light touch and pin-pricks in the territory of ophthalmic, maxillary, and mandibular divisions (see figure) (**care**: use a fresh pin for every patient).

To test the motor division of the trigeminal nerve inspection the muscles of mastication. Ask the patient to clench their teeth firmly and palpate the masseter

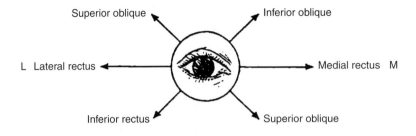

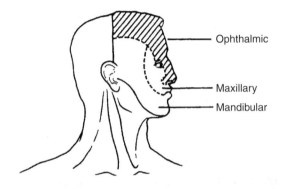

and temporalis muscles—these will be wasted on the side of a lower motor neuron lesion. The jaw will deviate to side of a lower motor neuron lesion when the patient opens the jaw against resistance.

Test the following reflexes:

- Corneal reflex: a blink elicited by a gentle touch of the cornea with a wisp of clean cotton wool. Touch the margin of the cornea from the side so that the patient does not see it approaching.
- Jaw jerk: ask the patient to open and relax their mouth so that it hangs half open. Place your thumb on the patient's chin and strike your thumb gently with a tendon hammer. The reflex is very variable but may be brisk in upper motor neuron lesions (see figure).

The facial nerve (VII)
The facial nerve supplies the muscles of facial expression. Ask the patient to grin, show their teeth, screw up their eyes against resistance, and wrinkle their forehead. Note the following:

- There is bilateral innervation of cortex for movement of the forehead.
- A LMN (lower motor neuron) lesion involves unilateral weakness of the whole of one side of the face.
- A UMN (upper motor neuron) lesion involves unilateral weakness of the lower face only.

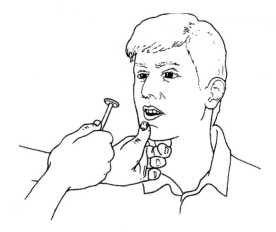

- The facial nerve also supplies taste to the anterior two-thirds of the tongue via the chorda tympani.

The vestibulocochlear nerve (VIII)

To test the function of the vestibulocochlear nerve inspect the ear and drum. Test acuity of hearing—use a watch and test whether it can be heard. Perform Rinne's and Weber's tests as deafness may be conductive (bone conduction better than air conduction, due to wax or middle ear disease) or neural (air conduction better than bone conduction, due to inner ear or acoustic nerve lesions). A lesion of the vestibular division of the vestibulocochlear nerve results in impaired balance. An acute lesion causes nystagmus (jerky movements of the eyes) with the fast phase towards the lesion.

The glossopharyngeal nerve (IX)

The sensation of taste to the posterior third of the tongue is supplied by the glossopharyngeal nerve.

The vagus nerve (X)

The vagus nerve is involved in the motor supply to the palate, pharynx, and larynx. Check that the palate and uvula move centrally when the patient says 'ah'—these are drawn to the opposite side when the vagus nerve is paralysed. Check that the patient can cough and swallow properly and check the gag reflex and posterior pharyngeal sensation.

The spinal accessory nerve (XI)

The accessory nerve is involved in the motor supply to the sternomastoids and part of trapezius. Ask the patient to turn their head away from the sternomastoid you are testing and also to shrug their shoulders against resistance.

> **BOX 4.1** Tests for vestibulocochlear nerve function
>
> **Rinne's test**
> - Use a 256 or 512 Hz tuning fork.
> - After striking the fork place it on the mastoid process, until the patient can no longer hear the sound.
> - The sound should still be audible when the tip is held over the meatus. When air conduction is perceived louder than bone conduction, the middle ear transmitting system is intact and healthy. The patient therefore does not have a conductive hearing loss. They may, however, have a neural deafness if the complaint of hearing loss is related to that ear.
>
> **Weber's test**
> - Strike the tuning fork (as above).
> - Place the fork over the midline.
> - The patient normally hears the sound in the middle or equally in both ears. Deafness may be conductive (bone conduction better than air conduction, due to wax or middle ear disease) or neural (air conduction better than bone conduction, due to inner ear or acoustic nerve lesions). In patients with hearing loss the Weber test will lateralize to the side with greater conductive hearing loss or, in cases of sensorineural loss, the ear with the better cochlea.

The hypoglossal nerve (XII)

The hypoglassal nerve is involved in the motor supply to the tongue. Look for wasting and fasciculation. Check to see if the tongue protrudes centrally—if the hypoglossal nerve is damaged the tongue will protrude towards the paralysed side. Check the side to side movement of the tongue.

Examination of the motor system

Inspect for:

- wasting or hypertrophy of muscles
- fasciculation
- deformity
- tremor—at rest and moving
- myoclonic jerks.

Palpation should enable a determination of **muscle tone** as normal, spastic (UMN lesion), rigid (extrapyramidal lesion) or hypotonic (LMN lesion).

Determine the **muscle power** of the extensors and flexors and record as normal, or with moderate or severe weakness.

Test **coordination**: remember loss of position sense may cause incoordination. Test for:

- finger/nose ataxia (past pointing, intention tremor),
- difficulty with rapidly alternating hand movement,

> **BOX 4.2** MRC muscle power scale
>
> - 0, no contraction
> - 1, trace of contraction
> - 2, active movement with gravity eliminated
> - 3, active movement against gravity
> - 4, active movement against gravity and resistance
> - 5, normal.

- any difficulty with fine finger movements,
- heel/shin ataxia.

Test the **reflexes**:

- biceps C5
- brachioradialis C6
- triceps C7
- knee L3,4
- ankle S1,2
- the Babinski reflex (i.e. plantar responses).

Grade the reflexes as follows:

- normal, +
- reduced, +
- absent, −
- increased, ++.

Examination of the sensory system

Ask if the patient has any lost or altered feeling anywhere and test for:

- Light touch—with a light finger touch.
- Superficial pain—using a new pin for every patient.
- Temperature—cold metal.
- Vibration sense—tuning fork 128 Hz.
- Proprioception.

Check the gait—check whether the patient can:

- stand with feet together,
- stand with feet together and eyes shut,
- walk normally,
- walk heel-to-toe,
- run.

HEADACHE AND FACIAL PAIN

Headache and facial pain are common presenting symptoms. Almost 99% of the population suffer facial pain or headache at some stage, and pain which becomes troublesome may afflict up to 40%. The commonest causes of facial pain are benign or primary headache and pain of dental origin. However, the pain may be symptomatic of some serious underlying pathology. A comprehensive history to differentiate the type of pain cannot be overemphasized. Important points in the history are:

- Age of the patient.
- Age and time of onset of pain.
- Character of the pain.
- Mode of onset of the pain.
- Precipitating and relieving factors.
- Aggravating and accompanying factors.
- Duration of pain.

Examination of a patient with facial pain or headache of non-dental origin is important. Patients with secondary headache or pain of non-dental origin may have physical signs. Headache due to raised intracranial pressure may have very little history. Once dental causes have been excluded, consider the surrounding structures and check the pulse and blood pressure. Examine the following:

- Examine the ears carefully. Look for any rashes, scaling, or erythema on the external auditory meatus. Examine behind the ears and over the mastoid process for tenderness.
- Examine the maxillary and frontal sinuses for any tenderness and look for post-nasal drip behind the fauces in the nasopharyngeal region.
- Examine the eyes for erythema, proptosis, abnormal eye muscle movement, papillary response to light, and accommodation. Ideally the disc needs to be visualized and the intraocular pressure measured, but very few dentists are competent at these procedures.
- Examine the neck for any restriction in movement and tenderness of both the neck and its supporting muscles.
- Examine the temporomandibular joint for any abnormalities of movement in opening and closing, limitation of opening, or clicks and pain on movement of the joint. Examination of the temporomandibular joint is usually carried out routinely as part of the dental examination.

The eye

Pain in and around the eye should be regarded seriously. Glaucoma may present with pain around the eye. Optic neuritis pain may occur before there is any visual loss, and pain occurs around the eye and with eye movement. Uncorrected or incorrect refraction of the eye may lead to bifrontal headaches.

The ear

Sepsis of the ear—caused either by bacterial or viral infection of the middle or outer ear—may give rise to pain which is difficult to localize.

> **BOX 4.3** International Headache Society classification of facial pain, headaches, and facial neuralgias
>
> **Primary**
> - Migraine.
> - Tension-type headache.
> - Cluster headaches and chronic paroxysmal hemicrania.
> - Miscellaneous headaches unassociated with structural lesion.
>
> **Secondary**
> - Headache associated with head trauma.
> - Headache associated with vascular disorders including subarachnoid haemorrhage.
> - Headache associated with non-vascular intracranial disorders including: benign intracranial hypertension, intracranial infection, intracranial neoplasm.
> - Headache associated with substances or their withdrawal including: alcohol-induced headache, chronic ergotamine-induced headache, chronic analgesic-induced headache, alcohol withdrawal headache (hangover).
> - Headache associated with non-cephalic infection.
> - Headache associated with disorders of the cranium, neck, eyes, ears, nose and sinuses, teeth including: cervical spine, acute glaucoma, acute sinus headache.
> - Cranial neuralgias including: Herpes zoster, trigeminal neuralgia.
> - Headache not classifiable.

Paranasal sinuses

The maxillary and frontal sinusitis may present with localized tenderness. The maxillary teeth may protrude into the antral floor and pain may mimic dental pain. When the sphenoidal or ethmoid sinuses are inflamed, pain may be localized behind the nose and give rise to feelings of both stuffiness and a generalized headache.

The neck

Arthritis may give rise to both localized and referred pain to both the occipital and frontal regions. Limitation of movement of the neck associated with pain may point to the origin of the pain being from the cervical vertebrae.

Neuralgia

Trigeminal neuralgia

Patients with trigeminal neuralgia are usually aged over 50, with more women than men affected. The aetiology is unknown; however, arterial distortion of the nerve along its pathway has been implicated in some patients. Trigeminal neuralgia occurring in younger patients should arouse the suspicion of multiple sclerosis or tumours:

- Very rarely meningiomas, nasopharyngeal tumours, or neurofibromas may involve the trigeminal nerve.

> **BOX 4.4** Treatment of trigeminal neuralgia
> - Carbamazepine is the drug of choice. Start with 100 mg twice a day (b.d.) and gradually increase the dose. The dose is titrated against symptoms and side-effects. The most disabling side effects are drowsiness, ataxia, and diplopia. However, patients tend to tolerate the side-effects in preference to the pain. The dose may increase to 200 mg three to four times a day before the pain is relieved.
> - Phenytoin 300 mg together with baclofen 10 mg three times a day (t.i.d.) may also be tried. Vigabatrin is also used in those patients who cannot tolerate carbamazepine.
> - Surgery is considered in those patients with intractable pain. Phenol injections into the nerve have also been tried. However, this technique is used infrequently.

- Both multiple sclerosis and tumours result in persistent severe pain, or mimic the pain of trigeminal neuralgia.

The pain of trigeminal neuralgia can occur in any division of the trigeminal nerve but is more frequent in the second or third divisions. The pain is characteristically described as a sharp, shooting pain. There is usually a trigger zone, which triggers a paroxysm of pain so severe that patients may pass out; they frequently describe suicidal feelings when trying to combat the pain. The pain may be triggered by various stimuli such as exposure to changes in ambient temperature, night breezes, chewing, talking, brushing the teeth, shaving, washing, or touching the face and smiling.

Herpetic neuralgia

Herpes zoster more commonly affects the trigeminal nerve than the glossopharyngal nerve. The pain is usually severe, occurs in the region of the distribution of the nerve, and occurs up to 3 days before the vesicles appear. Post-herpetic neuralgia can be very distressing and last for years. Early treatment of the herpetic infection decreases the extent and severity of the post-herpetic neuralgia.

Atypical facial pain

Analgesics with or without an antiemetic, beta-blockers, serotonin antagonists (pizotifen and methysergide) are used to prevent attacks. Other drugs which may provide benefit include amitriptyline, carbamazepine, phenytoin, and phenelzine all provide the same benefit.

Migraine

Classic migraine or migraine with aura

Classic migrane is a paroxysmal unilateral headache which is recurrent and varies in intensity and duration. It may be accompanied by nausea and focal cerebral symptoms. There is usually a positive family history. Vahlquist gives a 7.4% prevalence in 16–19 year olds. Females are more often affetced than males (female : male ratio 3 : 2). Onset may occur at any age, but onset over

40 years of age is unusual. Migraine diminishes in frequency and intensity with age. Migrainous variants of classic migraine or intercerebral structural causes must be excluded.

Clinical features
- Precipitating factors include: food, e.g. cheese, chocolate, coffee; hunger and particularly starvation; stress; hormonal changes; minimal trauma to the head; exhaustion.
- The prodrome lasts 20–30 min. Symptoms experienced may be visual, sensory, motor, mood, or language disturbance.
- Headache is unilateral. There is no preference and the opposite side may be involved in a subsequent attack. There may be nausea, vomiting, photophobia, and/or facial pallor. Headache lasts for 1 h to 4 days.

Migraine variants
In the hemiplegic variant, limb weakness develops during or at the beginning of an attack. The paralysis may last for several days following the headache. A small number of families carry a dominant gene for familial hemiplegic migraine. In ophthalmoplegic migraine the pain is usually associated with a transient, third cranial nerve palsy.

Treatment
For an **acute attack**: lie patient in a darkened quiet room. Give symptomatic treatment for nausea and vomiting and specific treatment for headache.

Prophylaxis includes: the avoidance of trigger foods; assessment of the hormonal cycle to either introduce or stop oral contraception; decrease stress—biofeedback has been used to increase relaxation.

Common migraine or migraine without aura
These are migraine attacks without an aura. Unilateral paroxysmal episodic headache. Precipitating factors may include relaxation after period stress menstruation. They should be differentiated from tension type headaches.

Facial migraine
This particular form of migraine is frequently seen in the dental surgery. The pain involves the lower half of the face. There may be an aura. It has the same precipitating factors as classic migraine and is frequently associated with nausea and vomiting. Facial migraine must be distinguished from migrainous neuralgia (see below) in which 'clusters' occur.

Other headaches

Migrainous neuralgia (cluster headaches)
This headache is also called cluster headache and, rarely, Hortons syndrome. It occurs in men and women (male : female 1 : 1), in their third decade or older.

The pain is unilateral and periorbital with radiation to the forehead, temple, and maxillary area:

- An attack lasts approximately 30–60 min. One to two hours after falling asleep, pain wakes the patient, who becomes agitated.
- Patients try displacement activity: they may pace the floor or bang their head against the wall.
- The pain is severe and non-throbbing, associated with conjunctival injection, lachrymation, and a blocked nose. This is followed by rhinorrhoea and sometimes ptosis, miosis, and flushing of the cheek.

There are a number of features differentiating migrainous neuralgia from facial migraine:

- It recurs nightly in clusters for 6–12 weeks, once every year or every 2 years.
- There is no nausea or vomiting.
- The face of a patient turns red (under infrared photography), unlike in facial migraine where the face remains pale.

Tension-type headaches

These occur more often in middle age. Males and females are equally affected. They are precipitated by life events, stress, and the menopause. There may be associated depression. The headache is bilateral with extension either over the top of the cranium or in the occipital area. The pain is described as a fullness or tight band of pressure. It is the only type of headache that is present continuously, day and night, for long periods of time.

Traction headache

This type of headache can occur in any age group. The onset is sudden, progressive, and usually wakes the patient from sleep. The pain is associated with intracranial arterial displacement caused by tumours or increased intracranial pressure. Headaches associated with angioma and aneurysms are of sudden onset and reach a peak in minutes. If haemorrhage occurs, the pain increases in intensity then localizes towards the occipital area and is of prolonged duration.

Meningitis

Meningitis is often missed in young children as it can be accompanied by what appears to be a trivial illness. In adults, the headache is generalized frontal,

---

BOX 4.5 Serious causes of headache

- Traction headache.
- Meningitis.
- Subarachnoid haemorrhage.
- Cranial arteritis.
- Herpes zoster of the ophthalmic division of the fifth cranial nerve.

radiating to the neck. There is accompanying fever and neck stiffness. Later the headache is accompanied by nausea and disturbance of consciousness. There are also systemic signs.

Subarachnoid haemorrhage

The headache may be diagnostic, with sudden onset of severe headache which increases in intensity. The patient feels as though they have been hit at the back of the head. However, the headache may also come on slowly, with neck stiffness taking some hours to develop. The dental surgeon should have a high index of suspicion and refer the patient urgently. Delay in diagnosis may have disastrous consequences.

Cranial arteritis (temporal arteritis)

Cranial arteritis is arterial inflammation of unknown aetiology, occurring in the elderly and more often in females (female : male 3 : 2). It rarely occurs in people under the age of 55 years. The dental surgeon should have a high index of suspicion in patients presenting with facial pain with pain localized in the temporal area. The temporal artery is usually involved, although any artery may be affected. It is extremely important to make a diagnosis of temporal arteritis as delay might lead to blindness.

Clinical features

Clinical features of cranial arteritis are both local and systemic:

- Always consider this diagnosis in an elderly patient with a headache of recent onset or who is complaining of facial pain.
- Systemic symptoms are fever and weight loss; muscle weakness may precede the pain.
- The pain is distributed in the temporal region. It is slow in onset, becomes constant, and may become severe.
- The scalp feels tender with the arteries appearing enlarged, pulsatile, and irregular.
- Vision may be lost due to the involvement of the central retinal or posterior ciliary arteries.

Investigations and treatment

Investigations show the erythrocyte sedimentation rate (ESR) to be very high.

A biopsy should be performed. The histology shows inflammation of the large and medium-sized arteries (not arterioles or capillaries). The media is involved, with fragmentation of the elastic fibres. The intima demonstrates histiocytes, epitheliod cells, multinucleated giant cells, lymphocytes, and plasma cells which accumulate in the intima adjacent to the internal elastic lamina, resulting in a thickened intima.

Treatment is high-dose steroids, which should be started immediately.

Headache and facial pain related to systemic problems and medication
The following factors can all be involved in causing headache and facial pain:

- Coffee, alcohol, and tobacco consumption.
- Hypertension, especially persistent diastolic pressures of more than 100 mmHg.
- Fever.
- Chronic lung disease with hypercaneoa (nocturnal headache).
- Cushing's disease.
- Diabetes.
- The oral contraceptive pill.
- Withdrawal of steroid medication.
- Exposure to carbon monoxide exposure.
- Vasodilator drugs (e.g. nifidipine, nitrates).
- Hypothyroidism.
- Depression.
- Addison's disease (rare).

Medication misuse headache
Medication misuse headache affects 1 in 50 people. It may occur daily. The mechanism is not completely understood but it results from chronic over-frequent use of analgesics. This type of headache first became apparent in patients abusing ergotamine. The headache is mistaken for recurrent migraine, and patients repeatedly use the drug, decreasing the periods between headache and drug intake. Frequent use of a 5-HT receptor agonist, e.g. sumatriptan, zolmitriptan, or naratriptan, may also result in daily headache.

Aspirin, paracetamol, and other NSAIDs are all causally associated. Slow elimination of the drug produces a withdrawal syndrome of sick headache.

PAIN

The terminology used to describe pain can be very confusing. A list of commonly used terms are defined in Box 4.6.

Classification of orofacial pain

Classification of facial pain helps us to understand the anatomy and physiology of this complex but very important symptom. It will also help in the diagnosis and management of pain. The main categories of pain are:

- somatic
- neurogenous
- deafferentiation
- psychogenic
- psychopathic.

> **BOX 4.6** Definition of terms used in the description of pain
>
> - Allodynia: pain without noxious stimulation at site of pain.
> - Analgesia: absence of the sensibility of pain.
> - Anaesthesia: absence of all sensation.
> - Anaesthesia dolorosa: pain in an area that is anaesthetized as a result of deafferentiation.
> - Causalgia: sensation of unremitting burning pain as a result of deafferentiation.
> - Deafferentiation: the effect of eliminating afferent neural activity due to interrupted neurons.
> - Denervation: resection of, or removal of, the nerves to an organ or part.
> - Dysaesthesia: unpleasant, abnormal sensation (note: paraesthesia is an abnormal sensation which may be pleasant or not).
> - Heterotopic pain: a pain that is felt in an area other than the true site of origin.
> - Hypoalgesia: diminished sensitivity to stimulation-evoked pain.
> - Hyperalgesia: increased sensitivity to stimulation-evoked pain.
> - Hyperaesthesia: increased sensitivity to stimulation.
> - Hypoaesthesia: diminished sensitivity to stimulation.
> - Neuralgia: neurogenous pain felt along the peripheral distribution of neural structures.
> - Neuropathy: term used to designate an abnormality or pathology in a peripheral nerve.
> - Nociceptor: a sensory receptor preferentially sensitive to noxious or potentially noxious stimuli.
> - Parasthenia: abnormal sensation occuring spontaneously or by induction.
> - Radiculopathy: abnormal function or pathology due to changes in one or more sensory roots.

Pain occurring in the region of the head and neck may fall into any one of these groups. Examples given here are from the oro-dento-facial area.

Somatic pain

Superficial somatic pain can be cutaneous or mucogingival.
   Deep somatic pain can be:

- Musculoskeletal pain: myofascial trigger point, muscle spasm and inflammation.
- Temporomandibular joint pain: disc attachment, retrodisc, capsule, arthritic, osseous, and periosteal.
- Periodontal and pain of dental origin: atypical odontalgia, visceral mucosal.
- Vascular pain: migrainous neuralgia, common migraine, classic migraine, salivary gland, ocular, and auricular pain.

Neurogenous pain

- Neuropathic pain: traumatic neuroma, paroxysmal neuralgia, idiopathic neuralgia.
- Neuritic neuralgia: peripheral neuritis in Herpes zoster, post-herpetic neuralgia.

Deafferentiation pain

Deafferentiation pain can be due to causalgia, anaesthesia dolorosa, or phantom tooth pain.

Psychogenic pain

An example of psychogenic pain in the oro-dento-facial area is chronic facial pain.

Psychoneurotic pain

Psychoneurotic pain can be delusional, neurotic, psychopathic, or due to conversion hysteria.

Clinical features of different catagories of pain

Clinical features of somatic pain

- Somatic pain has bright, stimulating quality.
- Subjective localization of pain is excellent and anatomically accurate.
- The site of the pain identifies the correct location of its source.
- The response to provocation at the site of pain is faithful in incidence, intensity, and location.
- The application of a topical anaesthetic at the site of pain temporarily arrests it.

Glossodynia ('burning mouth')

This condition is an example of superficial somatic pain. Localization of pain corresponds to the area of greatest movement. The cause may be the abrasive effect of tissues rubbing against themselves and the teeth. The tip and side of the tongue commonly involved. Aggravating and complication factors include infection, xerostomia, emotional problems, stress, dental appliances, and tongue thrusting.

The application of topical anaesthetic brings relief to the painful area, and this will enable a diagnosis to be made.

Clinical features of neurogenous pain

Neurogenous pain is due to an abnormality in nervous system itself rather than to noxious stimulation of otherwise normal neural structures. In neuropathic pain of the mouth and face:

- The pain has a bright, stimulating quality that provokes alarm in the patient.
- The site is accurately localized by the patient.
- The pain is disproportionate in intensity to the exciting stimulus.
- Topical anaesthesia of the site does not arrest the pain (except for muscosa-triggered neuralgia).

Traumatic neuroma

Traumatic neuroma occurs after a nerve is cut. The regenerating nerve tissue is disorganized and painless. Stimulation by pressure, stretching, or impinging on the area induces pain. Traumatic neuromas are found in scar tissue after facial fractures or deep lacerations. Pain due to traumatic neuroma is differentiated by:

- Painless except when compressed and/or stretched.
- Pain is of greater intensity than expected from the stimuli.
- There are no accompanying sensory or motor symptoms indicative of neural deficit.
- Pain is arrested by injection of local anaesthetic at the site of the pain.

Acoustic neuroma

Acoustic neuroma is indicated by the presence of signs and symptoms diagnostic of this condition. Reflex sympathetic dystrophy is very rare. It follows nerve injury incidental to trauma, surgery or infection and is described as anaesthesia or paraesthesia of the area which may be accompanied by dull, persistent, unremitting, variable, and diffuse sensation. Stellate blockade will remove the symptoms.

Post-herpetic neuralgia

Occurs after Herpes zoster infection. It is associated with a severe, persistent, intractable, chronic, burning pain. Pain is felt superficially in the area of an acute attack. The pain may be accompanied by other sensory symptoms such as hypoaesthesia or hyperaesthesia.

Paroxysmal neuralgia

Paroxysmal neuralgia has no known cause. Features of the pain include:

- A severe paroxysmal pain.
- Pain is accurately located by the patient.
- Pain occurs spontaneously with eating, talking, face washing, and shaving.
- Pain has a unilateral location.
- Triggering initiates pain: the trigger is by minor superficial stimulation of the peripherally distributed sensory (pain) fibres.
- The pain is bright and stimulating, burning, hot, shocking, electric.
- There may be delay of 15–30 s between the trigger and the sensation of pain.
- There may be a refractory period after the stimulatory impulse.
- There appears to be no neurological deficit in either sensory or motor function.

    Examples of paroxysmal neuralgia include:

- **Trigeminal neuralgia (tic douloureux):** Trigeminal neuralgia is more common in middle and old age, and is more frequent in women. Pain is unilateral. Pain remains in the anatomical distribution of the trigeminal nerve. The speed of spread suggests that this is a neuralgia. The character of the pain is of single shocks but it may be so frequent and repetitive that it seems to be nearly continuous. To arrest the pain the nerve needs to be blocked completely.

- **Glossopharyngeal neuralgia:** Glossopharyngeal neuralgia occurs in the distribution of the glossopharyngeal nerve. It may be accompanied by vagal symptoms. Watch for syncope, arrhythmia, and even cardiac arrest.
- **Symptomatic neuralgia:** Symptomatic neuralgia accounts for 20% of paroxysmal neuralgias. In the orofacial region it can result from pathological lesions. Characteristics include: prolonged or continuous paroxysms of pain, paroxysms with continuous aching/burning pain, bilateral neuralgic pain, involvement of two or more cranial nerves, neuralgia accompanied by other sensory disturbances such as hypoaesthesia, paraesthesia, anaesthesia, and dysaesthesia. Neuralgia may be accompanied by muscle weakness or autonomic symptoms. **Differential diagnosis**: multiple sclerosis (MS) can present in this way as can meningioma of Meckel's cavity and arteriovenous aneurysm. It is mimicked by post-traumatic pain.

Clinical features of deafferentiation pains of the mouth and face

Despite considerable regeneration, the sensory disturbances due to deafferentiation may persist. Causes include crushing and lacerating injuries to the mouth and face and surgery—even simple tooth extraction. Symptoms are anaesthesia, hypoaesthesia, paraesthesia, dysaesthesia, hyperalgesia, and spontaneous pain. The most frequent complaint is anaesthesia and paraesthesia following injury of the mandibular nerve.

Differential diagnoses are multiple sclerosis, syphilis, and anaesthesia dolorosa. **Anaesthesia dolorosa** is a complication of trauma or surgery, especially rhizotomy for control of facial pain. Deafferentiation normally induces anaesthesia but in this case it is accompanied by paraesthesia or hyperaesthesia.

Clinical features of psychogenic pain and psychopathic pain

Psychogenic pain is associated with depression and stress.

Psychopathic pain is a delusional anaesthesia and/or pain. The pain may be a manifestation of schizophrenic hallucination. It is recognized by the presence of other psychiatric symptoms.

DISORDERS OF THE CRANIAL NERVES

Patients with disorders of the cranial nerves often present in the dental practice. An appreciation of the associated disorder and underlying lesion is needed as these disorders frequently impact on dental care. Disorders of several cranial nerves may occur at the same time.

Disorders of the first cranial nerve (the olfactory nerve)

The olfactory nerve is formed by olfactory neuronal receptors in the nasal mucosa. The olfactory receptors pass through the cribiform plate. They synapse at secondary neurons that project in the cortex of the temporal lobe.

BOX 4.7 Points to note: papilloedema

Causes of papilloedema
- Accelerated hypertension.
- Raised intracranial pressure.
- Retinal vein occlusion.

Signs of papilloedema
- Pink or pale disc with blurred margins.
- Loss of central cupping.
- Engorged retinal veins.
- Flame shaped haemorrhages.

Smell is perceived in the temporal cortex. Lesions, usually secondary to trauma to the olfactory nerve, result in anosmia (loss of the sense of smell).

Disorders of the second cranial nerve (the optic nerve)

The optic nerve is formed by axons of cells in the retina. The axons converge from the entire retinal area to form the optic nerve. The nerve traverses the pituitary gland. Medial retinal fibres cross to the opposite side of the optic chiasma and travel to synapse in the thalamus. Some fibres traverse the midbrain to the reflex centres where the control of reflexes associated with turning of the head, neck, and eyes towards a visual stimulus reside. The thalamic axons transverse the occipital visual cortex where vision is perceived.

Lesions of the optic nerve result in blindness in the ipsilateral side. Lesions of the optic chiasma, e.g. a pituitary tumour in Cushing's disease or acromegaly, result in bitemporal hemianopia.

Disorders of the third cranial nerve (the oculomotor nerve)

The oculomotor nerve supplies most muscles that move the eyeball, and the muscle that raises the eyelid. It also conveys parasympathetic innervation for the control of pupil size and focusing by adjusting lens size. **Causes** of third nerve lesions include:

- Oculomotor compression caused by intracranial tumour, aneurysm of the posterior communicating artery, trauma after road traffic accidents.
- Oculomotor paresis caused by: sarcoidosis, diabetes, infarction due to ischaemia, demyelination.

The patient with a third nerve disorder presents with: the eye rotated outward and upward, giving a squint; ptosis; dilated pupil; inability to focus the eye; movements of the left and right eyes are not coordinated resulting in diplopia. An accompanying headache or change in the level of consciousness is an indicator of serious underlying pathology.

> **BOX 4.8** Points to note: causes of ptosis
>
> - Congenital.
> - Cervical sympathetic lesion.
> - Third nerve palsy.
> - Myasthenia gravis.
> - Dystrophia myotonica.

CT and/or MRI scans should be performed. Angiography is applicable when the pupil is involved with no history of head injury.

Disorders of the fourth cranial nerve (the trochlear nerve)

The fourth cranial nerve innervates the superior oblique muscle. Causes of fourth nerve disorders include trauma, especially a closed head injury (this is the most common cause). Uncommon causes include MS, aneurysms, and tumours.

In fourth nerve disorders there is diplopia and the eye is turned inward.

Disorders of the fifth cranial nerve (the trigeminal nerve)

The dentist must at all times consider the anatomy of the fifth nerve. Its branches affect the sensory and motor function of the orofacial area.

Causes of fifth nerve disorders include:

- Vascular malformations.
- Tumours.
- Ischaemia.
- Vasculitis.
- Multiple sclerosis.
- Sjögren's syndrome.
- Rheumatoid arthritis.
- Nerve compression by arterial or venous vessels as the nerve enters the brainstem.

The main problem affecting the fifth cranial nerve is trigeminal neuralgia which was considered in detail earlier in the section on headache and facial pain.

Disorders of the sixth cranial nerve (the abducens nerve)

The abducens nerve supplies motor fibres to the lateral rectus, which moves the eye.

Causes of sixth nerve disorders include:

- Nasopharyngeal tumour.
- Cavernous sinus thrombosis.

- Intracranial tumour.
- Diabetes.
- Trauma causing a basilar skull fracture.
- Infections.
- Wernicke's encephalopathy.
- Aneurysm.
- Multiple sclerosis.
- Hydrocephalus causing compression.

In sixth nerve disorders the eye is turned inward, i.e has a squint, and the patient has diplopia. **Investigations** are aimed at trying to determine the underlying aetiology: CT and MRI, lumbar puncture, check blood sugar, and do an autoimmune screen.

Treatment involves treating the underlying disorder.

Disorders of the seventh cranial nerve (the facial nerve)

The **anatomy** of the facial nerve is important:

- The facial nerve arises at the junction of the pons and medulla and crosses the following structures: posterior cranial fossa, internal auditory meatus, temporal bone in the facial canal.
- It exits the skull through the stylomastoid foramen.
- The parotid gland is the last large structure it traverses.
- The terminal facial motor branches are: temporal, zygomatic, buccal, marginal mandibular, cervical.

The **functions** of the facial nerve are:

- Motor: to the muscles of facial expression.
- Somatic sensory: from the geniculate ganglion to an area around the external auditory meatus.
- Taste: to the anterior two-thirds of the tongue via the chorda tympani and lingual nerve.
- Parasympathetic: secretomotor via the greater petrosal nerve to the lacrimal gland; secretomotor via the chorda tympani to the submandibular and sublingual salivary glands.

The main **causes** of facial nerve disorders are:

- Intracranial lesions including tumours, compression, and aneurysms.
- Vascultic disease.
- Sarcoidosis.
- Ramsey Hunt syndrome.
- Mastoid or middle ear infections.
- Petrous bone fractures.
- Lyme disease.
- Tumours of the cerebropontine angle.

- Chronic tuberculous meningitis.
- Idiopathic causes are the major problem affecting the extracranial course of the facial nerve.

The **clinical features** of the disorder depend on whether the lesion is intra- or extracranial:

- Intracranial lesions (suprabulbar) result in an upper motor neuron lesion.
- Extracranial lesions result in a lower motor neuron lesion.
- Lower motor neuron lesions affect the whole of one side of the face.
- Upper motor neuron lesions spare the forehead.

Bell's palsy

Bell's palsy is a lower motor neuron palsy of unknown aetiology. Viral or immune-mediated mechanisms cause ischaemia and swelling of the nerve, which becomes compressed along its course in the petrous–temporal bone.

The initial symptom of Bell's palsy is post-auricular pain. There is no sensory loss. Facial weakness begins within an hour of experiencing the pain. Facial weakness is unilateral on the side of the lesion. The affected side loses all creases and looks expressionless (students frequently mistake the affected side for the normal side as the patient looks younger without the facial creases).

On **examination** it can be seen that:

- Patients are unable to close their eyes completely.
- They have no forehead creases and are unable to grimace, show their teeth, or inflate their cheeks.
- There is hyperacusis, i.e. sensitivity to sound.
- Facial swelling is present.
- There is diminished or distorted taste.
- There is drooling with 'crocodile tears' when trying to eat due to muscle spasm.
- Salivation may be increased or reduced.

Appropriate investigations include CT and MRI (only when there is diagnostic difficulty), chest X-ray, serum angiotensin-converting enzyme (ACE) and full blood count (FBC).

Treatment is symptomatic:

- Prevent corneal drying and scarring by using an eye patch.
- A mouth splint is infrequently required.
- Patients become depressed and need psychological support.
- Specific treatment: corticosteroids within 24 h at 60–80 mg per day for 1 week and decrease over the next 7 days may reduce swelling and vasculitis.
- Surgery should only be considered in patients who have problems eating and speaking 12 months after the initial event.

Evidence-based reviews show that steroids are effective. Acyclovir combined with prednisone is probably effective in improving the facial functional outcome. There is no evidence that surgical facial nerve decompression is helpful.

The **prognosis** depends on the extent of nerve involvement and damage Complete recovery may occur with partial paralysis. Recovery is reduced to 15–20% if complete paralysis with no electrical excitability occurs.

Ramsey Hunt syndrome

Ramsey Hunt syndrome is a lower motor neuron facial nerve palsy due to Herpes zoster infection. It includes intense pain in the ear ipsilateral to the facial paralysis. The pain is much more intense than in Bell's palsy. There is a vesicular rash in front of the tragus of the ear together with: hearing loss; vertigo; tinnitus; taste loss in the tongue; and lymphadenopathy. There may be associated xerostomia and xerophthalmos.

Treatment is symptomatic; give analgesia for pain. Acyclovir for specific treatment.

Melkersson–Rosenthal syndrome

In Melkersson–Rosenthal syndrome the facial swelling is usually of the lips, which display granuloma on biopsy. The tongue has deep furrows and appears crenallated. A unilateral or bilateral seventh nerve palsy develops. The palsy is recurrent and occurs on the same or the opposite side at any time interval. It is important to consider sarcoidosis in the differential diagnosis.

Disorders of the eighth cranial nerve (the vestibulocochlear nerve)

The vestibulocochlear nerve is responsible for the sense of hearing, balance, and body position sense. The vestibular division contain the balance fibres and the cochlear division the auditory fibres. The vestibular fibres supply information from the inner ear to the brainstem regarding the position of the head. The cochlear fibres supply auditory information to the thalamus and ultimately the temporal lobe cortex: they are responsible for hearing.

Clinical features of eighth nerve lesions:

- Lesions of the eighth nerve can result in deafness, tinnitus, dizziness, vertigo, and vomiting.
- Lesions of the cochlear division of the nerve will result in deafness on the ipsilateral side.
- Lesions of the vestibular division result in nystagmus and vertigo.

> **BOX 4.9** Point to note: causes of facial paralysis
>
> The lesion may be at three different levels:
>
> - Supranuclear: stroke affecting the internal capsule.
> - Nuclear: poliomyelitis, pontine tumour.
> - Infranuclear: trauma, sarcoidosis, parotid trauma or neoplasm, meningioma, Bell's palsy, acoustic neuroma.

Disorders of the ninth cranial nerve (the glossopharyngeal nerve)

The glossopharyngeal nerve has five branches with distinct functions:

- The branchial motor branch supplies the stylopharyngeus muscle which elevates the palate when talking.
- The visceral motor branch supplies parasympathetic innervation of the smooth muscle and salivary glands, the pharynx, larynx, and viscera of the abdomen and thorax.
- The general sensory branch provides the sensations of pain, temperature, and touch from the cutaneous tissue of the external ear, the internal surface of the tympanic membrane, the posterior third of the tongue, and the upper pharynx.
- The visceral sensory branch carries visceral sensory information from the chemoreceptors of the carotid sinus and body.
- The special sensory branch provides taste sensation to the posterior third of the tongue.

The main disorder of the ninth nerve is **glossopharyngeal neuralgia** characterized by attacks of severe recurrent pain in the posterior third of tongue, middle ear, tonsil, and pharynx.

Disorders of the tenth cranial nerve (the vagus nerve)

The name 'vagus' comes from the Latin word meaning 'wandering'. The nerve travels from the brainstem to the splenic flexure of the colon. The vagus nerve consists of five branches all of which have separate functions:

- The branchial motor branch supplies the voluntary muscles of the pharynx, the larynx, and one of the extrinsic muscles of the tongue.
- The visceral motor branch supplies parasympathetic innervation of the smooth muscle and salivary glands, the pharynx, larynx, and viscera of the abdomen and the thorax.
- The general sensory branch supplies general sensory information from the skin of the periauricular area, the external auditory meatus, parts of the external surface of the tympanic membrane, and the pharynx.
- The visceral sensory branch supplies sensory information from the larynx, oesophagus, trachea, abdominal, and thoracic viscera. It also supplies the stretch receptors of the aortic arch and chemoreceptors of the aortic bodies.
- The special sensory branch is a minor branch which supplies taste sensation from the epiglottic region.

Isolated lesions to the vagus nerve are unusual and rarely occur in isolation. During thyroid surgery for thyrotoxicosis or tumour the recurrent laryngeal branch may be damaged, resulting in hoarseness of the voice.

Disorders of the eleventh cranial nerve (the spinal accessory nerve)

The spinal accessory nerve supplies the trapezius and sternocleidomastoid muscles. It controls movement of the neck and shoulder.

Lesions of the spinal accessory nerve result in paralysis of the trapezius and sternocleidomastoid muscles.

Disorders of the twelfth cranial nerve (the hypoglossal nerve)

The hypoglossal nerve supplies the muscles of the tongue.

Lesion of the hypoglossal nerve result in paralysis of the tongue muscles on the affected side. On protrusion the patient's tongue moves to the ipsilateral side.

Bulbar palsy

There is bilateral impairment of the function of the ninth, tenth, and twelfth cranial nerves. Occasionally the lowest part of the seventh cranial nerve may also be involved. The defect is of the motor nuclei and not the corticobulbar tracts.

Causes of bulbar palsy include:

- motor neuron disease
- poliomyelitis
- syringobulbia
- encephalitis
- Lyme disease.

The **clinical features** are of lower motor neuron origin:

- Dysarthria.
- Dysphagia with recurrent episodes of choking together with regurgitation of fluids.
- Dysphonia.
- Poor cough reflex.
- Aspiration pneumonia is common.
- Weak facial muscles with wasted fibrillating tongue.

Bulbar palsy is distinguished from pseudobulbar palsy by the presence of lower motor neuron signs.

Pseudobulbar palsy

Pseudobulbar palsy is due to impairment of the corticobulbar pathways to the nuclei of the fifth, seventh, tenth, eleventh, and twelfth cranial nerves. The nuclei of the third, fourth, and sixth nerves are spared.

Causes of pseudobulbar palsy include:

- motor neuron disease
- multiple sclerosis
- strokes
- ischaemia of the internal capsule.

The **clinical features** are of upper motor neuron origin:

- dysarthria
- dysphagia
- spastic tongue
- exaggerated jaw jerk
- emotional lability.

EPILEPSY

An epileptic attack is the clinical manifestation of an abnormal discharge of neurons. A seizure is a transient neurological deficit or dysfunction which may or may not result in loss of consciousness.

Seizures with loss of consciousness

Petit mal seizure (generalized absences)
Occurs between the ages of 4 and 13. Petit mal seizures are uncommon and account for 2% of all seizures in children. The child hyperventilates and the diagnosis is confirmed by a 3 Hz spike and wave formation. There is a brief episode of loss of consciousness (a few seconds) accompanied by eyelid blinks at a rate of 3 per second. A rare form with 2 per second motor and EEG pattern may be seen in sudden generalized myoclonic spasms of limb or sudden falls. Whatever the clinical type it is prudent to remember that young patients may during treatment suddenly become uncooperative, increasing the chances of untoward accidents in the dental setting.

Grand mal seizure
This type of seizure accounts for 50% of all seizures in school-aged children. There are three distinct clinical phases:

- The **aura:** these are brief and give clues to the aetiology and origin of the seizure. Olfactory, visual, auditory, and gustatory hallucinations indicate origin in either the frontal or temporal lobe. Intramuscular diazepam is slow and incomplete.
- The **convulsion:** this is the tonic and clonic motor activity which occurs during an epileptic seizure. During the tonic phase there is generalized spasm of

---

BOX 4.10 Clinical classification of epileptic seizures
- Grand mal seizure.
- Petit mal seizure.
- Partial (Jacksonian) seizure.
- Complex partial (temporal lobe seizure).
- Myoclonic seizure.
- Akinetic seizure.

all motor neurons including those of the respiratory muscles and jaw. The muscles of the jaw contract and the tongue may be bitten. The patient appears completely rigid and does not breathe. The patient may become cyanosed. The clonic phase then occurs, with powerful uncoordinated rhythmic movements of almost all the muscles. This phase may last 30 to 60 s and may be accompanied by the patient being incontinent of urine and faeces.

• The **post-ictal period:** after the convulsion the patient's breathing returns to normal and the patient becomes quiet and still. There is usually post-ictal confusion, accompanied by headache and drowsiness. A period of post-ictal amnesia also occurs. In rare cases there is a focal neurological deficit which may last up to 20–24 h, e.g. Todd's paralysis.

Investigations and treatment

The EEG shows focal spikes, sharp waves, and/or spike and wave discharges. Serum prolactin levels rise transiently (peak at 15–20 min) following a grand mal or temporal lobe seizure.

During a seizure the patient may become severely hypoxic. In a dental setting administer oxygen, making sure the patient is unharmed during the attack. After a second seizure it is worth considering the use of muscle relaxant. Diazemul 2–10 mg I.V. should be given, titrated against body mass and the patient's known drug history. Flumazenil should always be at hand as diazepam causes both cardiac and respiratory depression in patients who are already hypoxic.

After repeated attacks and at the establishment of a diagnosis counselling is invaluable.

Drug therapy is usually started after the second seizure within a 12-month period. All medication has side-effects. Medications include carbamazepine, phenobarbital, phenytoin, primidone, sodium valproate, and vigabatrin.

Status epilepticus

This is a persistent seizure activity which lasts for more than 30 min. It is more likely to occur with other forms of cerebral, discarded, or complicating systemic disease in epileptics. This is a medical emergency associated with a mortality of over 10% and a morbidity of up to 40%. In these patients the dental surgeon must try and maintain good oxygen, obtain intravenous access, and contact the emergency services. These patients will need admission to hospital.

The early use of rectal or intravenous diazepam will markedly cut down the risk of further seizures. If diazepam is not available or the dental surgeon is unable to obtain intravenous access, paraldehyde, adult dose 5–10 ml IM, into each buttock may be administered. The injection is very painful but highly effective. A glass syringe is needed. Paraldeyde can also be obtained for rectal administration. There are ethical problems surrounding the administration by a dental surgeon of rectal medication to patients who are unconscious. In children, parents and relatives are usually competent or can be guided to administer the medication. In adults who are known to have epilepsy the dental surgeon should discuss emergency treatment with all those patients who have a history of recurrent attacks.

Seizures without loss of consciousness

Simple partial seizures

These seizures account for 15–20% of all seizures in children. The seizure discharge remains confined to a small area of the motor cortex or temporal lobe and does not become generalized. There is no loss of consciousness. The clinical pattern localizes the focus.

A Jacksonian seizure may be experienced if the focus involves the lower or upper limb area resulting in a localized convulsion of part of the arm, leg, hand, or even finger or toe, on the contralateral side.

Temporal lobe seizure may result in '*jamais vu*' (the illusion or impression of never having experienced something that has actually been experienced many times before) or similarly *déjà vu* (when present events are felt as though they had been previously experienced). The sudden convulsive movement of an arm or leg may cause both disturbance and alarm to the dental surgeon. However, this is only transitory.

Myoclonic seizures

Myoclonic seizures are more common than petit mal and account for 5% of all seizures in children. These are commonly confused with petit mal and are multiple, sudden jerks of upper or lower limbs accompanied by 'absences'. The EEG shows epileptic waveforms.

Akinetic seizures

These are sudden falls resulting from loss of muscle tone. The patient is unable to move for a brief period. Akinetic seizures must be differentiated from vertebrobasilar syndrome and more rarely cataplexy.

DEMYELINATING DISEASES

Demyelination is a pathological process that destroys the myelin sheaths while sparing the neurons and axonal processes. Multiple sclerosis (MS) (disseminated sclerosis) is the most important. Other diseases include:

- Acute disseminated encephalomyelitis: occurs post measles, chicken pox, and also smallpox vaccination, in children aged 3–13 years. The clinical syndrome similar to MS.
- Neuromyelisis optica (Devic's syndrome): visual failure due to optic neuritis with spinal cord disease. Rapid blindness and paraplegia.
- Diffuse sclerosis (Schilder's disease): failure to form normal myelin. Fatal within 12 months.
- Subacute myelo-opticoneuropathy (SMON): occurs mainly in Japanese. Distressing, paraesthesia in legs, followed by weakness resulting in severe disability.

Multiple sclerosis (MS)

In MS episodes of demyelination occur at different sites within the CNS at different times. In the UK about 100 000 patients a year are diagnosed with MS. It is a disease of young adults with a peak age of 30 and a female : male ratio of 3 : 2. The risk of MS rises with increasing distance from the equator and is increased fifteen-fold in first-degree relatives.

Clinical features

There are many clinical features:

- Patients commonly experience eye problems.
- Optic neuritis occurs which ocular pain, abnormal movement, diplopia, and transient blindness.
- Fatigue and malaise may be pronounced.
- Sensory problems such as paraesthesia and hypoaesthesia occur frequently.
- An MS plaque in the spinal cord may cause the clinical feature called Lhermitte's symptom which is an electric shock which travels down the spine felt on flexion of the neck.
- Spasticity, particularly in spinal cord lesions, may lead to stiffness, flexor spasms, cramps, or spontaneous clonus.
- Cerebellar involvement will result in ataxia; the patient looks drunk when walking.
- Neuropathic pain may occur and may present as trigeminal neuralgia.
- Mood disturbance occurs; patients are often emotionally labile.
- Depression occurs, but is uncommon.
- Late-stage MS frequently has a euphoric effect.

Investigations and treatment

An MRI scan shows plaque anatomically distributed. Cerebrospinal fluid (CSF) shows the presence of oligoclonal bands which are not present in the serum; this indicates the presence of inflammation and is seen in almost all patients with MS. Visually evoked responses are unilaterally delayed.

Treatment is symptomatic. Interferon-β is disease modifying.

BOX 4.11 Dental relevance of general problems in MS

Social problems

- Relatives may be overprotective. The patient and family make frequent visits to hospital. The financial cost to the individual, family, and NHS is high.
- Anxiety in the family as there is a high risk for MS in first-degree relatives.

Medical problems

- Symptoms vary and are difficult to assess.
- There is rarely intellectual impairment, but mild memory impairment may interfere with the dentist–patient relationship.
- Patients are usually euphoric and can cope with arduous procedures well.

BOX 4.12 Dental relevance of specific problems in MS

- Trigeminal neuralgia.
- Recurrent facial palsies.
- Increased caries rate due to spasticity or ataxic movements of the upper limbs making oral hygiene difficult.
- Dental pain of no specific origin with no apparent underlying dental problem.
- Inability to tolerate dental procedures because of spastic movements of head, limbs, and even the tongue.
- Difficulty in swallowing and emotional lability due to pseudobulbar palsy.
- Oral dysaesthesia.
- Mobility—symptoms may be very mild and not present any problems or the patient may be severely incapacitated and unable to walk or talk because of spasticity or ataxia.
- Patients have recurrent urinary tract infections and are on frequent courses of, or are on long-term, antibiotics.
- Vision can be affected during active episodes of disease but often returns to normal. Visual loss can be sudden and occur during treatment in the dental surgery.
- Careful treatment planning is needed because a hot environment, anxiety, and stress can all exacerbate or precipitate active disease.
- Patients are usually prescribed numerous different medications which may interact with drugs used routinely in dentistry (see Table 4.1).

Table 4.1 Drugs interactions and side-effects in MS

Indication for drug	Drug	Point to note
Ataxia	Isoniazid	Drug metabolism may be a problem with general anaesthetic
	Clomazepan	Muscle relaxant—dental implication, care with sedation and general anaesthetic
Spaciticity	Baclofen	Muscle relaxant—care when considering sedation
	Diazepam	Muscle relaxant—care when considering sedation
Dysaesthesia	Carbamazepine	Aplastic anaemia
	Phenytoin	Gingival hypertrophy, acne hirsute, P-450 enzyme inducer—care with metronidizole, fluconazole, erythromycin
Injection	Antibiotics	This might induce resistant oral infections and increase the intraoral risk of candidosis

CEREBROVASCULAR DISEASE

Cerebrovascular disease may result in cerebrovascular accident (stroke), transient ischaemic attack (TIA), and multi-infarct dementia.

There are many risk factors for cerebral infarction:

- increasing age
- high blood pressure
- diabetes mellitus
- atrial fibrillation and other arrhythmias
- transient ischaemic attack
- oral contraception
- increased plasma viscosity
- cigarette smoking
- hyperlipidaemia
- peripheral vascular disease
- alcoholism
- syphilis
- HIV.

Cerebrovascular accident

A stroke is an episode of neurological dysfunction with clinical symptoms which persist for more than 24 h. The causes of stroke are shown in Table 4.2.

Clinical features

The clinical features of a stroke depend on the site of the infarct. The neurological deficit may increase with time due to continued haemorrhage, recurrent emboli, or propagation of the clot. If the neurological deficit improves rapidly this is called a transient ischaemic attack (TIA). The symptoms and signs last for less than 24 h. TIAs are almost always due to arterial thromboembolism.

Clinical features due to lesions affecting the anterior and middle cerebral arteries are:

- Contralateral facial paresis.
- Contralateral hemiparesis.

Table 4.2 Causes of stroke

Cause	Cases (%)
Cerebral infarction secondary to thrombosis or an embolus	80
Cerebral haemorrhage	10
Subarachnoid haemorrhage	5
Rare causes of cerebral infarction[†]	5

[†]Oral contraceptives, pregnancy and the puerperium, polycythaemia rubra vera, hyperviscosity syndrome, sickle cell disease, irradiation, arteritis (e.g. systemic lupus erythematosus, giant cell arteritis, polyarteritis nodosa etc.

> **BOX 4.13** Stroke outcomes
> - 20% of stroke patients die within the first month (25% within the first year).
> - 50% of patients who die have a pulmonary embolism.
> - 50% of all stroke patients have deep vein thrombosis.
> - There is a rate of recurrence of 10–15%.
> - 50% of survivors return to normal or near normal function.

- Transient blindness (amaurosis fugax).
- Blindness secondary to retinal infarction.
- Visuospatial disturbance (non-dominant lobe lesion).
- Dysarthria.
- Expressive and/or receptive dysphasia (dominant hemisphere lesion).
- Head moves towards the side of the lesion.

There are many complications with stroke. Try and avoid practical complication with good nursing care, e.g. urinary catheterization, physiotherapy, speech therapy. Death may occur due to localized oedema or haemorrhage. There may also be: bronchopneumonia, urinary tract infection, depression, limb contractures, dislocation of shoulder common secondary to hemiparesis.

Investigations

Appropriate investigations depend on both the patient's age and the severity of the stroke. Try to establish whether there is a treatable underlying cause and what risk factors are operating, which if treated may decrease the risk of recurrence:

- Haematology and serology: haemoglobin and haematocrit, white cell count and differential, platelet count, ESR and C-reactive protein (CRP), blood sugar, urea and electrolytes, treponemal screen, immunoglobulins and protein electrophoresis.
- General tests: examine the urine, chest X-ray, skull X-ray, ECG.
- Other tests which may be indicated: CT scan, MRI scan, cerebral angiography, blood culture, examination of the cerebrospinal fluid (CSF), EEG, anti-nuclear antibodies.

Treatment

- Acute management involves resuscitating the patient.
- Treat the underlying cause, e.g. giant cell arteritis, hypertension, cerebral embolus from the heart, diabetes, intracerebral haematoma.
- Treat complications of the stroke.
- Specialist help is required before considering whether to anticoagulate the patient. The risks and benefit of anticoagulation must be considered carefully. Patients with mild strokes with good recovery should be treated with aspirin.

Transient ischaemic attacks (TIAs)

TIAs are neurological deficits which last less than 24 h. Only 50% of patients develop a stroke or die after suffering a TIA. If examination reveals carotid bruit, carotid endarterectomy to remove artheroma at the carotid syphon should be considered. All patients should be given antiplatelet therapy (aspirin 85–300 mg/day). If the embolus originated in the left side of the heart full anticoagulation with warfarin should be instituted.

Myocardial infarction is the most common complication leading to death post TIA.

Multi-infarct dementia

Multi-infarct dementia occurs in both sexes over the age of 50 years. It is less common than Alzheimer's disease. it results in both intellectual and physical disability. It is caused by a succession of minor cerebrovascular events; each event may not be clinically obvious. Deterioration in the patient is usually slow and 'step-wise'. The condition has a poor prognosis.

Aspirin, 75–300 mg/day, is given if no treatable cause can be identified. This reduces the morbidity by 50%.

PARKINSON'S DISEASE (PARALYSIS AGITANS)

The clinical syndrome of Parkinsonism is characterized by tremor, rigidity, and hypokinesia. The clinical syndrome may be associated with:

- A number of neurological disorders which involve the substantia nigra.
- Drugs such as phenothiazines, butyrophenones, tetrabenazine and neuro-toxic chemicals MPTP (methylphenyltetrahydropyridine).
- Infections such as syphilis, flu virus, or the encephalitis lethargica agent may cause irreversible damage to the substantia nigra.

Idiopathic Parkinson's disease

Idiopathic Parkinson's disease is due to denervation of the dopaminergic nigro-striatal pathways. The prevalence in Europe is 1.5 in 1000. It affects all races and both sexes are affected equally. Patients are usually over 50 years of age.

Clinical features
- **Tremor** is the commonest presenting complaint. It is present at rest but disappears on voluntary movement. Tremor is increased by stress, infection, and fatigue. The tremor rate is four to eight cycles per second. The dental surgeon should be aware that besides the limbs the tongue and jaw may also be affected, making any intraoral operative procedure difficult, especially as patients also tend to drool saliva as the initiation of the swallowing reflex is delayed.

> **BOX 4.14** Parkinson's disease: clinical features of dental relevance
>
> - Drooling saliva and hypersalivation are early signs of disease.
> - Dysphagia.
> - Uncoordinated swallowing movement.
> - Hand deformities.
> - Postural disorders.

> **BOX 4.15** Differential diagnosis of tremor
>
> - Causes of tremor: postural tremor, thyrotoxicosis, anxiety, alcohol, drugs, heavy metal poisoning, benign familial essential tremor.
> - At rest in Parkinsonism.
> - Intention tremor: multiple sclerosis, vascular disease, spinocerebellar degeneration.

- **Rigidity:** the hypertension can be detected by resistance to passive movement ('lead type rigidity'). It results in a flexed position of the neck and occurs early in the disease process. Patients find difficulty in lying back in the dental chair. The flexed posture also contributes to the hurrying (festinant) gait. A patient may be helped from the dental chair to find themselves unable to stop at the door, as they have increasingly rapid steps.
- **Hypokinesia:** paucity of movement causes the most disruption to day-to-day activity. Dental surgeons may notice the mask-like faces of patients with very little apparent emotion expressed. The staring appearance is due to reduced blinking and monotonous speech.
- Other features are micrographia (writing becomes smaller) and reduced swinging of the arms while walking.
- Oculogyric irises—eyes are deviated upwards and outwards associated with facial flushing, hypertension, and tachycardia.

Treatment
- Early medication: anticholinergic drugs and amantadine—the efficiency of these drugs is limited.
- Later medication: levodopa combined with carbidopa—these should be taken with a snack. Levodopa plus carbidopa combined with bromocriptine.
- Surgery: transplants of foetal substantia nigra or sympathetic ganglia are effective. Adrenal autotransplants. Stem cell implants are undergoing evaluation at present.
- Field defects resulting from lesions to visual pathway. Direction of action of the external ocular muscles. Sensory divisions of the fifth cranial nerve. To elicit the jaw jerk.

5 | Renal disease and transplantation

RENAL FUNCTION

The main role of the kidney is the elimination of waste material and maintainance of the composition of body fluid. It receives about 25% of cardiac output every minute. Sixty to 80% of the filtered water and sodium are reabsorbed in the proximal tubule along with almost all the bicarbonate, potassium, glucose, and amino acids. In the distal tubule more water and some sodium are reabsorbed. The latter process is controlled by aldosterone. The total urine volume in health is 1–2 litres a day.

The kidney regulates electrolyte balance, acid–base balance, calcium metabolism, blood pressure, and the composition of body fluid. The kidney is a major site for the catabolism of many small-molecular-weight proteins and also has a number of endocrine functions:

- Erythropoietin is secreted by the kidney and is the major stimulus to the bone marrow to produce red cells.
- Prostaglandins are secreted by the kidney.
- Renin–angiotensin system: the cells of the juxtaglomerular apparatus secrete renin which converts angiotensinogen to angiotensin 1. Angiotensin 1 is subsequently converted to angiotensin 2 by angiotensin-converting enzyme (ACE), which is a potent peripheral vasoconstrictor.
- Vitamin D metabolism—vitamin D requires hydroxylation in the liver and then by the kidney to produce the active compound 1,25-hydroxyvitamin D.

BOX 5.1 Definition of common clinical terms

- Albuminuria: albumin in the urine.
- Anuria: no urine output.
- Bacteruria: bacteria in the urine (growth of 10^5 organisms/ml urine).
- Cystitis: bladder infection.
- Dysuria: pain or difficulty on urination.
- Frequency: increased rate of urination.
- Haematuria: blood in the urine.
- Nocturia: increase in night-time urination.
- Polyuria: excessive urine output.
- Proteinuria: protein in the urine.
- Pyelonephritis: kidney infection.
- Pyuria: pus in the urine.
- Urethritis: inflammation of the urethra, mainly in males.

Haematuria

Haematuria should always be considered as pathological and investigated. There are a number of causes of haematuria including:

- Anticoagulant drugs.
- Infection, including simple urinary tact infections and tuberculosis.
- Infective endocarditis.
- Renal tract and kidney stones.
- Tumours of the bladder, kidney, or prostate gland.
- Trauma to the renal tract and kidneys.
- Polycystic kidneys.
- Henoch–Schonlein purpura.
- Systemic lupus erythematosus (SLE) and polyarteritis nodosa.
- Malignant hypertension.

Proteinuria

Urine normally has a protein content of less than 150 mg/24 h (100 ng/l). This is increased in proteinuria. Proteinuria has a number of possible causes:

- pyelonephritis
- glomerulonephritis
- nephrotic syndrome
- obstructive nephropathy
- congestive cardiac failure
- postural proteinuria
- myeloma.

URINARY TRACT INFECTION (UTI)

UTIs are very common: every year 5–6% of all women develop a UTI. UTIs are 50 times more common in women than men and are uncommon in men less than 70 years of age. UTIs can be caused by bacteria, viruses, or fungi.

Bacteria causing UTIs

Bacteria are the most common organisms causing UTIs. Most urinary pathogens are bowel commensals:

- 70% of infection is caused by *Escherichia coli*.
- 15–30% of infections are caused by coagulase-negative staphylococci.
- Hospital acquired staphylococcal infections are associated with use of catheters and surgical instrumentation.
- 2% of infections are caused by enterococci.
- *Klebsiella pneumoniae*, *Proteus mirabilis*, and *Enterobacter* spp. also cause infection.

Predisposing factors

There are a number of reasons why females are more vulnerable to UTIs:

- Females have a short urethra which increases the chance of ascending infection.
- The urethral opening is nearer the rectum than in males.
- Vaginal secretions can harbour bacteria.
- Sexual intercourse may cause trauma to the urethra.
- In pregnancy the uterus presses on the bladder and urethra.

Other factors predisposing to UTIs are:

- Urinary reflux.
- Damage or infection by instrumentation during surgery or bladder catheterization.
- Vesicoenteric fistula.
- Polycystic kidney disease.
- Horseshoe kidney.
- Obstruction caused by prostatic hypertrophy and urethral stricture.
- Diabetes mellitus.

Clinical features

A third of patients present with haematuria. Other symptoms include dysuria, frequency, and urgency. Suprapubic or, more rarely, perineal pain may occur. The urine has an offensive odour and may be cloudy. Incontinence occurs in both the very young and in the elderly.

Investigations

Reagent strips are used to detect blood and protein in the urine. Nitrite shows the presence of pathogens as they convert nitrate to nitrite. Leucocyte esterase is a marker of urinary leucocytosis. Midstream urine culture can be used to ascertain the infective organism.

Prevention

A number of steps can be taken to prevent UTIs:

- A high fluid intake is essential; drink six to ten glasses of water per day.
- The pH of the urine can be lowered by drinking cranberry juice or citrate solutions.
- Correct toileting in females, wiping from front to back.
- Avoid tight fitting clothing such as jeans.
- Wear cotton underwear.
- Don't use perfumed soaps, douches, or deodorants in vaginal area.
- Wash before and after sexual intercourse.

Treatment

Trimethoprim is the first-line antibiotic. Cotrimoxazole bestows no additional benefit. Resistance has developed with a number of antibiotics used for treatment of UTIs: there is resistance to amoxicillin in 50% of cases, to oral cephalosporins in 10–30%, and to nitrofurantoin in 15%.

CONDITIONS AFFECTING THE BLADDER

Urinary incontinence

Urinary incontinence is caused by loss of control of the flow of urine. It is a common disorder affecting 45% of females over the age of 60.

Urinary incontinence has a number of causes, including:

- pregnancy
- childbirth
- menopause
- hysterectomy
- enlarged prostate in males
- stroke
- epilepsy
- urinary tract infection
- medication, e.g. antihypertensives, muscle relaxants.

Clinical features

Check the history for medication such as antihypertensives, muscle relaxants, antihistamines, and anxiolytic sleeping pills. Incontinence of urine may be associated with sleep disturbance, social isolation, depression, and loss of libido (as sexual activity may trigger incontinent episodes). There may be signs and symptoms of underlying systemic disease such as stroke or urinary tract infection.

Treatment

Symptomatic treatment

Females and males may wear adult diapers, incontinence briefs, or sanitary napkins. Males may also use external appliances, e.g. catheters.

BOX 5.2 Types of incontinence

- Stress incontinence: coughing, laughing, and sneezing all stress the bladder resulting in inability to hold urine.
- Overflow incontinence: the bladder does not empty completely when filled. Overfilling results in leaking.
- Urge incontinence: the bladder has a sudden uncontrollable urge to empty irrespective of the amount of filling.

Specific treatment
- **Stress incontinence**: exercises to strengthen the pelvic floor and muscles; bladder suspension; injection of collagen around the sphincter; oestrogen supplementation in females with low oestrogen levels.
- **Overflow incontinence**: self-catheterization; medication.
- **Urge incontinence**: bladder training by emptying the bladder hourly for 6–7 days then slowly lengthening the period between bladder emptying; exercises (e.g. pelvic floor exercises).
- **Post prostate surgery incontinence** is difficult to treat and further procedures may be necessary.

Carcinoma of the bladder

Bladder cancer is the most common carcinoma of the urinary tract. It is more common in males (males : female ratio 3 : 1) and usually occurs after the 7th decade of life.

The aetiology of bladder cancer is unknown, but associated risk factors are smoking (number over lifetime), exposure to industrial chemicals, and chronic cystitis.

Clinical features
Symptoms of haematuria, dysuria, and nocturia usually appear late in the disease.

Investigations and treatment
Cystoscopy can be used to view the bladder wall. A biopsy sample can be taken during cystoscopy for further investigation.

Treatment involves transurethral resection to remove the tumour or radical resection by cystectomy. Metastases are treated by radiotherapy and chemotherapy.

DISEASES OF THE KIDNEY

Pyelonephritis

Pyelonephritis is an infection of the kidney. There are a number of possible causes:

- Ascending infection caused by obstruction of flow through the ureters resulting in abscesses forming in the kidney and causing pyuria.
- Haematogenous spread of infection to one or both kidneys.
- Kidney stones.
- Pregnancy.
- Prostate enlargement.
- Tumours.

Pyelonephritis manifests with a sudden onset of fever with rigors, loin pain, and haematuria. Vigorous treatment of infection with antibiotics is necessary, together with treatment of the underlying cause. Repeated bouts of infection lead to kidney scarring, ureamia, and eventually kidney failure.

Glomerulonephritis

Glomerulonephritis is inflammation in the glomerulus; it can occur as primary glomerular disease or as part of a systemic illness. It is common in children and young adults. There may be a genetic component to the aetiology as a combination of genes control the immune response to environmental factors such as infective organisms, drugs, and chemicals.

There are a number of associated systemic conditions:

- Infections, particularly streptococcal infections.
- Other infections including hepatitis B, HIV, *Staphylococcus aureus*.
- Malaria.
- Systemic lupus erythematosus.
- Infective endocarditis.
- Drug reactions including reactions to non-steroidal anti-inflammatory drugs (NSAIDs), gold, and penicillamine.
- Malignant disease including carcinoma, myeloma, and lymphoma.

Glomerulonephritis is associated with the **clinical features** of malaise, flank pain, fever, loss of appetite, peripheral oedema, oliguria, haematuria, and signs associated with any underlying systemic problem.

Investigations include urine analysis for albumin and casts, midstream urine, full blood count and erythrocyte sedimentation rate, chest X-ray, blood cultures, viral serology, antinuclear antibodies and DNA antibodies, complement levels, and antineutrophil cytoplasmic antibody (ANCA).

Supportive **treatment** includes antipyretics and diuretic and dietary restriction of salt and protein. Fluids may need to be restricted. The associated infection, tumour, or autoimmune condition should be treated and any offending medication stopped. The immune response can be damped down with immunosuppressives.

Renal calculi or 'kidney stones'

These commonly form in the kidney, but stones can occur in the bladder. The kidney secretes organic molecules which form aggregates together with mucoprotein and calcium, phosphate, or oxalate salts. The calcium in the stones make them radio-opaque.

Kidney stones vary in size from minute to staghorn calculi which are so large that they fill the entire pelvis of the kidney. Bladder calculi occur mostly in patients from hot countries. They vary in size from a few millimetres to filling the whole bladder. They can cause problems with obstruction.

Small stones pass spontaneously without symptoms. Larger stones may cause haematuria or renal colic: renal colic is caused by spasm of the ureters and can be severe.

> **BOX 5.3** Types of urinary stones
>
> Calcium oxalate stones are the most common (70%). Approximately 50% of oxalate stones have a mixture of calcium phosphate in combination with apatite or calcium carbonate with apatite.
>
> Triple-phosphate stones (16–17%). These are composed of magnesium ammonium phosphate hexahydrate (also known as 'struvite'), combined with apatite. Staghorn calculi are formed from this type of stone.
>
> Uric acid stones (5–6%). These are usually very small and are able to be passed without causing obstruction.
>
> Cystine stones (2–3%). These are very small. They contain sulphur giving them a yellow-green colour.

Investigation of the condition should include an analysis of the stones if they are available. Midstream urine and urine culture should be done. An X-ray will show the size and position of the stones. Blood biochemistry should be checked.

Treatment can be by minimally invasive methods such as basket retrieval or lithotripsy. Surgical removal may be necessary.

Autosomal dominant polycystic kidney disease (ADPKD)

ADPKD is a common genetic disease affecting approximately 1 in every 800 people. It affects teenagers and young adults and is slowly progressive. In most patients the disease progresses to renal failure, and 20–30% of renal dialysis patients have ADPKD.

A gene for ADPKD was identified in 1994. It has autosomal dominant inheritance but shows genetic heterogeneity. A second gene has been identified and other additional genes may also play a part in the disease.

Clinical features

The kidneys enlarge and may fill the abdomen. The main symptoms are lumbar and loin pain, haematuria, and recurrent UTIs. There will be hypertension as the kidney fails, as well as later signs of renal failure. Features secondary to high circulating ammonia levels are present—high levels of circulating ammonia cause: skin pruritus and rashes; nausea, vomiting, and diarrhoea; pyuria; haematuria and glycosuria; breath which smells of urine; mental confusion, visual disturbances, drowsiness and coma.

Investigations and treatment

An intravenous pyelogram (an X-ray examination of the kidneys, ureters, and urinary bladder) can be used for investigation. Treatment includes dialysis or renal transplantation.

Kidney tumours

Wilms' tumour (nephroblastoma) occurs in children and renal cell carcinoma (renal adenocarcinoma, hypernephroma) in adults.

Wilms' tumour is the commonest renal tumour in children and accounts for 6–7% of all childhood malignancies Peak incidence is between the ages of 1–4 years. It is thought to arise from a mutation of the *WT1* gene on the short arm of chromosome 11.

Renal cell carcinoma is the commonest renal tumour. It accounts for 85% of all malignancies of the kidney in adults and is rare before the age of 40 years. It is more common in men, who have an incidence of 10/100 000, whereas the incidence in women is 5/100 000. Smokers have an increased risk of renal cell carcinoma. There may be autosomal dominant inheritance of renal cell carcinoma in von Hippel–Lindau syndrome.

Clinical features of renal tumours

Up to 40% of patients present with incidental mass and no symptoms. There is haematuria in 50%, abdominal pain in 40%, and an abdominal mass in 30%. Non-specific features include fever, malaise, weight loss, hypertension, and hypercalcaemia.

Investigations and treatment

There are a number of non-specific tests which show abnormal results: full blood count; serum urea and electrolytes; erythrocyte sedimentation rate; C-reactive protein; calcium and alkaline phosphatases. Specific tests include urine analysis for blood, protein, and casts, ultrasound, MRI scan, and biopsy.

Early referral to a urologist is necessary. Combined surgery, radiotherapy, and chemotherapy is usual.

Staging of renal tumours

The prognosis for both Wilms' tumour and renal cell carcinoma is dependent on staging (Tables 5.1 and 5.2). The overall survival in renal cell carcinoma is 60–65%.

Table 5.1 Staging of Wilms' tumour

Stage	Extent of spread	4-year survival (%)
I	Confined to kidney—complete excision	>95
II	Extends through capsule—complete excision	93
III	Residual tumour in abdomen. No blood spread	87
IV	Haematogenous metastases	73
V	Bilateral kidney tumours	76

Table 5.2 Staging for renal cell carcinoma

Stage	Extent of spread	5-year survival (%)
I	Confined to kidney	65–85
II	Through capsule but not fascia	45–80
III	To lymph nodes and or renal vein	15–35
IV	Distant metastases	0–10

Renal failure

Renal failure is the failure of the kidney to maintain homeostasis. Renal failure may be acute or chronic.

Acute renal failure (ARF)

Acute renal failure (ARF) occurs when the renal excretory function declines over a few hours or days. Causes of acute renal failure can be pre-renal, renal, or post-renal:

- Pre-renal—poor perfusion of kidneys.
- Renal causes:
  - Acute tubular necrosis secondary to poisons which are nephrotoxic, and severe sepsis.
  - Small and large vessel disease including obstructive and vasculitic problems.
  - Accelerated hypertension.
  - Scleroderma and systemic lupus erythematosus.
  - Glomerulonephritis.
  - Interstitial nephritis.
  - Acute cortical necrosis.
  - Myeloma.
  - Rhabdomyolysis.
  - Hepatorenal syndrome.
- Post-renal—obstruction.

The underlying cause must be treated to reverse acute renal failure. Dialyse will remove toxic wastes.

Chronic renal failure (CRF)

Chronic renal failure (CRF) is characterised by uraemia and a glomerular filtration rate (GFR) of about 15 ml/min. It is commonly seen in the latter stages of chronic renal disease. In the UK more than 500 patients/million population are currently receiving treatment for CRF. There has been a four-fold increase in the incidence of CRF in ethnic minority groups in the last 20 years.

The causes of CRF are shown in Table 5.3.

Table 5.3 Causes of CRF

Pathology	% of total cases
Diabetes	40
Hypertension	25
Glomerulonephritis	12
Pyelonephritis	0.9
Polycystic kidney disease	0.6
Renovascular disease	0.6

Table 5.4 Signs and symptoms of renal failure

Problems	Signs and symptoms
Acute failure	Excretory function declines over hours or days (see text)
Uraemia	Nausea and vomiting
Cardiovascular	Congestive cardiac failure
Gastrointestinal	Weight loss, nausea, and vomiting
Dermatological	Pruritus, yellow–green tinge to skin
CNS	Poor concentration and mental lassitude, clonus and asterixis
Respiratory (serositis)	Pleuritic chest pain

Clinical features

Patients with CRF are initially asymptomatic. The symptoms are related to the stage of renal failure. They begin with nausea, pruritus, and nocturia. As chronic renal failure progresses nausea becomes more severe and vomiting, oedema, dyspnoea, and impotence develop. The end stages of chronic renal failure are associated with confusion, fits, hiccoughs, and end in coma (see Table 5.4).

Treatment

Uraemic symptoms should be treated. It is best to institute dialysis, combined if possible with renal transplantation. Renal transplantation is the treatment of choice for most patients with end-stage renal failure (ESRF).

Renal transplantation

Renal transplantation has many advantages as a treatment for renal failure:

- Enhanced survival.
- Improved quality of life.
- No dialysis is needed.
- No dietary restrictions.

- Costs are less than for dialysis.
- Both anaemia and bone disease recover.

The donor kidney may be from a live healthy donor or a cadaver organ. During surgery the transplanted kidney is placed in the iliac fossa. The best results are seen in ABO compatible donors and patients with close matching for DR, A, and B major histocompatibility complex antigens. Medical treatment involves triple therapy with a tapering dose of corticosteroids plus cyclosporin and azathioprine. Prophylactic therapy includes: *Pneumocystis* prophylaxis with cotrimoxazole, antifungal prophylaxis; an amphotericin H2-receptor antagonist or proton pump inhibitor is also given to cover oral corticosteroids. Antituberculous prophylaxis is given for 1 year to African and Asian patients.

> **BOX 5.4 Survival in renal transplantation**
>
> - Graft survival at 1 year >85%.
> - Patient survival at 1 year 90%.
> - Graft survival at 5 years 70%.
> - Graft survival at 10 years 50%.

> **BOX 5.5 Dental relevance of renal disease and renal transplantation**
>
> - Patients may have hypertension being treated with antihypertensive drugs. These drugs present a myriad of problems for the dentist: e.g. hypotensive episodes when getting up from the chair, angioeodema associated with ACE inhibitors, nifedipine and gingival hypertrophy.
> - Patients may have associated cardiac disease and be prone to arrhythmias and cardiac failure.
> - Anaemia is normochromic, normocytic and the blood film is hypoproliferative due reduced production of erythropoietin. The anaemia may also be due to iron deficiency and haemolysis. Dental patients may present with oral ulceration, oral soreness, or in severe cases dyspnoea.
> - Renal osteodystrophy may be present. This is a bone disorder associated with secondary hyperparathyroidism. Patients have loss of the lamina dura around the teeth, and brown tumours may be present in the skull.
> - Osteomalacia is one of the bone disorders seen in chronic renal failure and dental patients may be prone to bone fractures.
> - Dialysis patients may be anticoagulated.
> - Dialysis patients they have an increased risk of contacting hepatitis B and C.
> - Transplant patients may be taking immunosuppressive drugs, which may include steroids suppressing the adrenocortical axis causing patients to require additional steroid cover, and ciclosporin which may cause gingival hyperplasia.
> - Transplant patients are also prone to infections including oral candida.
> - Patients are at risk of tuberculosis.
> - Impaired drug excretion occurs. It is important to modify the dose in patients with renal failure.

Complications of renal transplantation

Acute rejection develops in 30–50% of recipients within the first 2 weeks. It is usually treated with pulses of high-dose corticosteroids. Newer agents such as tacrolimus, antilymphocyte antibodies, and mycophenolate mofetil may be tried. Chronic rejection occurs in a large number of grafts without any obvious cause at any time after transplantation. Delayed primary function is usually due to prolonged cold ischaemia and may take a few days to several months to recover. Vascular complications include a thrombotic episode in a functioning graft rendering it non-viable—this presents with sudden onset of anuria. Other complications include: leakage of urine; lymphocele caused by a peri-nephric collection of lymph; infection with cytomegalovirus (this may be treated with ganciclovir).

6 Infections

FEVER

Fever is caused by the release of endogenous pyrogens from monocytes. Micro-organisms, endotoxins, drugs, tumours, sensitized lymphocytes, and immune complexes may all release pyrogens when triggered. The core body temperature varies between 37.0 and 37.5 °C and is controlled from the hypothalamus. Body temperature has a circadian rhythm with the core body temperature being 0.5–1.0 °C higher in the evening: an increase in temperature to above the normal core temperature is defined as fever. Incidence of fever is independent of sex, age, race, and geography.

Pyrexia of unknown origin

Pyrexia of unknown origin (PUO) occurs when a patient has been pyretic for 3 weeks or more. The body temperature is greater than 38.3 °C on several separate occasions. It can also be diagnosed if a hospital inpatient has no diagnosis after 1 week of investigation. The causes are varied (see Table 6.1).

Causes
- Infection: tuberculosis most common infection causing PUO. Others include: HIV, bacterial endocarditis, abscesses (including dental, intra-abdominal, and brain abscesses), urinary tract infection, brucellosis, cytomegalovirus, and Epstein–Barr virus.
- Neoplastic conditions: lymphoma (Hodgkin's and non-Hodgkin's), leukaemia, hypernephroma, hepatoma, and disseminated carcinoma.
- Autoimmune diseases: systemic lupus erythematosus and rheumatoid arthritis can both cause PUO.
- Drugs: NSAIDs, especially salicylates, iodine, phenytoin, and isoniazid can all cause PUO.

Investigations
Suitable screening tests include repeated temperature monitoring, blood cultures, full blood count, liver function tests, screening for acute antibodies, chest X-ray, and plain abdominal X-ray. Specific tests will depend on the initial results of the screening tests.

Table 6.1 Causes of pyrexia of unknown origin

Cause	Per cent of cases
Infection	35
Malignancy	20
Autoimmune disease	20
Other causes[†]	25

[†]Granulomatous conditions, inflammatory bowel disease, pulmonary emboli, hypothalamic lesions, thyroiditis, phaeochromocytoma, factitious illness.

BOX 6.1 Dental relevance of fever

- A patient with fever may present to the dental surgeon either in the dental practice or in hospital. Patients in practice may be young children, elderly, immunocompromised, or previously fit adults.
- Cross-infection control is very important. Special care should be taken with the use of latex gloves.
- Viruses adhere to gloves, which may be responsible for direct spread.
- Herpes encephalitis may result from cross-infection between the patient and dental staff.
- Herpetic whitlow can be spread by direct infection to the dental surgeon or assisting nurse.
- In patients with eczema, especially if they use topical steroids, herpes infection can result in eczema herpeticum which may cause dissemination of the virus or lead to bacterial superinfection.
- In immunocompromised patients, especially those with transplants, infection quickly becomes disseminated.

VIRAL INFECTIONS

Herpes viruses

The herpes viruses are a family of large DNA-containing viruses. Examples of herpes viruses are Herpes simplex virus, Varicella zoster virus, cytomegalovirus, and Epstein–Barr virus. The main properties of these viruses are their latency and their reactivity.

Herpes simplex virus

The main sites of infection with Herpes simplex virus (HSV) are the skin and mucous membranes. Infected deep epidermal cells balloon up to form giant cells with oedema. This results in thin-walled vesicles on an inflammatory base. The vesicles ulcerate then crust and heal. Intranuclear inclusion bodies are also found.

There are two types of this virus: HSV-1 and HSV-2. Infection with HSV-1 peaks at 5–15 years and HSV-2 infection peaks at the onset puberty. The virus is spread directly by infected secretions. The rate of infection depends upon socioeconomic group, and is higher in lower socioeconomic groups.

Primary infection

Most initial infections with HSV are asymptomatic. Primary herpetic gingivostomatitis occurs in symptomatic cases. Gingivostomatitis usually occurs in children but is also sometimes seen in young adults.

Children with primary herpetic gingivostomatitis usually start with a temperature, are fractious, and may have a sore throat. They complain of a sore mouth, which is very painful. They often refuse to eat or drink. Classical signs are foetor oris (bad breath) as well as drooling of saliva. Examination also reveals cervical lymphadenopathy. Intraorally there are vesicles on all the mucosal surfaces including the hard and soft palate, the buccal mucosa, the tongue, the gingivae, the floor of the mouth, and the lips. The disease is self limiting, lasting 10–14 days.

Treatment is symptomatic, and antivirals should not be used unless the child is also immunocompromised.

Primary infection in adults has slightly different clinical features. The initial presentation is usually with pyrexia and malaise. This is followed by the appearance of vesicles. The distribution of the vesicles in the mouth shows a few odd lesions on any of the mucosal surfaces. There is more widespread lymphadenopathy than in children.

Herpetic whitlow

Herpetic whitlow is an intense painful infection of the hand involving one or more fingers that typically affects the terminal phalanx. HSV-1 is the cause in approximately 60% of cases and HSV-2 in the remaining 40%. Dental surgeons and other healthcare workers are particularly at risk of this infection which can be caused by a combination of direct infection from patients and the presence of microscopic holes in surgical gloves, which provide a warm, moist area for incubation of the virus.

Ocular infection

This is also very important and presents as an ulcerated follicular conjunctivitis and photophobia. There is oedema of the conjunctiva with excessive tear production. Patients may have a dendritic ulcer. They need to be referred to an ophthalmologist urgently.

Genital and anal infections

Genital and anal lesions similar to oral lesions may be caused by either HSV-2 or HSV-1.

Recurrent infection

- **Herpes labialis** (cold sores): there is a short prodrome of tingling and/or itching which occurs at the site where the lesion will later appear. This is precipitated by sunlight, menstruation, stress, local trauma, immune suppression, or fever. Lesions commonly recur at the same site.
- **Recurrent gingivostomatitis and genital herpes**: these infections frequently recur. The clinical features are the same as in the primary infection. Prophylactic acyclovir may need to be given for 4–6 months if recurrences are frequent. The lesions will appear within hours to 2 days. It is important to note that the virus is only present before the vesicles ulcerate (within the first 24 to 48 h). Healing then occurs within 7 to 10 days.

Varicella zoster virus

Humans are the only host for this virus. There is only one serotype of Varicella zoster virus (VZV). The primary infection is **chicken pox** which usually occurs in late winter and spring. The virus is spread by two routes: airborne droplets from the respiratory tract and vesicle fluid. The incubation period is 14 days. There is a prodrome of a few hours to 2 days. This is followed by the appearance of an itchy rash on the trunk, scalp, limbs, and face. The rash begins as macules and develops into discrete oval vesicles. The vesicles are surrounded by an erythematous halo. A characteristic of chicken pox is that the lesions crop. This means all the lesions appear to be at different stages of development.

Reactivation of VZV

Reactivation of VZV causes herpes zoster (shingles). The reason for reactivation is unknown but may be related to factors which are known to cause immunosuppression, such as underlying malignancy, stress (emotional or physical), or trauma (local or generalized).

BOX 6.2 Dental relevance of primary VZV infection

- Scratching may give rise to secondary bacterial infection with streptococci or staphylococci in the head and neck area.
- Oral lesions are under-diagnosed. They may occur on any mucosal surface on an erythematous base.
- In children the mouth can be uncomfortable and painful.
- Care should be taken because of cross-infection from vesicles. Viral particles tend to sick to gloves.
- Infection may be complicated by bacterial pneumonia, acute meningitis, and encephalitis.
- Thrombocytopenia may occur as the rash is healing. This is a relatively uncommon complication and may be responsible for post-extraction bleeding.
- In the immunocompromised child infection carries a high morbidity.

BOX 6.3 Dental relevance of shingles (VZV reactivation)

- Mandibular, maxillary, or ophthalmic divisions of the fifth cranial nerve may be affected. This results in severe pain in the face. Patients are very distressed and sometimes think that the pain is of dental origin.
- Careful intraoral examination is required to exclude associated oropharyngeal lesions.
- The presence of vesicles on the nose indicates that the ophthalmic division is involved (the nasocilliary branch of the ophthalmic division of the fifth cranial nerve). It is an urgent indication for referral to ophthalmologist.
- Care must be taken with immunocompromised patients, including patients taking systemic immunosuppressive drugs such as steroids, azathioprine, or ciclosporin because of the risk of dissemination.
- Ramsay Hunt syndrome (herpes zoster oticus): this is due to herpes zoster affecting the geniculate ganglion of the seventh cranial nerve. It usually starts with severe pain in the ear and/or throat. Pain is followed by a vesicular rash, best seen on the tragus of the ear, and a few unilateral vesicles on the posterior aspect of the palate. The clinical signs are of a lower motor neuron seventh cranial nerve lesion and occur on the ipsilateral side of the face. The prognosis is good. Post-herpetic neuralgia is very difficult to treat and may be severe and confused with pain of dental origin.

The clinical features of shingles include:

- Malaise, anorexia, and low-grade pyrexia—these are the initial features.
- This is followed by severe radicular pain and hyperaesthesia over skin.
- The rash is always confined to a dermatome and is unilateral.
- The erythematous rash is followed by large vesicles which increase in size and number.
- The vesicles ulcerate and become crusted over the next 8 to 12 days.

Mononucleoses

This is a group of infections with similar clinical features caused by three different organisms. The resulting infections are infectious mononucleosis, cytomegalovirus infection, and toxoplasmosis (this latter is not a viral but a protozoan infection).

Infectious mononucleosis (glandular fever)

The Epstein–Barr virus (EBV) is responsible for infection. The incidence in the United Kingdom is 4 per 10 000 population. The primary infection occurs between the ages of 5 to 15 years in underdeveloped countries and 14 to 24 years in developed countries. In the professional socioeconomic classes (1 and 2) primary infection may occur as late as 30 years of age.

The virus is excreted into the oropharynx during infection and for 3 to 4 months afterwards, resulting in the occurrence of case-to-case spread. The virus may also be spread directly by sputum (glandular fever is commonly known as 'the kissing disease'). After infection the B lymphocytes remain chronically infected. The Epstein–Barr DNA is incorporated into that of the host cells. In a few cases infected cells are not eliminated and chronic latent infection or progressive disease becomes established: this occurs more commonly in adults over 30 years of age.

Clinical features

There are a number of symptoms of infection with EBV, although subclinical infection is common in younger children:

- Malaise and low-grade fever are common.
- Sore throat.
- Anorexia, nausea, and vomiting.
- Jaundice.
- About 90–100% of patients develop a pruritic maculopapular rash with ampicillin, either during its use or after the drug has been stopped.

Signs of EBV infection include:

- Lymphadenopathy, especially the cervical nodes.
- Pyrexia, which may be intermittent.
- Oropharyngeal inflammation, which may be severe.
- Palatal petechiae may occur at the junction of the hard and soft palate; less commonly palatal petechiae may be more widespread.
- There is usually periorbital oedema.
- Splenomegaly.
- Skin rash—a maculopapular rash which becomes confluent.

Investigations and treatment

There is a raised white blood cell count, with atypical peripheral lymphocytes in more than 20% of cases. The Paul Bunnell test shows the presence of heterophil antibodies (this may be initially negative, and should be repeated). The Monospot test for heterophil antibodies is also positive. Liver function tests and antibody titre virus detection are also done.

Treatment is symptomatic and complications should be treated as required.

Cytomegalovirus infection

Cytomegalovirus (CMV) is a DNA herpes virus. It is found in 6% of pre-school children and 50% of children have antibodies to CMV by the age of 5 years. Peak incidence is between 25 and 35 years. The incubation period is between 4 and 6 weeks. Virus transmission is by direct contact, e.g. by kissing; this is an important mode of transmission. In the dental context aerosol spray is a potential cross-infection risk.

Virus is secreted in the saliva, vaginal and cervical secretions, seminal fluid, and urine. Virus is secreted for prolonged periods in congenitally acquired

> **BOX 6.4 Dental relevance of EBV infection**
> - The dental surgeon must be wary of oropharyngeal involvement.
> - The oropharynx may have widespread erythema, occasionally severe, oropharyngeal oedema may threaten the airway. This is usually treated with prednisolone 10–20 mg per day for 5 days.
> - Ampicillin given for dental treatment may induce a skin rash.
> - Patients frequently become depressed during convalescence and may develop facial pain.
> - Cranial nerve palsies may occur and infectious mononucleosis should be kept in mind (as well as multiple sclerosis) in any young patient presenting with cranial nerve palsy.
> - Headaches and facial pain may be secondary to meningoencephalitis.
> - Post-extraction bleeding may result from thrombocytopenia.
> - Drug metabolism may be affected by renal involvement.
> - Almost 100% of patients have subclinical or frank hepatitis. Rarely patients may have an initial presentation with jaundice. This will affect drug metabolism, postoperative bleeding (vitamin K-dependent factors not metabolized), and potentiation of drugs, especially P-450 dependent metabolism.
> - Patients may be short of breath and unable to lie flat in the dental chair because of myocarditis or pericarditis.

infection and immunosuppressed patients. The virus can also be transmitted by blood products or transplantated organs.

Clinical features
Symptoms of CMV infection are like those of glandular fever: malaise, anorexia, and pyrexia. Most primary infections are subclinical.

Signs of infection are varied:

- Palpable liver with jaundice is more common than in infectious mononucleosis but lymphadenopathy is less common.
- Mononucleosis.
- Tonsillitis is unusual.
- Palpable spleen is uncommon.
- Complications include ampicillin-induced rash, encephalitis, pericarditis, arteritis, and rarely pneumonitis and haemolytic anaemia.

Investigations and treatment
Investigations show a rise in the CMV IgM titre. Peak titres occur 4–6 weeks after primary infection. The virus can be isolated by direct culture. Treatment is symptomatic.

Human immunodeficiency virus (HIV) infection

HIV is a member of the lentivirus group of retroviruses. The virus is lymphotropic and neurotropic. It binds to CD4 receptors on lymphocytes, macrophages, and monocytes. These secrete an enzyme which is a reverse transcriptase allowing viral RNA to be transcribed to mimic the host DNA and become incorporated into the host genome. One incorporated into the host genome the host seroconverts.

Acute infection may be asymptomatic or with an illness resembling glandular fever, which occurs 4–6 weeks after the initial infection. The symptoms include sore throat, fever, myalgia, lymphadenopathy, and headache. The course thereafter is variable. The patient remains asymptomatic from 1–10 years after the initial infection.

Acute infection progresses to chronic infection and symptoms of immune deficiency appear. The first of these may be oral candida. The final stage is characterized by opportunistic infections, classically *Pneumocystis carinii* pneumonia and later tumours.

HIV can be transmitted between humans by a number of routes:

- By unprotected sexual intercourse with an infected partner.
- By vertical transmission from an infected mother to her fetus or neonate.
- By transplantation of organs from an infected individual.
- In blood or blood products.
- By needle sharing between intravenous drug abusers.
- By needlestick injury in healthcare personnel (a low risk but transmission has occurred in this way).
- By infected saliva when there are breaks in the mucosa such as oral ulceration and tonsillitis.

Clinical features of HIV/AIDS

The clinical features of HIV infection are dependent on the disease stage/Centers for Disease Control (CDC) group:

- Stage 1/CDC group I: Acute infection (transient lymphadenopathy). CD4 count low normal.
- Stage 2/CDC group II: Asymptomatic. CD4 count (350–8000) $\times$ 10^9/l.
- Stage 3/CDC group III: Persistent generalized lymphadenopathy/recurrent bacterial infections. CD4 count (200–350) $\times$ 10^9/l.
- Stage 4/CDC group IV: AIDS, with opportunistic infection. Mucocutaneous disease, respiratory, gastrointestinal, and neurological disease. Malignancy. CD4 count <200 $\times$ 10^9/l.

Symptoms, problems and complications are listed below according to the body system affected:

- Generalized symptoms: weight loss (more than 10% of normal body weight); malaise, night sweats; fever which lasts longer than 1 month; diarrhoea.
- Respiratory problems: pneumonia caused by bacteria, e.g. tuberculosis, *Pneumocystis carinii*, or viruses, e.g. cytomegalovirus.
- Neurological problems: depression, dementia, psychosis, encephalitis, progressive multifocal leucoencephalopathy, motor, sensory, or autonomic neuropathy.

- Haematological complications: lymphopenia, anaemia, neutropenia, thrombocytopenia.
- Tumours: non-Hodgkin's lymphoma, Hodgkin's lymphoma, Kaposi's sarcoma, anorectal carcinoma.
- Gastrointestinal problems: any part of the bowel may be affected from the mouth to anus; diarrhoea is common; abdominal pain; malabsorption; candidosis.
- Common oral problems: candidosis (erythematous or pseudomembranous); hairy leucoplakia caused by EBV; periodontal conditions include necrotizing ulcerative gingivitis and/or rapidly progressive periodontitis; severe aphthous-like ulceration or change in frequency and/or change in the morphology of aphthous ulcers.
- Less common oral problems: necrotizing ulcerative gingivostomatitis; human papilloma virus (HPV) warts; Herpes zoster; Herpes simplex; Kaposi's sarcoma; non-Hodgkin's lymphoma; salivary gland disease, primary or secondary to other viral infections.

Investigations and treatment

Polymerase chain reaction (PCR) and Western blotting techniques are definitive. Confidentiality at all stages of investigation is important.

The main aim of treatment is to help the patient maintain good physical and psychological health. The patient should be educated to decrease risk of cross-infection. In women of childbearing age risks of vertical transmission and choices for feeding their baby should be discussed. Specific medication includes:

- Nucleoside analogue reverse transcriptase inhibitors: zidovudine (AZT), didanosine (DDI), zalcitabine (DDC).

BOX 6.5 Dental relevance of HIV/AIDS

Oral problems are common in patients with HIV and cause considerable morbidity. 40% of those with HIV and 80% of those with AIDS have one or more problems in the mouth.

Post-exposure prophylaxis

There is a reduction in the rate of infection by more than 80% if prophylaxis is given after exposure. Protocols can be obtained from local virology or health and safety departments.

Point to note

Although generalized lymphadenopathy is found in AIDS other causes should be considered. Treatable causes of persistent generalized lymphadenopathy include: sarcoidosis, infectious mononucleosis, cytomegalovirus infection, Epstein–Barr virus infection, toxoplasmosis, tuberculosis, secondary syphilis, lymphoma, auto-immune disease, drugs effects.

- Non-nucleoside reverse transcriptase inhibitors: nevirapine, delavirdine, loviride.
- Protease inhibitors: saquinavir, ritonavir, indinavir, nelfinavir.

Measles

Measles is caused by an RNA paramyxovirus. The virus is transmitted through nasopharyngeal and oropharyngeal droplets, with transmission increased in winter (or the dry season). In the developing world it most commonly occurs between the ages of 4 months and 2 years. In the developed world peak incidence is around pre-school and school entry, age 3–6 years; there is a decreased incidence due to the use of vaccination with live attenuated virus. WHO figures show that in Africa, South America, and Asia there are around 800–1000 reported cases per year of which 10 to 20 are fatal. Infectivity or communicability lasts 7 days from the onset of the prodrome to just before the rash occurs.

Clinical features

The **prodromal stage** begins 10 days after infection and can last for another 4–5 days. It is characterized by cough, nasal stuffiness, and conjunctivitis. Koplik's spots appear during last 48 h. These are pathognomic for measles and last a few days. They are pinhead-sized red spots with white centres found on the buccal and labial mucosa. The overall appearance resembles grains of salt on an erythematous background.

In the **exanthematous stage** a maculopapular rash begins behind the ears and spreads to the face and trunk. It disappears after 72 h leaving a brown stain on the skin which may last for 6–8 weeks. Fever decreases after 3 days.

Complications

There are a number of complications which can arise after infection with the measles virus:

- croup (laryngotracheobronchitis)
- pneumonia—secondary bacterial

BOX 6.6 Dental relevance of measles

- Careful examination of the mouth in the prodromal phase may reveal Koplik's spots.
- Rash occurs first in head and neck area.
- Take care to avoid cross-infection, especially to children on steroids or who are immunocompromised.
- Immunosuppressed children may develop gingivostomatitis in the post-measles state. Always check in children that they have followed the recommended immunization schedule. If the live attenuated vaccine was contraindicated there must be a careful regime to prevent putting the child at risk through cross infection.
- In under-developed countries, especially if children are malnourished, cancrum iris may occur in the post-measles state, resulting in massive destruction and gangrene of the perioral tissues.

- encephalitis
- late complications: encephalopathy (has a high mortality), subacute sclerosing panencephalitis (SSPE) (occurs up to 7 years later and is always fatal).

Failure to recover occurs in a small group of patients (known as 'post-measles state'):

- Patients stay immunosuppressed.
- There is recurrent diarrhoea.
- Gingivostomatitis.
- Measles predisposes to Herpes simplex encephalitis.
- Corneal ulcers.
- There may also be reactivation of tuberculosis, candidosis, cancrum oris, and gangrene of the digits.

Rubella (German measles)

Rubella is caused by an RNA virus of the togavirus family. Virus is excreted from the nasopharynx, blood, urine, and stool. Epidemics can occur every 6–8 years. Spread is usually via respiratory droplets during acute systemic infection.

Clinical features

The majority of people infected (60%) are asymptomatic. Symptomatic cases show:

- Mild systemic symptoms, with low-grade fever.
- Nasal stuffiness and mild conjunctivitis.
- Lymphadenopathy—postauricular, cervical, and suboccipital.
- A rash which begins on the face and spreads to the trunk and extremities. It is a maculopapular rash with discrete lesions. The lesions remain discrete and do not become confluent.
- Arthralgia in several joints.

BOX 6.7 Dental relevance of rubella

- Congenital rubella may result from maternal infection in the first trimester.
- If a pregnant woman is exposed to rubella establish her immune status immediately. If she has a positive antibody status there is no risk. If she has negative antibody status a three- to four-fold increase in the IgM antibody titre indicates infection.
- Morbidity due to congenital rubella is high, with problems that may impact on dental care: congenital heart disease, mental retardation, cataracts, deafness.
- Patients with young children should be advised to inform dental staff of childhood infections and not be given appointments with pregnant patients.
- Do not confuse primary infection with a booster response. Most young women are now immunized at school or on entry into employment.

Mumps

Mumps is caused by a paramyxovirus. It is spread by droplets from the oro- and nasopharynx. The incubation period is 2–3 weeks. The infectious period lasts for a few days before the start of clinical symptoms and signs until parotid swelling subsides. Epidemics occur every 7 years or so. Lifelong immunity occurs after primary infection.

Clinical features

Forty to fifty per cent of cases are asymptomatic. Two to three weeks after infection the child develops fever, malaise, and discomfort over the angle of one or both jaws.

Signs:

- The parotid swells and becomes very painful as the capsule stretches, with oedema in the cervical area of neck below the gland.
- The ear is pushed forward because of swelling of the tail of the parotid. The swelling may be bilateral or unilateral.
- Both the parotid and the submandibular glands may be swollen.

Complications

A number of complications can arise:

- Aseptic meningitis, with 50% of patients having a cerebrospinal fluid (CSF) lymphocytosis. The prognosis is good.
- Orchitis occurs in 25% of post-pubertal males; infertility is very rare.
- Breast and pancreatic complications (serum amylase is raised—this is both pancreatic and salivary gland derived).
- Arthritis in adults.

Investigations and treatment

The virus can be isolated from saliva or CSF. There is a four-fold rise in antibody titre.

Treatment is symptomatic. Antipyretics may be used. Emphasize good oral hygiene and oral toiletting.

BOX 6.8 Dental relevance of mumps

- Recognize other causes of parotid swelling. These are: Meal time syndrome associated with parotid calculi, sarcoidosis, toxoplasmosis, autoimmune disease, salivary gland tumours, bulimia, hypersensitivity reaction to iodides, mercury, lead, hypersensitivity to drugs, thiouracil, phenothiazines, hypersensitivity to toothpaste, food additives.
- Remember almost all patients with mumps have asymptomatic meningitis.
- The pain associated with mumps is due to stretching of the parotid capsule.
- Instruct patients on careful oral toileting to prevent secondary bacterial infection (ascending sialoadenitis).

Hand, foot, and mouth disease

Hand, foot, and mouth disease is caused by infection with the coxsackie A16 virus. It is spread by droplets from coughing and sneezing. It is common and occurs mainly in schoolchildren in small epidemics. The incubation period is between 3 and 7 days.

Clinical features

Children are more frequently affected than teenagers or adults, and infected children should be kept from school. Clinical features last for 10–14 days. There is a short prodrome followed by systemic infection with fever, malaise, and anorexia and associated sore throat. Vesicular lesions appear in the anterior oral cavity.

Treatment is supportive with antipyretics and analgesics such as paracetamol.

BACTERIAL INFECTIONS

Escherichia coli O157:H7

Escherichia coli O157 is a bacterium that lives in the gut of animals, including cattle, sheep, deer, and goats. *E. coli* serotype O157:H7 is an emerging cause of disease. *E. coli* O157 is unusual in that very few individual organisms are needed to cause infection in humans.

The main source of infection has been contaminated food, particularly meat. Infection can also be acquired by direct contact with animals or contact with animal dung, e.g. on a farm visit, when camping on a farming, and by person-to-person spread.

In the UK 18 general outbreaks of *E. coli* O157 infection occurred between 1992 and 1994 and 106 outbreaks between 1995 and 2000. The clinical effects are caused by a cytotoxin produced by the bacterium. The toxin responsible is a verotoxin (O157 VTEC).

Clinical features

O157 VTEC can cause a range of symptoms from a mild diarrhoea to severe bloody diarrhoea (haemorrhagic colitis) and haemolytic uraemic syndrome

---

BOX 6.9 Oral lesions in hand, foot, and mouth disease

- Lesions are more frequent on the labial mucosa and heal with crusting.
- Occasionally discrete lesions appear on the palate, gingivae, and tongue.
- These lesions can be distinguished from herpetic gingivostomatitis as they are fewer in number and usually appear on a less erythematous base.
- The discrete lesions are surrounded by an erythematous halo with a central white ulcer.
- Careful examination of the hands and feet will reveal similar vesicular exanthema.

(HUS). There may also be thrombocytopenic purpura. The incubation period is 1–4 days and patients can become acutely unwell. Mortality can be very high in the elderly. The clinical features are identical to those of ischaemic colitis.

Treatment

There is no specific treatment for *E. coli* O157:H2 infection. All clinical problems are treated symptomatically. Antimicrobial treatment may not be beneficial. Haemolytic ureamic syndrome and thrombocytopenic purpura require specialized care. An antitoxin to absorb free verotoxin is been appraised.

Borrelia burgdorferi (Lyme disease)

Burgdorfer described an organism responsible for an outbreak of disease in Lyme, Connecticut, USA. The organism is a spirochaete bacterium *Borrelia burgdorferi*. The bacterium is transmitted by the bite of an infected *Ixodes* tick. Deer are the main source of infection.

Ticks transfer the spirochaetes to other deer, humans, and dogs after a blood meal on an infected animal. In humans and other animals, including dogs, infection with *Borrelia burgdorferi* results in the pathology of Lyme disease.

Clinical features

Clinical features appear a few days to weeks after the bite:

- Stage 1: rash—erythema chronicum migrans. The rash appears around the area of the bite. Develop fever and ache.
- Stage 2: headache, malaise, chills and fever, arthropathy and muscle pain, lymphadenopathy, secondary annular skin lesions.
- Stage 3: persistent infection. Arthritis occurs in 60% of patients months to years after the bite. Neurological involvement occurs in 15% of patients, including meningitis/encephalitis and facial palsy. Cardiac disorders, including pericarditis and arrhythmias, occur in 5% of patients.

Investigations and treatment

Lyme disease is difficult to diagnose. The Gundersen Lyme test (GLT) uses flow cytometry to detect borreliacidal antibodies in the sera of infected individuals. The drug of choice for treatment is doxycycline. Penicillin and erythromycin may also be used. A vaccine, LYMErix®, is now available.

Anthrax

Anthrax occurs in the animal population of Africa, South America, and the Middle and Far East. In these regions there are 10 000–20 000 cases in humans per year. In the UK there have only been four reports since 1990.

The causative organism is *Bacillus anthracis*, a large, Gram-positive spore-forming bacillus. Anthrax is usually a disease of herbivorous animals, but humans may become infected if bacterial spores are acquired via skin lesions while handling dead animals or hides (cutaneous anthrax; this is the most common route of infection), are eaten in contaminated meat (gastrointestinal anthrax, less common) or breathed in (pulmonary anthrax, uncommon). In the UK those at risk are handlers of dead animals, such as abattoir workers and tanners.

Clinical features

Cutaneous anthrax

The incubation period is 1–5 days. Symptoms of cutaneous anthrax infection include:

- Small itchy papules on the face, neck, arms, or hand. Non-painful papules form larger blisters without pus. These are surrounded by erythema and oedema.
- The area ulcerates followed by a black scar called an eschar.
- The lesion reaches diameter of 2–6 cm in 6 days.
- Systemic symptoms include fever, rigors, and malaise.

The following signs are observed:

- The temperature may become increasingly raised, up to 40 °C in some patients.
- In a few cases the organism spreads to regional lymph nodes.
- If there is lymphadenopathy blood-borne dissemination may occur to give a severe illness.
- If patients develop septicaemia the morbidity is high. Mortality is 20% in untreated cases.
- Cutaneous lesions usually heal within 10–30 days.

Intestinal anthrax

Intestinal anthrax is caused by the consumption of contaminated meat. Symptoms are those of a severe food-poisoning, with fever and septicaemia. Intestinal anthrax is frequently fatal.

Respiratory anthrax

Respiratory anthrax is caused by aspiration of spores. It starts with flu-like symptoms which worsen rapidly. Respiratory and cardiovascular collapse occur within 2–6 days of the initial symptoms. It is frequently fatal.

Investigations and treatment

Gram staining of the vesicle fluid, culture swabs, blood culture, and toxin-neutralizing antibodies can all be used to identify the infection.

Treatment is by 2.5–3.5 g of benzyl penicillin IV for 10–12 days with or without streptomycin or tetracycline or chloramphenicol. Untreated cutaneous anthrax is fatal in 20% of patients. With treatment the mortality falls to less than 1%.

> **BOX 6.10** Dental relevance of anthrax infection
> - Take care with the differential diagnosis of cutaneous anthrax.
> - The lesions are typical but may be confused with: erysipelas if the eschar is small or absent; furuncle, but anthrax has no pus; primary syphilis.
> - Care with cross-infection as the bacterium is spread by direct contact with vesicular fluid.

Whooping cough (pertussis)

Whooping cough is caused by the organism *Bordetella pertussis* which is a Gram-negative coccobacillus. It is highly infectious and is spread by airborne droplets from the respiratory tract; rarely it may also spread on clothes, instruments, and toys. The disease is most contagious during the cold-like initial phase (catarrhal phase). It affects children and occasionally young adults. All children should be immunized. Children below the age of 3 months are at risk before immunization.

Clinical features
The incubation period is 7–14 days. There are three stages of the disease:

- Catarrhal stage: slight pyrexia, cough and rhinorrhoea, symptoms and signs are non-specific.
- Paroxysmal cough stage: cough slowly becomes more persistent severe and paroxysmal. The child may become cyanotic during paroxysms followed by a typical 'whoop'. This may be followed by vomiting. Up to 50 episodes may occur daily. This stage may last from 2–4 weeks and the child becomes increasingly debilitated. There will be feeding problems.
- Convalescent stage: lasts 2–4 weeks; the paroxysms gradually decrease.

Note that the cough may be associated with prolonged apnoea and cerebral anoxia. Conjunctival or cerebral haemorrhage may occur. Secondary bacterial infections include sinusitis, otitis media, and bronchopneumonia.

There may be complications including bronchopneumonia, acute encephalopathy or long-term brain damage as a result of cerebral hypoxia. There is increased morbidity in infants under the age of 1 year.

Investigations and treatment
Culture of nasal pharyngeal swabs can identify the infective organism. Full blood count may show lymphocytosis. Treatment is with erythromycin, 50 mg/kg/24 h.

Vaccination against whooping cough is offered to all children in the UK in the early months of life. Whooping cough in the community occurs in 85% of all unimmunized children.

> **BOX 6.11** Dental relevance of whooping cough
>
> - Children may be brought to the surgery with frenal ulcer: this is usually traumatic.
> - Remember: whooping cough is highly infectious, so protect other patients.
> - Prophylactic erythromycin may be beneficial when in contact with a child with whooping cough.

> **BOX 6.12** Dental relevance of legionnaires' disease
>
> - *Legionella* can survive and increase in dental units. Good cross-infection control and sterilization of equipment is needed.
> - *Legionella* can be spread by aerosol from handpieces.

Legionnaires' disease

Legionnaires' disease is caused by *Legionella pneumophila* which is a Gram-negative bacterium. In their normal environment *Legionella* bacteria do not cause infections but man-made water systems (e.g. air conditioning and industrial cooling systems) sometimes provide environments that let *Legionella* bacteria increase to large numbers. The number of confirmed cases in England and Wales per year is between 129 and 211, but the real incidence is almost certainly higher than this. Two per cent of cases of pneumonia requiring hospital admission are due to legionnaires' disease.

Although *Legionella pneumophila* is water borne no infection occurs from drinking infected water, but only if *Legionella* is inhaled in aerosol form. The most susceptible to infection are those of middle-age and older, especially smokers, the immunosuppressed, or those with chronic disease. A number of outbreaks have been associated with hospitals although 80% of cases are sporadic.

Clinical features

The incubation period is 2–10 days, followed by fever and rigors, muscle aches and pains, vomiting and diarrhoea, headache, and sometimes confusion. Patients become short of breath and coughing occurs. Haemoptysis may occur in 25% of patients. A non-pneumonia form of infection called Pontiac fever may occur instead of legionnaires' disease. This presents as a flu-like illness.

Investigations and treatment

The *Legionella* organism can be cultured from secretions. Serum antibodies show a four-fold increase in titre. *Legionella* antigen is present in the urine.

Treatment is with antibiotics such as erythromycin, clarithromycin, or ciprofloxacin. The earlier that treatment is begun, the better the outcome.

Tuberculosis

Tuberculosis (TB) is an infection which is increasing in incidence (see Chapter 10).

Syphilis

Syphilis is caused by infection with *Treponema pallidum*. It is spread by direct contact or by vertical transmission to the fetus. In the UK the incidence in 1996 was 0.82 per 100 000 in males and 0.35 per 100 000 in females. In Germany the incidence is 3.7 cases per 100 000.

Acquired disease

In acquired disease the primary lesion is the chancre. This appears 14–90 days after infection and develops at the site of infection (usually on the genitals, but may occur on the lips, in the throat, or in any part of the oral cavity). The appearance is a red or pink macule which becomes papular and then ulcerates. The ulcer is painless, but the base of the ulcer is teeming with spirochaetes and is highly infectious. The ulcer is accompanied by regional lymphadenopathy with discrete, mobile, rubbery and non-tender nodes. Ulcers usually heal in 7–10 days.

Secondary syphilis

Secondary syphilis begins 6–8 weeks after the appearance of the chancre. The patient systemically unwell with fever and malaise.

- A characteristic rash appears on the trunks, with papullar, discrete, non-itchy lesions which become scaly. The rash may also be seen on the plantar-palmar surfaces, which should be examined.
- There is generalized lymphadenopathy.
- Condylomata lata (flat flower-like papules) may appear around the genitals, perineum, and anus.
- Intra-oral lesions occur in approximately 30–40% of cases: snail track ulcers appear most commonly on the buccal mucosa and palate; the lesions are usually discrete and 1–2 mm across, forming a line before coalescing to form a snail track. The bases of the ulcers are infective.

Latent syphilis

If no treatment is given in the secondary stage there is resolution and the disease enters a latent stage. Cases may be identified by routine serological testing and can be successfully treated.

Tertiary syphilis

Tertiary syphilis develops after 2–15 years. Patients may present with oral lesions. The characteristic gumma is caused by granuloma which affects the hard and soft tissue and may cause a cavity to appear between the oral and sinus cavities or the oral cavity and nares. Syphilitic leucoplakia may be seen on the tongue, which may also be small and atrophic.

Quaternary syphilis

Neurosyphilis may affect the patient's ability to accept or present themselves for dental treatment. Care should be taken as cardiovascular syphilis may necessitate changes in the dental treatment plan.

> **BOX 6.13** Dental relevance of syphilis
> - Congenital syphilis gives rise to characteristic facies and tooth malformation.
> - Syphilitic ulceration is highly infectious: the base of the chancre is teaming with spirochaetes.
> - Gumma frequently produces palatal erosion with consequent nasal collapse. 'Donald Duck' speech results from the resultant oronasal fistula.
> - There may be peripheral sensory neuropathy.
> - Confabulation in Wernicke's encephalopathy may resemble that due to tertiary syphilis.

Congenital syphilis

Congenital syphilis is caused by vertical spread from an infective mother to her fetus. The severity of infection varies from still birth to latent disease. At birth the baby may have mucosal ulcers and later develops Hutchinson's incisors and moon-shaped molars. The children have a characteristic facies with small head, ragades (creases) around mouth, and a flat bridge to the nose giving the appearance of increased spacing between the eyes. Other organ systems, e.g. the liver and kidney, may also be involved.

Investigations and treatment

There are a number of specific serological tests for syphilis:

- TPHA: *Treponema pallidum* haemagglutination assay.
- FTA-ABS: fluorescent treponemal antibody absorption test.
- ELISA: treponemal linked immunosorbent assay.

Swabs from lesion demonstrate the presence of *Treponema pallidum*.

Treatment is with penicillin. Patients who are penicillin hypersensitive patients may receive tetracycline. Penicillin-resistant cases are treated with ciprofloxacin or cefotaxime.

FUNGAL INFECTION

Candidosis

Candida albicans is the most common organism in the oral cavity causing infection. It is a saprophytic yeast and usually exists as a commensal in the mouth, gastrointestinal tract, and vagina. When infection occurs it is usually superficial but may be systemic.

Factors influencing the conversion from commensalism to infection include reduced immunocompetence, prolonged use of immunosuppressive drugs, AIDs, diabetes mellitus, and damaged mucosa, especially due to the use of dentures.

Superficial oral candidosis is common. However, candidosis can occur in the genital area, eyes, and ears as well as the skin. Oral candidosis is pseudomembranous, erythematous, hyperplastic, and mucocutaneous. Chronic superficial oral candida is usually associated with oral leucoplakia and chronic mucocutaneous candida is associated with endocrinopathies. In the mouth candida may also be associated with mucosal barrier breaches in conditions such as median rhomboid glossitis, angular cheilitis, and denture stomatitis.

Systemic candidosis is seen in immunocompromised patients—those on immunosuppressive drugs, patients with either primary or secondary immuno-deficiency (frequently in patients with AIDS), and in transplant patients. It can also occur after surgery or antibiotic therapy, in the presence of underlying sys-temic disease (e.g. diabetes, hypothyroidism), and with the use of intravenous catheters or lines. Disseminated invasive candida may develop in severely immunosuppressed patients. **In rare cases** candida can cause an endocardi-tis. In these cases the vegetations on the heart valves are very large.

Investigations and treatment

Candida is simple to culture. Any body fluid, including saliva, tears, blood, or urine can be cultured. Serological testing and typing may also be helpful in patients with systemic disease.

Superficial candidosis may be treated with topical nystatin, amphotericin B, or miconazole (especially for angular cheilitis as it has an antistaphylococcal effect). Systemic disease should be treated vigorously using fluconazole, itra-conazole, or in severe cases intravenous amphotericin B.

Histoplasmosis

Histoplasmosis is caused by the fungus *Histoplasma capsulatum*. It is found in soil, bird, or bat droppings and can also be isolated from lesions in an affected individual. *H. capsulatum* is endemic in Canada, the east coast of the USA, South America, India, the Far East, Australia, and parts of Africa. In endemic areas up to 95% of the population may have a positive skin test.

Clinical features

If symptoms occur, they will start within 3 to 17 days after exposure; the aver-age is 10 days (many infected people show no apparent ill-effects). The patient is systemically unwell with severe malaise, pyrexia, breathlessness, and cough, with or without erythema nodosum- or erythema multiforme-like lesions. Patients usually recover spontaneously. Chronic infection is associated with pulmonary emphysema, weight loss, malaise, chest pain, cough and fever.

Disseminated histoplasmosis is a chronic form of infection which may develop in previously healthy individuals years after leaving endemic areas. The patient may present to the dentist with oral ulceration with associated cer-vical lymphadenopathy. The ulcer is indolent and not usually painful, but the cervical swelling slowly enlarges and may eventually ulcerate. Other foci of dis-semination should be excluded by bone marrow, blood cultures, and chest X-ray (one must be careful to exclude AIDS).

African histoplasmosis: patients from Central and West Africa may present with painless oral ulcers, cervical nodules, or nodules or ulcers on any area of the skin. X-rays of the jaw must be taken as lytic bone lesions may be present.

Treatment of histoplasmosis is with oral itraconazole or intravenous amphotericin B followed by oral itraconazole.

Antifungal therapy

The main antifungal agents are: polyenes, imidazoles, triazoles, and flucytosine.

Polyenes

The polyenes nystatin and amphotericin are commonly used by dental surgeons. Nystatin is frequently used topically as a gel or suspension in the mouth, 100 000 units/ml, or as lozenges. Amphotericin B is used topically as a 10 mg lozenge sucked four times a day. Amphotericin B is also used systemically for serious life threatening infection: it can be administered intravenously with a dose of 0.3–1.0 mg/kg/day in 5% dextrose over 2–4 h. There are no circumstances in which a general dental practitioner would be required to administer intravenous amphotericin B.

The advantages of amphotericin B is that it penetrates the CSF, urine, and peritoneal fluid. It is excreted by the liver. Amphotericin has numerous side effects including:

- Rigors, nausea and vomiting.
- Hypochromic anaemia.
- Hypokalaemia.
- Renal impairment. This is the most serious side effect. It is dose dependent. The clinical involvement is reversible but damage may be permanent.
- Thrombophlebitis may occur at the site of the lesion.

Toxoplasmosis

Toxoplasmosis is a common infection found worldwide. It is caused by a protozoan parasite *Toxoplasma gondii*. In the UK 20% of the population are seropositive for *Toxoplasma* whereas in France or Greece 60–70% of the population are seropositive. The sexual phase of the life cycle of *Toxoplasma gondii* occurs in cats, and infection is often from accidental ingestion of *Toxoplasma* sporozoites developed from the oocytes passed in cat faeces. Infection can also occur by drinking unpasturized milk, eating undercooked meat, and, rarely, from a blood transfusion.

Clinical features

Clinical features depend on whether the infection is recently acquired or a recurrence of previous infection.

The incubation period of **acquired disease** varies between 3 days and 3 weeks. Patients present with flu-like symptoms of malaise, headache, fever, and myalgia. The infection may also be subclinical, with 25% of patients being

> **BOX 6.14** Dental implications of toxoplasmosis
> - Severe malaise prevents patients seeking treatment.
> - Persistent cervical lymph node hypertrophy should alert one to the diagnosis (the differential diagnosis is HIV and lymphoma).
> - Parotid hypertrophy may occur: these patients have tender bilaterally enlarged glands. Ultrasound or MRI may show cystic spaces within parotid tissue. PCR of saliva enables one to identify infection within the glands.

asymptomatic. Signs are:

- Lymphadenopathy of the cervical lymph nodes, which may be tender and firm for 3–6 months.
- Ocular involvement of the retina to give retinochoroiditis.
- The salivary glands may be affected, giving enlarged parotids.
- The heart and central nervous system may rarely be affected.
- If disease occurs in pregnancy congenital toxoplasmosis is associated with retinochoroiditis and CNS involvement.

Reactivation and recurrence of disease may occur because cysts remain dormant in the body after resolution of active disease. If reactivated, acute symptoms recur and resemble chronic fatigue syndrome. In patients who are immunocompromised reactivation may cause serious disease including encephalitis.

Investigations and treatment

The *Toxoplasma* dye test uses methylene blue to stain live organisms. There will be antibodies present, both IgG and IgM in adults and IgA in neonates. MRI scan is necessary in patients with suspected cerebral disease and ultrasound examination in suspected parotid disease (PCR of saliva can identify infection). Current infection is indicated by a four-fold increase in titre compared to control in the dye test, raised IgG and raised IgM.

No treatment is needed in asymptomatic patients. Those who are pregnant, who have chronic active infection, or who are immunocompromised should be treated. Drugs used for treatment are pyrimethamine 200 mg followed by 50–75 mg/day. Add sulfadiazine 1–2 g four times a day and folic acid 15 mg/day. Treatment lasts for 6 weeks. In neonates spiramycin should be used. Corticosteroids are kept for ocular disease.

MENINGITIS

Meningitis is an infection of the meninges, which are the covering layers of the brain and spinal cord. Infective meningitis can be caused by viruses, bacteria, or fungi.

- **Viral meningitis** is a common complication of viral infections and is usually not a serious clinical problem.
- **Bacterial meningitis** includes:
  - Streptococcus pneumoniae
  - Haemophilus Influenzae type b (Hib)
  - Neisseria meningitidis

Most cases of meningitis in the UK are B and C serotypes. Group B accounts for 60% of cases and Group C 40%. However, with increasing travel type A serotype should be looked for in patients from sub-Saharan Africa and Southeast Asia.

Clinical features

Symptoms include:

- fever
- photophobia
- neck stiffness
- rash (petechial)
- change in the level of consciousness.

Viral meningitis is usually less aggressive than bacterial meningitis.

Complications can include fits, especially in children, multi-organ failure (which may result in death), intra-cranial abscesses, and hydrocephalus in the long term.

Investigations and treatment

General investigations show a raised white cell count, C-reactive protein, and erythrocyte sedimentation rate. Specific investigations include blood culture. Examination of cerebrospinal fluid shows positive Gram stain or Zhiel–Nielson stain, a high neutrophil count in bacterial infection, and a high lymphocyte count in viral infection.

Treatment should be undertaken in close consultation with microbiologists or virologists. Drugs that may be used include the antibacterials benzylpenicillin, chloramphenicol, and cefotaxime and the antiviral acyclovir. Supportive management of cases is important.

When there have been two or more cases in a specific group (e.g. nursery, school, dormitory) prophylactic antibiotic treatment (rifampicin or ciprofloxacin or ceftriaxone) should be given to the wider target group as well as 'kissing' or household contacts within 7 days of diagnosis of the index case.

Meningitis vaccination policy

Childhood immunization against meningitis C and *Haemophilus influenzae* (Hib meningitis) is recommended. There is no vaccine available against Group B meningococcus. For travellers to sub-Saharan Africa or Southeast Asia the old vaccine covering both meningitis A and C is recommended. Travellers to

Mecca or other areas where these groups are common should receive cover against serotypes A,C, Y, and W135 (the quadrivalent vaccine). Pneumococcal vaccine is available for those susceptible to pneumococcal pneumonia, i.e. those with an absent or non-functioning spleen, the immunocompromised, patients with diabetes mellitus, and those with chronic heart, lung, renal, or liver disease. Two different vaccines are available against pneumococcal meningitis.

Encephalitis

Encephalitis is inflammation of the brain caused by bacteria or viruses. Occasionally no organism can be identified; this is called aseptic encephalitis.

Viral encephalitis includes:

- Measles
- Varicella
- Mumps
- Rubella

West Nile fever virus and Herpes simplex can both cause severe disease. The other viruses tend to be associated with mild disease.

Clinical features include:

- Fever
- Headache
- Anorexia
- Malaise

Fits may occur either at the beginning or during the illness.

Investigations may be difficult. CT or MRI scans may be helpful, especially in herpes encephalitis. Lumbar puncture to try and identify an organism. Serology for organisms.

Treatment is symptomatic and supportive.

TRAVEL-ASSOCIATED INFECTIONS

When diagnosing infections acquired abroad the details of time spent abroad, areas travelled to, and whether the patient was immunized or used chemoprophylaxis are all important. A careful history may indicate exposure to an infective source, contact with animals or animal products, occupational hazards, trauma, and previous surgery.

Symptoms of fever, jaundice, diarrhoea, and rashes should be assessed:

- Causes of pyrexia: malaria, legionnaires' disease, typhoid fever, tuberculosis, dengue fever, lassa fever, amoebic abscess.
- Causes of jaundice: hepatitis A, non-A and non-B hepatitis, leptospirosis, secondary syphilis.
- Causes of diarrhoea: *Giardia lamblia* (giardiasis), *Campylobacter, Shigella*.
- Causes of rashes: tick borne infections (e.g. Lyme disease).

Signs of the above carefully explored. In young children look for signs of childhood infections, both intra- and extraoral signs. In the elderly infection may frequently be occult but intraoral signs of candida, pallor, or erythema may all indicate underlying immunosuppression. In fit young adults always look for local sepsis.

Examination of the head and neck area is of particular importance. Carefully examine the eyes, ears, nose, throat, and sinuses. Perform a careful intraoral examination of all hard and soft tissues, and examine all the cervical nodes and all exposed skin surfaces. If no cause for fever is found in the head and neck area, the patient must be referred to a general physician for further investigation. All other orifices must be examined by a general physician.

SEXUALLY TRANSMITTED INFECTIONS

Sexually transmitted diseases (STDs) are endemic. Dentists and their patients are at increased risk from these due to changes in lifestyle (e.g. increased promiscuity) as well as exposure to an ever-increasing variety of pathogens (e.g. due to increasing travel). The risk begins with the first sexual exposure.

Risk factors for STDs include:

- unprotected sexual intercourse
- risk increases with increasing number and type of sexual contact
- drug abuse
- travel abroad
- previous STD

There are many types of STDs:

- Chlamydia is the most common.
- Gonorrhoea.
- Non-specific urethritis (NSU): *Ureaplasma urealyticum, Bacteroides, Mycoplasma*, Herpes simplex virus (HSV).
- Non-specific vaginosis: *Gardnerella, Bacteroides, Mycoplasma*, trichomoniasis.
- Syphilis.
- Molluscum contagiosum.
- Genital warts.
- Chancroid.
- Lymphogranuloma venereum.
- Granuloma inguinale.

The commonest symptom is either vaginal or urethral discharge:

- Causes of urethral discharge:
  - Infective: *Neisseria gonorrhoea, Chlamydia trachomatis, Ureaplasma urealyticum, Mycoplasma, Trichomonas vaginalis*, HSV, urethral warts, *Treponema pallidum*.
  - Non-infective: urinary tract infection, trauma.

- Causes of vaginal discharge:
  - Infective: *Candida albicans, Trichomonas vaginalis*, bacterial vaginosis, *Neisseria gonorrhoea, Chlamydia trachomatis*, HSV.
  - Non-infective: cervical polyps, neoplasia, retained products of conception, foreign bodies, chemical irritation, e.g. creams, soaps, and deodorants.
- Common causes of orogenital ulceration:
  - Trauma
  - Infection: HSV, syphilis, herpes zoster
  - Behçet's syndrome
  - Reiter's syndrome
  - Stevens–Johnson syndrome
  - **do not forget** carcinoma

Chlamydia

Chlamydia is the most common STD caused by *Chlamydia trachomatis* which is an obligate intracellular parasite.

Symptoms include discharge from the vagina or penis, but infection is often asymptomatic. Penile or vaginal discomfort can occur, including itching. There may also be urethritis, dysuria, and genital ulceration. In untreated cases neonates may become infected, with resulting conjunctivitis or pneumonia.

Treatment is with tetracyclines for 7 days or single-dose azithromycin.

Gonorrhoea

Gonorrhoea is the second most common STD and is caused by a Gram-negative intracellular diplococcus, *Neisseria gonorrhoea*, which infects the epithelium of the urogenital tract, rectum, pharynx, and conjunctivae (in neonates). The incubation period is 2–14 days and humans are the only host.

Symptoms are the general symptoms for STDs (see above) plus fever, malaise, arthritis, a purple macular rash, and ophthalmia neonatorum.

Treatment is with a single dose of antibiotic using either ceftriaxone, cefixime, or ciprofloxacin.

Non-specific urethritis (NSU)

Causes of NSU may be infective (e.g. urinary tract infection) or non-infective (e.g. foreign bodies).

Symptoms are the general symptoms listed above plus conjunctivitis, and arthritis. Reiter's syndrome (reactive arthritis) is a triad of urethritis, conjunctivitis, and arthritis and is thought to occur as a reaction to an infection that began elsewhere on the body (either an STD or an infection of the GI tract).

Treatment is with tetracyclines.

Bacterial vaginosis

Bacterial vaginosis is the equivalent in females of non-specific urethritis.

Symptoms are the general symptoms listed above plus a fishy smelling grey to white vaginal discharge. Bacterial vaginosis is diagnosed by the characteristic vaginal discharge, a raised vaginal pH (above 4.7), the fishy odour which occurs on mixing the discharge with 10% potassium hydroxide, and the appearance of 'clue' cells on microscopy (squamous epithelial vaginal cells with adherent bacteria). Three of these features must be present to make a diagnosis.

Treatment is with metronidazole for 7 days.

Trichomoniasis

Trichomoniasis is caused by *Trichomonas vaginalis* which is a flagellated protozoan.

Trichomoniasis is often asymptomatic, or there may be the general symptoms plus a frothy yellow discharge which is characteristic. The cervix typically has a 'strawberry' appearance. Microscopy of discharge shows the characteristic organisms.

Treatment is with metronidazole for 7 days or as a single dose.

Molluscum contagiosum

Molluscum contagiosum is a viral infection which is common in the immuno-suppressed and patients with HIV patients. It may also be transmitted by direct contact (non-sexual) in children.

Lesions are found on the neck, trunk, arms, and legs. They are raised pink papules. Treatment is with cryotherapy. The lesions can be burst with a needle dipped in phenol or removed by curettage.

Genital warts

Genital warts are caused by the human papilloma viruses (HPV) 6 and 11.

Symptoms are general plus warts on the anogenital region. HPV is also found in neonates, characterized by anogenital warts and laryngeal papillomas.

Treatment involves painting the warts with podophyllin extract (except in pregnancy), cryotherapy, or laser therapy.

Pediculosis pubis

Pediculosis pubis, known as crabs or crab lice, is an infestation with the crab louse (*Phthirus pubis*). The louse lays eggs at the base of the hair follicle.

Infestation does not cause urethritis or discharge. The main symptom is itching, which may be intense.

The lice and eggs can be eliminated using 1% benzene hexachloride or 0.5% malathion. This should be applied all over the body from neck down and left for 24 h.

7   Eyes and ears, taste and smell

EYES

Red eyes

Patients with red eyes are frequently seen by dental surgeons. The problem may stem from minor pathology to life-threatening disease or impending blindness. Common causes of red eye/s include:

- corneal trauma
- conjunctivitis
- episcleritis
- scleritis
- uveitis
- angle-closure glaucoma.

The dentist must be able to recognize and advise whether a referral to a specialist is urgent or routine, but should always err on the side of caution. Examination of the conjunctiva may give clues to the underlying pathology. The physical sign to recognize is the arrangement of the pattern of redness of the conjunctiva:

- Localized redness: episcleritis, marginal keratitis.
- Generalized redness: corneal trauma, acute conjunctivitis, angle-closure glaucoma, scleritis.
- Redness surrounding the cornea: acute iritis.

Trauma: corneal abrasion and erosion

The cornea is prone to the affects of trauma because it is the outermost covering of the eye. Corneal trauma may be caused by a retained foreign body under lid, damaged contact lenses, or physical trauma such as accidentally poking a finger into the eye.

Clinical features of corneal trauma are an acute onset of pain (but this may be 10–15 h after the insult). The cornea has no sensory fibres and the pain felt comes from the inside of the eyelid. An acute onset of abrasive scratchy pain indicates abrasion. Excessive production of tears may indicate corneal trauma.

Investigation is by a specialist using fluorescein and **treatment** is with chloramphenicol and/or an eye protection pad. The case should be reviewed after 24 h to exclude infectious keratitis.

Subconjuctival haemorrhage

Subconjuctival haemorrhage can be caused by trauma (e.g. a foreign body under the eyelid or physical contact), can occur spontaneously, or can be due to hypertension (in recurrent cases) or acute viral haemorrhagic conjunctivitis.

Investigation is necessary only in recurrent or severe cases: full blood count, erythrocyte sedimentation rate, blood pressure measurment, clotting studies, virology. **Treatment** consists of reassuring the patient and referral if there is any concern about severe or recurrent episodes.

Conjunctivitis

Conjunctivitis is an inflammation of the conjunctiva (the pink membrane lining the inner eyelids). Both bacterial and viral conjunctivitis pose problems of cross-infection for the dentist and dental staff, who should recognize the condition and defer dental treatment.

Conjunctivitis can be caused by environmental exposure to bacteria, viruses, or *Chlamydia*, and environmental antigens (e.g. dust, sun, chemical allergens).

Bacterial conjunctivitis

Bacterial conjunctivitis is commonly caused by staphylococci and is highly infectious. The patient complains of itching, pain, excessive tears, and burning Examination reveals:

- One or both eyes may be affected.
- There is a mucopurulent discharge.
- Visual acuity is normal.
- The pattern of inflammation shows uniform engorgement of conjunctival vessels.
- The eye appears pink ('pink eye').

After swabbing treatment is with chloramphenicol with review at 24 h and 7 days.

Viral conjunctivitis

Viral conjunctivitis is usually associated with upper respiratory tract infection (adenovirus). It is highly infectious and occurs in epidemics. Patients complain of 'grittiness' or scratchy soreness of one or both eyes. This is caused by very mild keratitis. Examination may reveal aggregations of lymphocyte follicles in the tarsal conjunctivae. In Herpes simplex keratitis, the lesions are superficial or branching 'dendritic' lesions are present.

Patients should be referred for a specialist ophthalmic opinion. The disease is self-limiting after 4–6 weeks. Strict face hygiene and cross-infection control are necessary.

Chronic conjunctivitis

Chronic conjunctivitis is commonly seen by dentists as these patients often present asking for medical advice. Chronic conjunctivitis is frequently allergic in origin. Patients often have a personal or family history of atopy and may have used eye lotions containing preservatives. Patients complain of itching of both eyes and examination reveals a diffusely red conjunctiva with chemosis (oedema). The tarsal surface shows round swellings called papillae which become large as the disease persists and look like cobblestones.

Treatment is with mast cell stabilizers, e.g. sodium cromoglicate and nedocromil sodium.

Keratitis

Keratitis is an inflammation of the cornea and is caused by trauma, infection, and autoimmune disease, e.g. Sjögren's syndrome. It is usually unilateral but may be bilateral in Sjögren's syndrome. Infection is usually secondary to herpes labialis or herpes zoster infection of the fifth cranial nerve. Herpes simplex keratitis has superficial 'dendritic' lesions which may cause scarring and in severe cases blindness.

Clinical features of keratitis include:

- photophobia
- only one eye affected
- pain, which may be severe
- excessive tear production.

Urgent referral to an ophthalmologist is required. Antibiotic drops may be used to prevent secondary infection.

Episcleritis

Episcleritis is a restricted area of inflammation beneath the conjunctiva. Patients complain of a feeling of bruising or a dull ache in the eye. Localized redness of the conjunctiva occurs. Episcleritis is self-limiting and responds to NSAIDs, e.g. ketorolac or trometamol.

Scleritis

Scleritis is serious and may result in blindness and perforation. Patients present with severe pain in the eye. The conjunctiva is diffusely red. Urgent referral is important as there may be serious associated systemic pathology.

Uveitis (iridocyclitis, iritis)

Uveitis is caused by inflammation of the uveal tract. It can occur in:

- Behçet's disease
- inflammatory bowel disease
- ankylosing spondylitis
- Reiter's syndrome.

The patient may have a history of photophobia, discomfort, and pain which is exacerbated by reading, sewing, painting, or using a computer. Examination of the eye reveals the following:

- Visual acuity may be normal.
- Pus in the anterior chamber may be seen by the naked eye. A fluid level is seen where the cells are deposited and settle. This is called a hypopyon.
- Other signs need slit-lamp examination by a specialist.

   Treatment should always be carried out by a specialist who may prescribe mydriatics and immunosuppressive drugs.

Acute angle-closure glaucoma

Acute angle-closure glaucoma occurs in 1/1000 people over the age of 40. It is more common in women. Associated risk factors include:

- family history
- previous episode
- long-sightedness (hypermetropia).

   The **clinical features** are:

- The eye is very painful and red.
- There is a history of previous attacks which began in the evening.
- There is impaired vision with rainbow haloes around bright lights.
- Sleep gives relief from symptoms.

Examination reveals a hazy-looking cornea. The pupil may be oval and intraocular pressure is raised.

   Immediate referral is vital. In the acute phase the ophthalmologist will prescribe topical pilocarpine 4% and acetazolamide, 500 mg, injected intravenously.

Visual loss

Visual changes, with slowly deteriorating vision, begin in the fifth decade and are part of the normal physiological ageing process. Blindness is defined as the lack or loss of the ability to see. Most blind people are elderly (over 65 years of age). A person is registered as blind if they have a corrected acuity of less than 3/60 in the better eye. In the UK more than 2 million people are visually disabled to some degree; of these 25% are registered blind.

   The WHO has published the following definitions:

- Profound blindness is the inability to distinguish fingers at a distance of 3 m or less.
- Partial sight is the inability to distinguish fingers at a distance of 6 m.
- The preferred terminology is people with sight problems.

   Loss of vision can be:

- of sudden onset with bilateral loss of sight or of sudden onset with unilateral loss of sight;

- of gradual onset with bilateral loss of sight or of gradual onset with unilateral loss of sight.

Sudden loss of vision

Any patient with sudden painless loss of vision requires specialist review unless the cause of visual loss is migraine. Care should be taken in differentiating patients who suddenly become aware of long-standing visual loss.

Sudden loss of vision can be due to:

- acute glaucoma
- massive vitreous haemorrhage
- retinal arterial occlusion
- central retinal vein occlusion
- amaurosis fugax
- retinal detachment.

Acute glaucoma

Clinical features of acute glaucoma are:

- pain, with or without vomiting
- a red eye
- corneal oedema
- semi-dilated pupil
- a stiff hard eye.

Massive vitreous haemorrhage

A characteristic feature of massive vitreous haemorrhage is loss of the red reflex on fundoscopy.

Retinal arterial occlusion

Central occlusion of the retinal artery will result in complete visual loss and branch occlusion will result in partial visual loss.

Central retinal vein occlusion

Extensive fundal haemorrhage occurs in central retinal vein occlusion. Elderly patients tend to be more seriously affected as an added problem is atherosclerosis of the retinal arterial supply. Central retinal vein occlusion is of slower onset than central retinal artery occlusion and is characterized by the onset of sudden painless visual loss.

Amaurosis fugax

Amaurosis fugax is a common clinical symptom indicative of transient retinal ischaemia. Patients describe a transient loss of vision. Visual loss is painless. The causes are cardiac or carotid artery emboli or stenosis of the ipsilateral carotid artery.

Clinical features of amaurosis fugax are:

- Sudden transient loss of vision.
- Visual loss, described as a curtain which appears to descend over the vision for minutes. This results from an embolus transiently lodging in the vessel. The embolus may be visible on the retina.
- A carotid bruit may be heard.

Retinal detachment

Retinal detachment is the separation of the outer retinal pigment epithelium from the inner neuro-retina. It occurs secondary to tears in the retina. Retinal tears can be caused by:

- congenital defects
- trauma
- a thin retina in severe myopes.

In all cases except the macula, when the retina becomes detached its blood supply remains intact. In these cases prompt surgical treatment may restore the sight.

When detachment of the macula occurs patient will start seeing flashing lights and floaters. The visual field loss will spread centrally.

Gradual loss of vision

Gradual loss of vision is the most common cause of visual loss, especially in the elderly. Loss of vision may be socially isolating and patients may not seek treatment. Rarely, the visually impaired dental patient has dependent behaviour which impacts on dental treatment (see Chapter 15 on disability).

There are a number of cause of gradual visual loss (see Table 7.1).

Dry eyes (xerophthalmia)

There are numerous cause of xerophthalmia:

- Ageing results in a reduced tear film.
- Sjögren's syndrome, where there are problems with dry eyes and a dry mouth.

Table 7.1 Causes of gradual visual loss

Disease	% of cases of visual loss
Macular degeneration	50
Glaucoma	12
Diabetes mellitus	10
Cataract	3–4
Optic atrophy	3–4

> **BOX 7.1** Dental relevance of ocular disease
>
> - Diseases that may present to the dental surgeon can also have ocular manifestations, many of which may need urgent treatment.
> - Dry eyes (xerophthalmia) may present to the dentist with a dry mouth in Sjögren's syndrome, or in cases due to side-effects of medication.
> - Vesiculobullous disease affecting the oral mucosa may cause conjunctival scarring as in cicatricial pemphigoid.
> - Behçet's disease may present with oral ulcers and at the same time patients may have uveitis and hypopyon affecting the eyes.
> - Herpes zoster of the ophthalmic and maxillary division of the trigeminal nerve may present to the dentist.
> - Dental patients as well as the dentist and dental assistant should all wear protective glasses during dental procedures to protect the eyes from infective material, trauma, and foreign bodies.
> - An acute red eye may be of highly infectious aetiology.
> - The dentist may recognize signs of serious ocular pathology and urgently refer patients for assessment by a specialist.
> - Visual loss makes oral hygiene difficult.
> - Pituitary tumour in Cushing's disease and acromegaly may cause peripheral visual loss, e.g. bitemporal hemianopia.

- Infection.
- Irritation from contact lenses.
- Allergies.
- The menopause with associated hormonal fluctuation, especially lack of oestrogen.
- Dry warm air, e.g. hot dry countries, central heating.
- Drugs such as tricyclic antidepressants, oral contraceptive pills, diuretics, antihypertensives.

HEARING

Loss of hearing

In the UK there are nearly nine million deaf or hard-of-hearing people. Thirteen out of every 1000 children are born deaf or develop deafness when they are very young. Of these four out of the 13 are profoundly deaf. The commonest cause of deafness in adults is age related: deafness or loss of hearing related to ageing is called presbycusis and is more common in men. Presbycusis is due to degenerative changes in cochlear and cochlear hair cells, which may become damaged, bones of the middle ear, and damage to the eighth cranial nerve. High-frequency hearing loss can start as early as 40 years of age. High-pitched sounds are lost initially, followed by gradual loss of low-pitched sounds.

> **BOX 7.2** Dental relevance of hearing loss
>
> - Patients have difficulty communicating problems to the dentist.
> - Loss of hearing may affect personality, behaviour, and attitudes, and may result in social isolation. This in turn leads to less frequent visits to the dentist.
> - Children who are deaf have delayed speech. The frustration of trying to communicate frequently results in behavioural problems.

Types of deafness

Conductive deafness is due to problems that disrupt the conduction of sound through the outer and middle ear, affecting hearing before the sound reaches the cochlea and the nerve receptors of the inner ear. **Sensineural deafness** is due to damage to the cochlea or to the eighth cranial nerve. It is often due to exposure to loud noises such as in clubs and pop concerts or industrial settings. Damage to the hearing is usually permanent. Sensineural deafness should be investigated using audiometry.

Causes of hearing loss

- In the outer ear: otitis externa, obstruction by wax.
- In the middle ear: glue ear (ear filled with fluid which thickens), chronic middle ear infection, otosclerosis (bony overgrowth of the stapes).
- In the inner ear: age-related presbycusis, rubella, meningitis, mumps, cytomegalovirus, trauma, ototoxic drugs (e.g. aspirin, streptomycin, gentamicin), noise (509 000 people in the UK have suffered hearing loss as a result of exposure to noise at work.

SMELL AND TASTE

The sense of smell is our most primitive sense and modulates the sense of taste. The sense of smell is most accurate between the fourth and seventh decades and then begins to decline. Women of all ages are better at identifying odours than men. A large proportion of elderly people lose their smelling ability. Peripherally the sense of smell is mediated by the nose.

The olfactory cells to detect odours (the olfactory sense) are present in the upper third of the nose. The nasal epithelium contains specialized olfactory cells which are responsible for the sense of smell. These are very sensitive, particularly to chemicals such as mercaptans. Vapour is directed directly over the olfactory cells. Aroma accommodates—it is most potent initially then fades away.

Nerve cells detecting taste (the gustatory sense) are stimulated by the food and drinks, and can distinguish sensations such as sweet, sour, and bitter. The taste papillae contain nerve cells which are distributed on the surface of the tongue in taste buds. Approximately 10 000 taste buds are present in the mouth. They send information about the different flavours in food along their nerve fibres.

BOX 7.3 Definitions of abnormalities associated with Smell and Taste

- **Anosmia**: complete loss of the sense of smell.
- **Hyposmia**: partial loss of the sense of smell.
- **Parosmia**: phantom smell or smell misrepresentation.
- **Ageusia**: complete loss of the sense of taste.
- **Hypogeusia**: partial loss of the sense of taste.
- **Dysgeusia**: persistent abnormal taste.

BOX 7.4 Dental relevance of disorders of taste and smell

- Smell and taste disorders can have a serious impact on patient's lives. These disorders result in more than 100 000 patient visits per year to doctors, with a substantial number of these patients also visiting dentists.
- The dentist may see a patients complaining of ageusia, hypogeusia, or dysgeusia, although the complaint of hypoguesia is most common.
- A careful history should be taken to try and identify both local and systemic problems.
- Careful examination of the mouth should be made to exclude dental problems and oral candida.
- Patients may be depressed, stop socializing, and focus all their problems on the mouth.
- Older patients are more likely to present with multiple underlying causes.

The common chemical sense detects the irritating properties of substances. It plays a part in the ability to taste and smell. There are specialized nerve endings which are present on the mucous membranes of the eyes, nose, mouth, and throat.

These three senses combine to contribute to the perception of 'flavour' which defines the different types of foods.

Loss of smell and taste

Causes of loss of and/or abnormal smell and taste include:

- Genetic disorders, e.g. Kallman's syndrome (a disorder of sexual differentiation).
- The normal ageing process.
- Thickened mucous membranes, e.g. due to allergy, nasal polyposis, or sinusitis.
- Anatomical problems, e.g. abnormal or distorted anatomy.
- Infections, e.g. adenovirus causing upper respiratory tract infection.
- Dental problems.
- Smoking.
- Trauma to the head.
- Brain and intranasal tumors.
- Endocrine disorders, e.g. diabetes mellitus, hypothyroidism, and Addison's disease.
- Degenerative diseases, e.g. Alzheimer's disease and Parkinson's disease.

- Drugs, e.g. streptomycin, gentamicin, penicillamine, chemotherapy.
- Radiotherapy and chemotherapy for head or neck cancer.
- Nutritional deficiencies, e.g. thiamine, zinc, and vitamin A.
- Exposure to potent chemicals, e.g. formaldehyde and organic solvents.
- Psychiatric illnesses, e.g. depression, schizophrenia.
- Idiopathic causes.

8 Reproductive system

The reproductive system is multifaceted, both anatomically and physiologically, with functions at endocrine and reproductive levels. Problems of the reproductive system may occur at any age.

DISORDERS OF THE FEMALE REPRODUCTIVE SYSTEM

Vaginal discharge

Vaginal discharge may be caused by vaginosis or cervicitis, the main cause in either case being of infective aetiology. Other causes of vaginal discharge include retained tampons or other foreign objects.

Vaginosis

Vaginosis or vaginitis is inflammation of the vagina. It can be caused by infection (trichomoniasis, *Candida* vaginosis, bacterial vaginosis). Atrophic vaginitis also occurs.

Clinical features of vaginosis include itching, burning, and discharge, the colour and consistency of which is dependent on the infecting organism.

Trichomoniasis

Trichomoniasis is caused by infection with *Trichomonas vaginalis* and is sexually transmitted. It is associated with co-infection with *Neisseria gonorrhoeae*. The discharge is copious, frothy, yellowish-green, and foul smelling. Treatment is with metronidazole (both partners should be treated).

Bacterial vaginosis

Bacterial vaginosis is commonly caused by *Gardnerella vaginalis* together with *Mycoplasma* and anaerobic organisms. Infection is associated with complications of pregnancy. The discharge is fishy smelling and opaque white-grey in colour. Treatment is with metronidazole but recurrences are common.

Candidal vaginosis

Candidal vaginosis is commonly caused by infection with *Candida albicans*, but other subtypes may be implicated. The discharge is thick and white, with the consistency of cottage cheese. Treatment is with antifungal drugs, e.g. imidazoles.

Atrophic vaginosis

Atrophic vaginosis is due to withdrawal of oestrogen from the vaginal mucosa. There is usually no discharge but pruritus, burning and erythema may be present. Treatment is with lubricants and hormone replacement therapy.

Menstrual problems

Menstruation begins between the ages of 9 and 15 years of age in females. There is evidence of a decrease in the age of onset of menstruation in the West. This is probably due to better nutrition but may also be due in part to by-products of hormone replacement therapy (HRT) and contraceptive medication in drinking water.

Amenorrhoea

Primary amenorrhoea is the absence of periods in a woman who has never menstruated. If the menses has not started by the age of 18 years amenorrhoea is considered to be primary. Causes of primary amenorrhoea are:

- Turner's syndrome
- chemotherapy or radiotherapy
- absent or malformed reproductive organs
- anorexia
- malnutrition.

Secondary amenorrhoea is the absence of menstruation for more than 6 months in a female with previously normal menstrual cycles (at least one period). Causes of secondary amenorrhoea are:

- pregnancy
- the oral contraceptive pill
- polycystic ovary syndrome
- hyperprolactinaemia
- hormonal imbalance
- severe emotional stress
- anorexia
- excessive exercise
- ovarian tumour.

Dysmenorrhoea

Dysmenorrhoea is difficult or painful menstruation. Causes of dysmenorrhoea are unknown in most cases but can include:

- endometriosis
- pelvic inflammatory disease
- cervical stenosis.

Clinical features are a cramping pain in the pelvic and low back area. This pain may be severe in endometriosis.

Treatment depends on the underlying cause. The pain of endometriosis and cervical stenosis often decreases after pregnancy. Oral contraceptives may decrease pain and NSAIDs (non-steroidal anti-inflammatory drugs) are helpful.

Menorrhagia

Menorrhagia is excessive or prolonged menstrual bleeding. Causes of menorrhagia are:

- hormone imbalance
- pelvic inflammatory disease
- uterine fibroids
- uterine malignancy
- bleeding diasthesis.

Treatment again depends on the cause. Dentists should take note of a patient's menstrual history as menorrhagia is a common cause of iron deficiency which can cause glossitis and ulceration.

Polycystic ovary syndrome

Polycystic ovary syndrome is due to increased secretion of androgen from the ovaries, resulting in chronic anovulation and amenorrhoea. Clinical and biochemical features include:

- Obesity.
- Hirsuitism due to increased testosterone levels.
- Hyperglycaemia secondary to Type 2 diabetes mellitus.
- Hyperlipidaemia, increasing the risk of coronary artery disease.
- Raised levels of luteinizing hormone.

Treatment is as follows:

- Treat hirsuitism with an antiandrogens, e.g. cyproterone.
- Regulate the menstrual cycle if necessary with combined oral contraception.
- Induce ovulation with antioestrogens, e.g. clomifene citrate.
- Treat diabetes and hyperlipidaemia.

Endometriosis

Endometriosis is the atypical extrauterine growth of endometrial tissue. It commonly occurs between the ages of 30 and 40 years. The mechanism of spread of endometrial tissue is unknown. Proposed pathways are via the bloodstream or lymphatics.

Clinical features include:

- Dysmenorrhoea, which may be severe.
- Intermenstrual pain which is relieved for a few days after the onset of bleeding.

- Dyspareunia (pain on sexual intercourse).
- Menorrhagia.
- Infertility.
- Ectopic pregnancy.

Endometriosis can be **treated** by:

- Hormonal therapy to inhibit gonadotrophin release from the pituitary.
- Laser removal of extrauterine tissue.
- In severe cases, total hysterectomy.
- Pregnancy gives relief from symptoms.

Pelvic inflammatory disease (PID)

PID is inflammation of part or all of the pelvic reproductive organs due to ascending spread of infecting organisms from the vagina. It is common and affects between 10 and 15% of women by the age of 45 years. Infective episodes may occur with the first sexual contact.

Organisms commonly associated with infection in PID are *Chlamydia trachomatis*, *Neisseria gonorrhoeae*, and *Mycoplasma* spp.

Risk factors for PID are:

- Increased number of sexual contacts.
- Increased frequency of sexual activity.
- Presence of sexually transmitted disease in the patient or partner.
- Use of intrauterine device.
- Drug abuse.

PID has the following **clinical features**:

- fever
- rigors
- vaginal discharge
- pelvic pain
- dyspareunia.

Untreated adhesions of reproductive tissue may lead to infertility and chronic pelvic pain.

Treatment is with bed rest, analgesia, and antibiotics.

Toxic shock syndrome

Toxic shock syndrome is an acute syndrome consisting of pyrexia, vomiting, diarrhoea, confusion, hypotension, renal failure and erythrodermia. Toxic shock syndrome is caused by toxins from *Staphylococcus aureus* phage group I strain entering the bloodstream. Heavy staphylococcal infection of high-absorbancy tampons is one of the causes, but fewer than half of reported cases are now seen in menstruating women using tampons (in the 1980s around 90% of cases occurred in menstruating women).

Clinical features are variable and may be very mild or severe with renal failure and circulatory collapse. These include:

- Rash – which is macular, diffuse, and erythrodermic.
- Hypotension – patients are dizzy and feel faint. Systolic blood pressure is <90 mmHg (in adults).
- Systemic abnormalities – all major systems are affected.
- Ruptured blisters on the mucous membranes of the mouth make it painful to eat or even drink.

Treatment involves removal of the tampon in tampon-associated cases, supporting vital functions, especially transfusion to restore the blood volume, and antibiotic treatment to help prevent reccurrence (as bacterial toxins have already entered the bloodstream antibiotic treatment has little effect on the immediate course of the illness).

The menopause

The menopause is defined as beginning 12 months after the last menstrual cycle. It is part of the natural biological ageing process. Early menopause may be precipitated by autoimmune disease, chemotherapy or radiotherapy, and hysterectomy.

The main **clinical features** of the menpoause are:

- Changes in the menstrual pattern. Periods may become irregular, lighter, or longer.
- Hot flushes during the day or night, which last for 20 s to 5–6 min.
- Sexual intercourse may be painful because of a thinner drier vagina.
- Increased propensity to urinary tract infections and stress incontinence.
- Sleep patterns disturbed by nocturia or hot flushes.
- Emotional lability due to fluctuations in oestrogen levels.
- Osteoporosis with an increase in loss of bone mass.
- Change of body shape to increased waistline, decreased muscle mass, and increased laying down of fat.

Unpleasant effects of the menopause, especially mood swings, hot flushes, and vaginal mucosal dryness, can be treated using hormone replacement therapy. This provides a low dose of oestrogen with progestogen. Patients who have had a hysterectomy have oestrogen alone; most other women have combined oestrogen and progestogen.

Combined oestrogen–progestogen treatment has a number of side-effects with **increased risk** of coronary artery disease (relative risk (RR) 29%), breast cancer (RR 26%), blood clots (RR 111%), cerebrovascular accident (RR 41%), and dementia in women over 65 years (RR 105%) and **decreased risk** of cancer of the colon (RR 37%), bone fractures (RR 33%).

Treatment with oestrogen alone also has risks above but increases the risk of ovarian cancer, which doubles after 10–19 years' treatment.

Table 8.1 Variation in maternal death rates

Country	Maternal deaths per 100 000 pregnancies
UK	12.2
Developed countries	27
Underdeveloped countries	480

Disorders of pregnancy

World Health Organization figures indicate that more than half a million women die every year from complications of pregnancy and childbirth (i.e. around 1600 deaths a day). More than 90% of these deaths occur in Asia and sub-Saharan Africa (see Table 8.1). In addition 50 million women experience long-term complications, such as infertility and permanent urinary incontinence.

Eating disorders in pregnancy

Eating disorders which may occur in pregnancy are anorexia, compulsive eating, and bulimia:

- Anorexia: anorexics are often infertile due to amenorrhoea, but if they do become pregnant they are likely to have small babies. Cardiac arrhythmias may lead to sudden death.
- Compulsive eating: obese women have an increased risk of gestational diabetes and high blood pressure. Babies born to women who are obese in pregnancy are more likely to be of high birthweight (with consequent risks of caesarean delivery).
- Bulimia: bulimics may have chemical imbalances giving rise to arrhythmias.

Nausea and hyperemesis gravidarum

Nausea occurs in 50% of pregnant women and varies in severity. Severe nausea with protracted recurrent vomiting which results in dehydration and excessive weight loss is called hyperemesis gravidarum.

Treatment of nausea and hyperemesis gravidarum involves:

- Simple measures such as small more frequent meals, dry crackers in the morning, and avoidance of fatty meals.
- If simple measures are ineffective antihistamines may be beneficial. However, care should be taken as their safety profile has not been fully determined in pregnancy.
- Acupuncture may also be beneficial.
- Use of vitamin B6 as an antiemetic should be avoided because of its toxic side-effects in overdose.
- Ginger is often used but its efficacy is not known.

Seizures in pregnancy

One in 40 women with epilepsy will have an affected child. Poorly controlled epilepsy may result in hypoxia during seizures and affect fetal development, but in 90% of patients the outcome is good. It is important to monitor blood levels of medication carefully and avoid phenytoin and sodium valproate in pregnancy and breastfeeding. Antiepileptic drugs during pregnancy increase the risk of learning difficulties in the child: sodium valproate increases the risk of the child having special educational needs by 50%.

Congenital abnormalities caused by drugs used to treat epilepsy include:

- spina bifida
- cardiac defects
- cleft lip and palate
- hypertelorism
- intellectual impairment
- malformation of the digits of the upper and lower limbs, which may be fused
- malformation of the bladder and sexual organs.

The British Epilepsy Association issue a list of drugs used in treatment of epilepsy and the associated risk to mother and fetus (Table 8.2). If it is possible medium- or high-risk drugs should be withdrawn before pregnancy.

Table 8.2 Drugs used in treatment of epilepsy and the associated risk to mother and fetus (list prepared by Dr Tim Betts and Lyn Greenhill, an Epilepsy Specialist Nurse from the Women's Preconception and Pregnancy Service of the Birmingham University Seizure Clinic)

Level of risk to fetus	Drug
High risk	Sodium valproate
	Phenytoin
	Phenobarbitone
	Primidone†
Medium risk	Carbamazepine
	Oxcarbazepine
	Topiramate
	Vigabatrin
	Clobozam
	Clonazepam
	Ethosuximide
Low risk	Lamotrigine
	Gabapentin
	Tiagabine
	Levetiracetam

†Primidone has recently been withdrawn in the UK.

Depression in pregnancy

Depression may occur at any time during pregnancy and during the post-natal period. Ten per cent of women become depressed during pregnancy. Those most at risk are women with anxiety disorders who discontinue medication during pregnancy.

During depression in pregnancy mood changes are very common. Clinical signs are similar to a depressive state not related to pregnancy. Post-natal depression occurs in 10–15% of mothers, and 2 in 1000 mothers develop post-natal psychosis which occurs within the first 6 weeks of delivery. The clinical signs of post-natal psychosis are:

• Sleep disturbance.
• Marked mood changes which may be elevated or depressed mood or mood swings a very high or elevated mood.
• Thought processes are perturbed.
• Auditory or visual hallucinations.

Treatment of depression during and after pregnancy is as follows:

• There is no indication to stop tricyclic antidepressants or selective serotonin re-uptake inhibitors (SSRIs) in pregnancy.
• Benzodiazepines should not be used in the first trimester as they are associated with major congenital malformations.
• The use of lithium was thought to be associated with severe fetal malformation. However, the risk has been overestimated and withdrawal of the drug has more serious consequences for the health of the mother and fetus.
• During the post-partum period lithium is excreted in breast milk and may affect the neonate.
• Neonates suffer withdrawal syndromes from psychotropic medication used in the last trimester of pregnancy.

Diabetes in pregnancy

In known diabetics:

• Counselling prior to pregnancy is important and referral for specialist care should be made early in pregnancy.
• Careful blood sugar monitoring before and during pregnancy is very important, as good blood sugar control will give the best outcome.
• Fetal growth should be monitored carefully using ultrasound.
• In the third trimester monitoring for pre-eclampsia is important.
• Encourage carriage of the fetus to full term in an otherwise healthy pregnancy and monitor insulin post-partum.

Patients with **Type 1 diabetes** tend to be insulin resistant. They are managed using mixtures of short- and medium-acting insulin two or three times a day before meals.

It is important for patients with **Type 2 diabetes** to have glycaemic control. This will require early transfer to insulin usage. The use of sulphonylureas should be avoided as they cross the placenta to stimulate beta pancreatic cells which in turn produce insulin and hypoglycaemia in the neonate.

Gestational diabetes

Gestational diabetes occurs in 2–4% of pregnancies in the later part of the second trimester. It is due to inadequate insulin reserves. Diagnosis of gestational diabetes is made using the WHO guidelines—a blood sugar level of ≥7.8 mmol/l 2 h after a 75 g sugar glucose tolerance test is diagnostic. Treatment in mild cases is by dietary measures and counselling but if levels are consistently high then short-acting insulins are used. Babies of mothers with gestational diabetes are usually large, are hypoglycaemic at birth, and may be jaundiced. Women should be advised that the risk of developing diabetes is 50% over 15 years after the pregnancy.

Hypertension and pre-eclampsia in pregnancy

Gestational hypertension

Gestational hypertension is hypertension which usually develops after the 20th week of pregnancy. There is no protein in the urine.

Treatment:

- As long as there is no protein in the urine careful home monitoring may avoid the need for hospital admission.
- Antihypertensives may be used to reduce blood pressure. The drugs most commonly used are methyldopa and labetalol but both have side-effects.

Pre-eclampsia

Pre-eclampsia is hypertension associated with proteinuria. It occurs around the 30th week of pregnancy. The incidence in the UK is 1 in 2000 pregnancies. Risk factors for pre-eclampsia are:

- Poor antenatal care and nutrition.
- First pregnancy.
- Pre-pregnancy hypertension, systemic lupus erythematosus, and diabetes.
- Multiparity of more than five children.
- Family history of pre-eclampsia.
- Personal history of pre-eclampsia.

Clinical features of pre-eclampsia are headaches, peripheral (feet and hands) and facial oedema, weight gain, abdominal pain, and blurred vision. Ten to 12% of women with pre-eclampsia develop HELLP syndrome. This consists of haemolytic anaemia (H), elevated (EL) liver enzymes, and low platelet (LP) count. They experience nausea, vomiting, headache, and upper abdominal pain. The consequences of hypertension and pre-eclampsia can be a small-for-dates fetus or placenta abruptio. Pre-eclampsia may lead to eclampsia which is life-threatening and may result in coma and death.

Investigations of pre-eclampsia consist of:

- Measuring the blood and protein content in the urine.
- Platelet count.
- Measuring blood pressure.
- Weighing the patient.

Treatment:

- Diuretics do not prevent the onset of pre-eclampsia.
- The antihypertensives hydralazine and labetalol are commonly used to lower the blood pressure.
- In pre-eclampsia: early delivery together with medication is essential to prevent maternal cerebral encephalopathy and haemorrhage; magnesium sulphate reduces the risk of seizures more than either diazepam or phenytoin.
- Calcium supplements may result in significant reduction in blood pressure in pregnancy but it is not known if there is a decrease in morbidity associated with pre-eclampsia.

Thromboembolism in pregnancy

Pregnancy increases the risk of thromboembolic problems such as deep vein thrombosis (DVT) and pulmonary embolism: 1 in 1000 pregnancies are affected. Most deaths occur in the first week after delivery. The causes of thromboembolism are:

- Obstruction in venous flow.
- Prothrombotic changes in the endothelium.
- Changes in haemostatic and fibrinolytic proteins.

Risk factors for thromboembolism are:

- Personal previous thrombotic episode.
- Family history.
- Patients with: antiphospholipid syndrome, hyperemesis gravidarum, pre-eclampsia, pneumonia, or multiple-fetus pregnancy.
- Prolonged labour.
- Prolonged immobilization, e.g. epidural, caesarean section, or operative procedure during pregnancy.
- Prolonged bed rest or immobilization following delivery.

Accurate **diagnosis** is vital. Inappropriate anticoagulation carries a risk to the mother's immediate and long-term health and the health of the fetus. For suspected DVTs real time Doppler ultrasound is investigation of choice and for suspected pulmonary embolism use CT scan or nuclear medicine ventilation/perfusion scan.

Treatment is with:

- Heparin, especially low-molecular-weight heparin used as thromboprophylaxis.

> **BOX 8.1** Recommendations of the Royal College of Obstetricians and Gynaecologists regarding thromboembolism
>
> Suggested protocols are as follows.
>
> **Prophylaxis against thromboembolic disease following caesarean section**
> Risk assessment and treatment:
>
> - **Uncomplicated pregnancy**: only early mobilization and attention to hydration are required.
> - **Patients at moderate risk**: administer subcutaneous heparin or use mechanical methods (stockings).
> - **Patients at high risk**: administer heparin prophylaxis and, in addition, leg stockings. Prophylaxis should continue for 5 days.
>
> The use of subcutaneous heparin in patients with an epidural or spinal block remains contentious. Current evidence from general surgery does not point to an increased risk of spinal haematoma.
>
> **Prophylaxis against thromboembolism in pregnancy**
> - Patients with a past history of thromboembolism in pregnancy or the puerperium (and no other risk factor) should receive thromboprophylaxis for 6 weeks post-partum.
> - Patients at high risk (multiple previous thromboembolism) may require anticoagulation in pregnancy.

- Wafarin should not be used between 6–12 weeks and after 36 weeks of pregnancy.
- The duration of anticoagulation is likely to be for a minimum of 3 months.

Miscarriage in pregnancy

One in six pregnancies miscarry, usually before 12 weeks of pregnancy. Recurrent miscarriage is defined as three or more miscarriages. Causes of miscarriage are:

- Parental chromosome abnormality.
- Factor V Leiden increases the chances of miscarriage by 40%.
- Thrombophilic defect.
- Polycystic ovaries with increased production of luteinizing hormone.
- Anatomical abnormality in the mother, e.g. abnormal uterus with cervical incompetence.
- Ectopic pregnancy.
- Miscarriage in the later stages of pregnancy may be due to poor fetal nutrition and abnormal growth or infection.

Investigations must include transvaginal ultrasound for confirmation or otherwise of an on-going pregnancy. If there is any doubt the examination should be repeated in 3 days.

Treatment:

- There is no evidence that bed rest is beneficial for threatened miscarriage.
- There is no evidence that hormonal therapy with progestogens or human chorionic gonadotrophin (HCG) is of benefit. Diethylstilbestrol is not effective and is contraindicated because of the risks from side-effects (see below) and later development of cancer.
- In antiphospholipid syndrome a combination of aspirin and heparin increases the chances of pregnancy going to term by 70%.
- In cases of cervical incompetence a stitch can be placed over the os of the cervix.
- With polycystic ovaries suppress the production of luteinizing hormone.
- In cases of thrombophilic defect give antithrombophilic prophylaxis.

Medication in pregnancy

About 1% of birth defects may be linked to drugs taken by the mother. Drugs used in the third trimester may interfere with labour, or the well-being of the baby at birth, e.g. dyspnoea or arrhythmias.

Special care is needed with drug dosages in the neonatal period because of the immaturity of enzyme systems for drug metabolism and excretion. Dosage in children is based on body weight or given according to the following age ranges: neonate 0–1 month; 1 month to 1 year; 1–5 years; 6–12 years. Where not specified the child dose is calculated from the adult dose:

child dose $=$ (body surface area (in m^2) $\times$ adult dose)/2.

The body surface area is calculated from the child's weight and height using a nomogram.

Daughters of women who took **diethylstilbestrol** during pregnancy are at increased risk of certain cancers, infertility, and pregnancy problems. Sons too may have reproductive and urinary tract problems. Five thousand children were affected with phocomelia after their mothers took **thalidomide** during pregnancy. Thalidomide is now being used increasingly for treatment of ulceration in HIV and in Behçet's syndrome so special care must be taken.

Disorders of the breast

Fibrocystic disease of the breast

Fibrocystic disease of the breast is a common condition affecting up to 40% of women. It occurs between the ages of 30 and 50 years and stops at the onset of the menopause. The name refers to the histological changes of increased fibrous stroma and epithelial elements in the ducts and lobules. These changes are caused by fluctuations in endogenous ovarian hormones.

Fibrocystic disease of the breast has the following **clinical features**:

- Cyclical discomfort which may be severe.
- Patients may experience some pain, which increases prior to menstruation.
- Lumps may or may not be associated with cystic lesions.
- Lumps recede after the menopause.

Recurrent breast cysts

Recurrent breast cysts are rare below 25 years of age. Cysts fill with fluid and increase in size towards the end of menstrual cycle. After a period the swollen cells slowly disappear. These cysts can be treated by aspiration of the contents.

Fibroadenoma or 'breast mouse'

Fibroadenoma cccurs in young women in their early 20s. It presents as a mobile lump or 'breast mouse', and is a benign tumour consisting of fibrous and glandular tissue. Fibroadenomas do not recur and should only be removed if the lump increases in size, becomes increasingly painful, or if the patient is over 30 years of age.

Carcinoma of the breast

Breast cancer is the commonest cause of death in women between the ages of 35 and 54 years. In the UK 1 in 9 women will develop breast cancer and there are 40 000 new cases each year with 13 000 deaths.

Risk factors for breast cancer are:

- Female sex.
- Genetic: two breast cancer genes *BRCA1* and *BRCA2* have been found in approximately 85 per cent of families with four or more cases of breast cancer diagnosed under the age of 60. These cancers account for 5% of all breast cancer cases, i.e. fewer than 2000 per year.
- Age is the most important risk factor (see Table 8.3).
  - Family history, especially an affected mother or sibling.
  - Personal history of previous breast, ovarian, uterine, or colonic cancer.
  - Diet, especially diets rich in saturated fat.
- Early menarche (at less than 12 years of age).
- Late menopause (at more than 54 years of age).
- Late first pregnancy (over 30 years of age).
- No pregnancies.
- Existing use of hormone replacement therapy or oral contraceptives.
- Obesity (for post-menopausal women only).
- Excessive consumption of alcohol.

Table 8.3 Risk of breast cancer increase with age

Age (years)	Risk
≤25	1 in 15 000
≤40	1 in 200
≤50	1 in 50
≤70	1 in 15

Breast cancer is histologically an adenocarcinoma of the duct tissue, with 85–90% of cases occuring in the ductal system and 10–15% in the lobular structures. The earliest stage is ductal carcinoma *in situ* (DCIS).

Staging of breast cancer:

- Stage I – The tumour is <2 cm with no spread outside the breast.
- Stage II – Tumour is:
  - <2 cm with spread to axillary nodes.
  - 2–5 cm with or without spread to axillary nodes.
  - >5 cm but no axillary node spread.
- Stage III is divided into IIIA and IIIB.
  - Stage III A – Tumour >5 cm with spread to axillae, and nodes attached to other structures.
    Tumour >5 cm with axillary spread.
  - Stage III B – Tumour has local spread to skin, chest wall, and muscles.
    Tumour has spread to surrounding chest nodes.
- Stage IV – metastatic spread.

Clinical features of breast cancer:

- Mass or lump in breast which is usually firm and painless.
- The nipple may be retracted and or have a discharge or clear serous, blood-stained, or purulent discharge.
- Skin may display dimpling or a 'peau d'orange' effect and in later cases frank ulceration.
- Pain in the breast over the affected region.
- May present as an axillary mass or swollen proximal upper arm.
- General symptoms include weight loss and malaise.
- Signs of metastatic disease.

Mammography is used for **investigation**. Mammography uses low-penetrating X-rays to image breast tissue. Any suspicious areas may be biopsied under ultrasound control.

The earlier the stage at which **treatment** occurs the better the outcome:

- Surgery: lumpectomy with sampling of the axillary lymph nodes or mastectomy, with or without axillary clearance, and which may be followed by breast reconstruction.
- Radiotherapy or chemotherapy if required.
- Hormonally dependent tumours may require anti-oestrogen, e.g. tamoxifen.

Breast examination should be carried out regularly to detect breast abnormalities at an early stage. Breast screening programmes have reduced the number of deaths from breast cancer.

Life expectancy after treatment for breast cancer is shown in Table 8.4.

Table 8.4 Five-year survival after treatment for breast cancer (no axillary node involvement)

Stage	5-year survival (%)
1	85
2	66
3	41
4	10

If the axillary nodes are involved survival is reduced to 45–50% at 5 years and 25% at 10 years.

DISORDERS OF THE MALE REPRODUCTIVE SYSTEM

Prostate disorders

The prostate is the most commonly affected organ in the male reproductive system.

Benign prostatic hyperplasia (BPH)

Benign prostatic hyperplasia is caused by hypertrophy of normal prostatic tissue. The cause is unknown but sex hormones have been implicated. It is thought to be due to variations in testosterone and oestrogen levels in elderly men. Age is the main risk factor: It affects 50% of those aged 60 years or more and 90% of men at the age of 90 years.

Benign prostatic hyperplasia affects the bladder by causing obstruction of outflow resulting in:

- hesitancy
- urgency
- frequency
- poor stream
- dribbling
- nocturia.

Rectal examination will reveal an enlarged prostate

Investigations:

- Urea and electrolytes to check renal function.
- Ultrasound to exclude hydronephrosis.
- Uroflowmetry.
- Serum prostatic specific antigen (PSA).

Treatment:

- Symptomatic relief by reducing obstruction to the bladder outflow.
- Surgical treatment: transurethral prostatectomy (TURP) or interstitial laser prostatectomy.

Carcinoma of the prostate

Carcinoma of the prostate is the second most common cancer in men after carcinoma of the lung. There are 10 000 cases per year in the UK and it accounts for 8500 (4%) of deaths each year. It affects men over 50 years of age, with 50% of men being affected by the age of 60 years. During operative procedures for benign hypertrophy 5–10% of cases are found to have malignant disease.

Carcinoma of the prostate is an adenocarcinoma which arises in the anterior part of the prostate. The **clinical features** are:

- Symptoms of outflow obstruction similar to BPH in most cases.
- A small percentage of patients have bone pain or renal failure.
- Rectal examination will demonstrate loss of the central sulcus and/or a hard nodule.

Investigations:

- Prostate-specific antigen (PSA): PSA is a kallikrein-like protein produced by the prostatic cells. Normal levels are up to 4 ng/ml. Levels above 10 ng/ml are highly indicative of carcinoma of the prostate. Care should be taken in the interpretation as the PSA may also be considerably increased in BPH.
- Urea and electrolytes.
- Transrectal ultrasound and biopsy in doubtful cases.
- Bone scan to exclude metastases.
- Pelvic MRI or CT scan to stage the disease.

Prostate cancer spreads directly through the capsule, via the lymphatic system, and may spread to the bones via the blood. Common sites for metastases are the pelvis and spine.

Treatment options will depend on the age of the patient and the stage of the disease:

- Local disease: no treatment may be necessary.
- Local spread without metastases: radical prostatectomy or radical radiotherapy which aims to cure the disease; radical radiotherapy; hormonal therapy.
- Disease with metastases: hormonal therapy (most prostate tumours are hormone dependent); androgen blockade or depletion provides good palliative care; bilateral orchidectomy; luteinizing hormone releasing hormone (LHRH) agonists, e.g. goseraline; anti-androgens, e.g. cyproterone acetate, flutamide; oestrogen hormones, e.g. diethylstilbestrol.

Testicular tumours

Testicular tumours are the commonest malignancy in young adult males. There are approximately 1500 new cases a year in the UK. Histologically the tumours are teratomas (50% of testicular cancers) with a peak incidence in men at 25 years and seminomas (40% of testicular cancers) with a peak incidence at 35 years. The remaining tumours are yolk sac tumours. Staging of testicular tumours is dependent on differentiation. The cause is unknown but several risk factors have been recognized:

- cryptorchidism
- maldescended testis
- Kleinfelter's syndrome.

Clinical features:

- Painless testicular mass.
- Some cancers of the testicle produce chemical markers, e.g. alpha fetoprotein or beta human chorionic gonadotrophin (βHCG).
- Symptoms of metastases: teratomas spread to the bone, brain, liver, and lung; seminomas metastasize to paraortic nodes and may produce bone pain.

Investigations include:

- Ultrasound to show the tumour mass.
- CT scan of the thorax and abdomen to stage the disease.
- Orchidectomy to confirm the diagnosis.
- Elevated tumour markers such as βHCG, elevated in both teratomas and seminomas, and alpha fetoprotein elevated teratomas.

Treatment for teratoma is orchidectomy plus chemotherapy and for seminoma orchidectomy plus radiotherapy. Metastases are treated by chemotherapy.

9 Rheumatology

Rheumatological disease is common and increases with age.

AUTOIMMUNE DISEASE

Autoimmunity occurs when the body's ability to maintain non-reactivity against self components breaks down, resulting in autoimmune disease. Autoimmune disease can be organ specific or non-organ specific:

- Organ-specific autoimmune diseases: autoimmune thyroid disease (see Chapter 14), pernicious anaemia (see Chapter 3), Addison's disease (see Chapter 14), pemphigus, pemphigoid.
- Non-organ-specific autoimmune diseases: systemic lupus erythematosus (SLE), rheumatoid arthritis, systemic sclerosis, Behçet's disease. Autoimmune disease is associated with:
- A defect in immunological tolerance.
- The presence of sequestrated antigen.
- Infection.
- Drugs, e.g. procainamide, methyldopa.
- Human leucocyte antigen (HLA) association: HLA-B5 Behçet's disease, HLA-DR3 Addison's disease, HLA-B8 Graves' disease, HLA-B8 DR3 myasthenia gravis, HLA-B8 DR3 HLA-B15 DR4 diabetes mellitus.

Systemic lupus erythematosus

Systemic lupus erythematosus is a multisystem disorder occurring mainly in young women (female : male ratio 9 : 1). It is characterized by flares and remissions. Onset is between the ages of 15 and 45 years.

The aetiology of SLE is unclear, but sex and genetic background are important. It is increased in Afro-Caribbeans in the UK with 206 per 100 000 population as well as in Blacks in the United States and the Caribbean. Associated genetic factors are an are increase in HLA-B8 DR5 and a decrease in HLA-C4.

Clinical features of SLE

The presenting features of SLE are variable and frequently non-specific:

- Arthritis/arthralgia present in most patients. It is polyarticular, flitting and symmetrical.
- Lymphadenopathy, fatigue, fever, malaise.
- Cutaneous lesions—butterfly rash, alopecia.

- Raynaud's phenomenon.
- Thrombocytopenic purpera.
- Haemolytic anaemia.
- Recurrent thrombophlebitis.
- Oral lesions: ulcers and lichenoid type lesions occur in 60% of patients.
- Sjögren's syndrome resulting in parotid enlargement, increased caries, periodontal disease, and candidosis.

Major organ involvement and clinical features in SLE

Cardiovascular system

- Pericarditis occurs in 25% of patients. Accelerated atherosclerosis occurs in this group.
- Conduction abnormalities are less common, with congenital heart block occurring in children whose mothers are anti-Ro or anti-La antibody positive.
- Myocarditis is rare.
- Libman–Sacks endocarditis.

Respiratory system

- Pleuritic pain is common and is seen in 50% of patients. This may be accompanied by pleural effusion.
- Patients with lupus anticoagulant are at risk of pulmonary embolism.
- Shrinking lung syndrome is characterized by progressive shortness of breath, basal crackles, small lung volumes, and diaphragmatic weakness.

Renal system

Thirty per cent of SLE patients develop renal complications. Symptoms are usually minimal until extensive disease develops. Renal complications are a major cause of death in SLE.

Neurological manifestations

Neurological manifestations are a major problem in both the treatment and diagnosis of SLE. They may affect both the central and peripheral nervous system:

- Central nervous system manifestations: neuropsychiatric SLE is a major cause of serious morbidity. The diagnosis is clinical and very difficult; headache; aseptic meningitis; fits; confusional states; psychosis; cerebrovascular disease; demyelinating disease.
- Peripheral nervous system manifestations: cranial and peripheral neuropathy; mononeuritis multiplex; Guillan–Barré syndrome.

Cutaneous lesions

- Malar butterfly rash on the face.
- Alopecia is common.
- Erythema nodosum, usually on the shins.

> **BOX 9.1** American Rheumatism Association criteria for diagnosis of SLE (1982 recommendations, amended 1997)
>
> A diagnosis of SLE requires four of the 11 criteria to be present:
>
> - Malar rash.
> - Discoid rash.
> - Photosensitivity.
> - Oral ulcers.
> - Non-erosive arthritis.
> - Serositis (pleuritis/pericarditis).
> - Renal disease (persistent proteinuria > 0.5 g/day or 3+ if not quantified); cellular casts.
> - Neurological disorders (seizures/psychosis in the absence of metabolic derangements or offending drugs).
> - Haemolytic anaemia, leucopenia, lymphopenia, thrombocytopenia.
> - Immunological disorder, abnormal anti-DNA titre, anti-Sm antibody, anti-phospholipid antibodies.
> - Antinuclear antibody. Antibodies to dsDNA, antibodies to extractable nuclear antigens/anticardiolipin antibodies.

- Maculopapular discoid lesions may occur on any body surface.
- Vasculitic lesions on the digits may be painful.
- Lipo-atrophy secondary to necrosis and inflammation, causing lupus panniculitis.

Other clinical features

Arthritis in SLE is mainly non erosive.

Investigations

A number of **immunological tests** help in diagnosis of SLE:

- Antibodies to double-stranded DNA in 90% patients.
- Antinuclear antibodies in 60% of patients.
- Antibodies to extractable nuclear antigen Sm in 25% of patients.
- Ribonuclear protein (RNP), Ro, and La antibodies.
- Antibodies to phospholipids.
- Platelet antibodies.
- Raised immunoglobulin G (IgG).
- Low complement C3/C4 levels.
- Cryoglobulinaemia.
- Skin biopsy for IgG, C3, C4 in a clinically unaffected site.

 Haematological tests show:

- Raised erythrocyte sedimentation rate (ESR)
- Low white blood count (WBC).

- Negative direct Coombs' test.
- Lupus anticoagulant.

Treatment

Treatment depends on symptoms, disease activity, and tissue damage.
  General treatment includes:

- Lifestyle modification by increasing exercise, stopping smoking, and stress management.
- Reducing exposure to the sun and using sun-block.
- If steroids are used carry out regular bone density scans and give calcium, vitamin D, and biphosphonates.
- Reduce the risk of infection.

  The mainstay of **specific treatment** is immunosuppression and prevention of major organ damage.

Rheumatoid arthritis

Rheumatoid arthritis is a common systemic condition which occurs in up to 3% of the population and is increasing in developed countries. The predominant

---

BOX 9.2 Dental implications of SLE

- Steroid therapy and the use of other immunosuppressives.
- Oral manifestation of disease: oral ulcers may look like non-specific aphthae or may mimic lichen planus.
- Sjögren's syndrome.
- Other drugs such as methotrexate can cause oral ulceration.
- Head and neck signs, e.g. butterfly rash, lymphadenopathy, alopecia, may be the initial presentation noticed by dentist.
- A low blood count may increase the risk of oral sepsis and post-extraction bleeding.

BOX 9.3 American Rheumatism Association revised diagnostic criteria (1988) for rheumatoid arthritis

Four of the seven criteria are needed to make a diagnosis. The first three have to be present for at least 6 weeks:

- Morning stiffness.
- Arthritis of three or more joints.
- Arthritis of hand joints (at least one of wrist, metacarpo-phalangeal joint, or proximal interphalangeal joint is swollen).
- Symmetrical arthritis.
- Rheumatoid nodules.
- Serum rheumatoid factor positive.
- X-ray changes typical of rheumatoid arthritis on an antero-posterior hand X-ray.

feature is a synovitis associated with widespread involvement of systemic tissues. It is characterized by a symmetrical polyarthritis resulting in joint deformity with extra-articular features and acute or chronic relapsing phases. Rheumatoid arthritis is more common in women than men (female : male ratio 3 : 1).

The aetiology of rheumatoid arthritis is unknown. There is sometimes a family history and a genetic association with HLA DR4. Microorganisms, e.g. *Mycoplasma*, have been associated.

Clinical features

Symmetrical arthritis is a particular feature. There are a number of common abnormalities of the hands: ulnar deviation, swan-neck deformity, Boutonnière deformity, Z deformity, thin skin secondary to steroid use, muscle wasting, and nail-fold infarcts.

Extra-articular features

Extra-articular features occur in 75% or more of patients:

- **General features:** malaise and weight loss, fever, lymphadenopathy, splenomegaly (Felty's syndrome—rheumatoid arthritis, leucopenia and splenomegaly), hepatomegaly, amyloidosis.
- **Pulmonary features:** pleurisy/pleural effusion, recurrent chest infection, rheumatoid lung nodules, Caplan's syndrome (lung nodules with fibrosis), fibrosing alveolitis.
- **Haematological features:** anaemia (iron deficiency, chronic disease and bone marrow suppression), hypergammaglobulinaemia resulting in hyperviscosity.
- **Cardiovascular features:** rheumatoid pericardial nodules, pericarditis, mesenteric and digital ischaemia (Raynaud's phenomenon), arteritis causing leg ulcers and nail-fold infarcts.
- **Ocular features:** keratoconjunctivitis sicca, episcleritis, scleromalacia perforans.
- **Neurological features:** carpal tunnel syndrome, peripheral neuropathy, nerve root compression.

Investigations

X-rays play an important role in diagnosis and monitoring. Immunological and haematological tests show:

- Rheumatoid factor is positive in high-titre IgM in 40% of cases.
- Positive antinuclear antibody.
- Complement C3 and C4 are normal or high.
- Skin biopsy is negative.
- Serum IgG is normal.
- Erythrocyte sedimentation rate and C-reactive protein are high.

> **BOX 9.4** Dental implications of rheumatoid arthritis
> - Problems of steroids (often long-term use) and immunosuppressive drugs.
> - Xerostomia secondary to drugs.
> - Xerostomia associated with secondary Sjögren's syndrome.
> - Temporomandibular joint involvement.
> - Atlanto-axial dislocation.
> - Osteoporosis.
> - Drugs used causing lichen planus and altered taste.

Treatment

Treatment is both symptomatic and disease modifying:

- Symptomatic treatment: pain relief with analgesics, e.g. non-steroidal anti-inflammatory drugs (NSAIDs). Severe pain may need more potent drugs and other strategies such as transcutaneous nerve stimulation. General immunosuppression with corticosteroids.
- Disease modifying drugs: gold, penicillamine, more effectively tumour necrosis factor-alpha (TNF-α).

Sjögren's syndrome

This is an autoimmune condition characterized by increased B-cell activity and antibodies leading to destruction of the salivary and lachrymal glands. It was originally described by Sjögren who described a syndrome of dry eyes and mouth in five patients with rheumatoid arthritis. It is more common in females (female : male ratio 9 : 1).

The terms Sjögren's disease or primary Sjögren's is now used to describe the dry mouth and dry eyes with extraglandular disease but no additional auto-immune rheumatic disease. Sjögren's syndrome or secondary Sjögren's describes xerostomia and dry eyes in association with non-organ-specific autoimmune disease, e.g. rheumatoid arthritis, SLE, or systemic sclerosis.

The aetiology of Sjögren's syndrome is unknown. Genetic factors include HLA-DR3 in primary and HLA-DR4 in secondary disease. Environmental viruses, e.g. Epstein–Barr or cytomegalovirus may act as a trigger.

Clinical features

Besides dry eyes (keratoconjunctivitis sicca), xerostomia, and dysphagia, symptoms are variable and may affect many organ systems. There is also swelling of the salivary glands and lymphadenaopathy.

Diagnostic features in primary Sjögren's are:

- dry eyes and mouth
- pharyngeal irritation
- renal tubular acidosis and glomerular nephritis

> **BOX 9.5 Causes of xerostomia**
>
> Saliva lubricates the mouth and starts the process of digestion of complex carbohydrates. Saliva protects against infection and protects the teeth from decay. Xerostomia results from reduced or absent saliva and may have a structural cause as in Sjögren's or a functional cause.
>
> **Functional xerostomia**
>
> Functional xerostomia can be due to:
>
> - Fear and anxiety.
> - Dehydration and mouth breathing.
> - Hypovolaemia.
> - Drugs: tricyclic antidepressants, antihistamines, phenothiazines, antiemetics, diuretics.
> - Parotid duct stones.
> - Radiation injury to the salivary glands.

- pulmonary fibrosis
- primary biliary fibrosis
- liver disease
- gastric atrophy
- mild anaemia
- Raynaud's phenomenon
- lymphoid malignancy.

In Sjögren's syndrome or secondary Sjögren's, besides dry eyes, dry mouth, and dysphagia symptoms are related to the specific primary disease.

Twenty per cent of cases progress to B-cell lymphoma derived from mucosal associated lymphoid tissue. The risk factors for developing lymphoma are as follows:

- Anti-Ro/anti La positive.
- Younger age of onset.
- Anaemia and lymphopenia.
- Salivary gland enlargement.
- Evidence of monoclonality in labial gland biopsy and extraglandular disease.
- Splenomegaly.
- Lymphadenopathy.
- Skin vasculitis.
- Peripheral neuropathy.
- Leg ulcers and peripheral neuropathy.

Investigations and treatment

Table 9.1 summarizes the various findings in Sjögren's syndrome.

Treatment is symptomatic. Lubricants can be prescribed for the eyes and mouth. Stimulation of salivary glands using an antimuscarinic, either pilocarpine or cevimeline (which is thought to have fewer side-effects and be more effective than pilocarpine). Good preventative dentistry is imperative to try and maintain the patient's own dentition. Immunosuppressive drugs may also be used.

Table 9.1 Findings of investigations in Sjögren's syndrome

Test	Finding
ANA	Positive
ENA	Positive
Ro(SS-A)	Positive in 55% of cases in primary disease
	Positive in 10% of cases in secondary disease
Ro(SS-B)	Positive in 40% of cases in primary disease
	Positive in 5% of cases in secondary disease
Rheumatoid factor	Positive in 95–100% of cases
Rheumatoid precipitins	Positive in 5% of cases in primary disease
	Positive in 85% of cases in secondary disease
Anti-salivary gland antibodies	Positive in 25% of cases in primary disease
	Positive in 70% of cases in secondary disease
IgG	Raised
IgA	Raised
IgM	Normal
ESR	Raised. May be very high in primary disease
Labial gland biopsy	Lymphocytic infiltration around and replacing acinar tissue in minor salivary gland. Lymphoepithelial lesions of chronic inflammatory cell infiltrate involving epithelial and myoepithelial cells and glands
Sialogram	Snowstorm appearance

Abbreviations: ANA, antinuclear antibodies; ENA, extractable nuclear antigens; Ig, immunoglobulin; ESR, erythrocyte sedimentation rate.

BOX 9.6 Dental implications of Sjögren's syndrome

- Xerostomia is a major problem.
- Patients are prone to oral candida infection.
- Salivary gland enlargement.
- Anaemia.
- Examine the mouth carefully, including major and minor salivary glands, for signs of development of lymphoma.
- Lymphopenia predisposes to increased oral infection.

Systemic sclerosis (scleroderma)

Systemic sclerosis is a disease which mainly affects women (female : male ratio 4 : 1) between the ages 30 and 60 years. Environmentally induced disease is more common in men. The prevalence is 1–2 per 10 000 population. It is characterized by persistent and continuous sclerotic changes in mucocutaneous tissues and blood vessels. The defect is in collagen fibres which initially swell before becoming sclerotic.

Systemic sclerosis has a multifactorial aetiology. Environmental factors have been implicated, including organic chemicals, epoxy resins, drugs, e.g. appetite suppressants, bleomycin, and the materials used in mammoplasty. There is an HLA association and linkage with the fibrillin 1 (*FBN1*) locus. Systemic sclerosis involves a combination of vascular, connective tissue, and immunological abnormalities.

Clinical features

Clinical features of systemic sclerosis are variable ranging from a limited syndrome to widespread systemic involvement resulting in life-threatening disability.

General features

General features of systemic sclerosis are weight loss, fever, fatigue, and malaise. There may also be progressive renal failure.

Cutaneous involvement
- Morphea, which is a localized sclerodermatous lesion on neck, limbs, or the trunk. It rarely proceeds to systemic sclerosis.
- Raynaud's phenomenon with telangiectasia and sclerodactyly.
- Early changes include waxy, smooth of skin which later becomes tight. This affects the face to give a mask-like facies, and the hands.
- Later the skin becomes thin, atrophic, and sclerotic.
- Subcutaneous calcification.

Gastrointestinal tract
- Mouth—limited opening (microstomia), oral ulceration.
- Oesophagus—dysphagia due to stricture formation and decreased motility.
- Stomach—dyspepsia due to gastric paresis and ulceration.
- Small bowel—abdominal pain and distension, steatorrhoea due to hypomotility, bacterial stasis, and malabsorption.
- Large bowel—diarrhoea and constipation due to sigmoid and rectal hypomotility and sphincter involvement.

Lung involvement

Lung involvement presents a major therapeutic problem:

- Diffuse interstitial fibrosis results in respiratory failure.
- Pneumonitis due to oesophageal overspill.

Heart involvement
- Restrictive cardiomyopathy and heart failure.
- Hypertension in some cases.
- Pericardial effusion.

Investigations and treatment

Serologyinvestigations are needed to discover the antibody profile:

- Antinuclear antibodies are present.
- Sclo-70 (recognizes the nuclear enzyme DNA topoisomerase) is present in 20% of patients.
- Anticentromere antibody is found in 30% of patients.
- Anti-RNA polymerase I and III found in 20% of patients.

Other investigations depend on specific organ involvement:

- Renal function.
- Lung function, e.g. CT or DTPA scan.
- Cardiac function, e.g. echocardiography.
- Endoscopy and barium meal and enema.

BOX 9.7 Dental implications of systemic sclerosis

- Widening of the periodontal membrane. The space between the tooth root and the lamina dura is widened around the tooth. The lamina dura is preserved.
- The patient may be taking steroids or other immunosuppressives.
- Patients may have renal failure causing delayed clearance of drugs used in dentistry, especially analgesics.
- Penicillamine causes abnormalities of taste.
- Microstomia makes it difficult for the dentist to gain access for dental treatment or for the patient for oral hygiene.
- Intraoral telangiectasia and petechiae.

BOX 9.8 Raynaud's phenomenon

Raynaud's phenomenon results from paroxysmal ischaemia of the fingers and or toes. Clinically a sequence of characteristic colour changes occurs. The digits turn white then blue followed by red. The fingers are most painful when they become red.

Causes of Raynaud's phenomenon

- Vasoconstriction caused by Raynaud's disease and when using vibrating machinery.
- Arterial occlusion caused by atheroma, Buerger's disease, and thoracic outlet syndrome.
- Increased blood viscosity caused by cryo- or macroglobulinaemia, polycythaemia, leukaemia, and lymphoma.
- Autoimmune disease, rheumatoid arthritis, SLE, and systemic sclerosis.
- Neurological disease, e.g. syringomyelia.

Treatment is symptomatic for Raynaud's phenomenon, hypertension, and oesophageal reflux. Physiotherapy is useful as is immunosuppression, e.g. D-penicillamine, cyclosporin, interferon α and γ.

Behçet's disease

Behçet's disease is a chronic multisystem disease characterized by intermittent episodes of active disease due to an enhanced inflammatory response and vasculitis. It was first described by Hippocrates and later in 1937 by Behçet a Turkish dermatologist. The incidence of Behçet's disease is increased in Mediterranean countries and those of the Silk Route. There is a high incidence in Japan and Korea. The male:female ratio varies geographically:

- Mediterranean and Middle East, male : female ratio 8 : 1.
- Japan, male : female ratio 2 : 1.
- Europe, male : female ratio 1 : 1.

The aetiology of Behçet's disease is poorly understood. There appears to be a genetic association with HLA-B51. Environmental factors such as infection, and immunological mechanisms may play a part in triggering the disease.

Clinical features
Behçet's disease has a large number of clinical features.

Mucocutaneous involvement
- Oral ulcers are the most consistent feature. The ulcers are aphthous in morphology and may be of the minor, major, and herpetiform type. Unlike aphthous ulcers found in the healthy population the ulcers are usually surrounded by erythema and swelling of the adjacent mucosa.
- Palatal ulceration is not uncommon.
- Genital ulcers, having the same morphology as the mouth ulcers. In females the entrance to the vagina and the perineal area are usually affected. The skin overlying the labia majora frequently has folliculitis and papulopustular lesions.
- In males papulopustular lesions cause scarring of the scrotum. The glans penis is less frequently affected. When lesion do occur they are usually ulcerations similar to the mouth lesions.
- Cutaneous lesions include folliculitis and pustules seen on the front of the chest, back, and outer thighs. They may due to the disease and also secondary to steroid usage. Erythema nodosum is also common and found on the shins, arms, and hands. They are very painful and occasionally have a central ulcerative area.

The **pathergy test** is an excessive reaction to injury and is seen in patients after venesection or venous cannulation. The test can also be demonstrated as part of the clinical diagnosis by insertion of a 20-gauge needle into the skin of the forearm. A papule appears at the site 24–48 h later. The pathergy reaction is common in Middle Eastern and Mediterranean patients but is only seen in 8–10% of UK patients.

Ocular involvement
- Uveitis may be both anterior and posterior and can cause loss of vision.
- Hypopyon is said to be pathognomonic of Behçet's disease. It is due to neutrophils in the anterior chamber of the eye.
- Iridocyclitis, cataracts, and secondary glaucoma also occur.

Neurological features
- Headaches, which may be debilitating.
- Brainstem syndromes, organic confusional states, upper motor neuron syndromes.

Vascular involvement
Vascular involvement occurs in 20–25% of patients, both sexes are affected but is more common in young males. Features commonly include:

- Thrombophlebitis and venous thrombosis.
- Arterial and venous vasculitis.
- The morbidity associated with arterial thrombosis is very high.
- Aneurysms of large vessels occur but are uncommon.

Arthritic features
- Musculosketal problems are common.
- Polyarthropathy and polyarthritis occur in 50% of patients.
- The arthritis is a non-erosive monoarthritis.

Gastrointestinal involvement
Problems associated with the gastrointestinal tract are being increasingly recognized:

- Irritable bowel syndrome secondary to ulcers anywhere along the gastrointestinal tract.
- A Crohn-like syndrome occurs. It has been suggested that there might be an overlap syndrome between Crohn's and Behçet's.

BOX 9.9 International Study Group criteria for diagnosis of Behçet's disease

To make a diagnosis oral ulcers plus two of the other four signs must be present:

- Recurrent oral ulcers: minor, major, or herpetiform aphthous ulcers which occur at least three times a year.
- Recurrent genital ulcers: ulcers or scarring.
- Eye lesions: anterior and posterior uveitis or cells in the vitreous on slit-lamp examination. Retinal vasculitis.
- Skin lesions: erythema nodosum, pseudofolliculitis, papulopustular lesions, or acneiform nodules in post-adolescent patients not on corticosteroid treatment.
- Positive pathergy test read by physician at 24–48 h.

BOX 9.10 Dental relevance of Behçet's disease

- The most important fact is that all patients with Behçet's have oral ulcers.
- The ulcers may be any of the subgroups of aphthous ulcers—major, minor, or herpetiform.
- Oral ulcers may appear before systemic complications.
- Dental surgeons must always take a systemic medical history.
- It is important to remember that the ocular, vascular, and central nervous system complications may be associated with an increased morbidity.

Investigations and treatment

There are no specific tests for Behçet's disease. The erythrocyte sedimentation rate may be raised and there may be hypergammaglobulinaemia. HLA status should be checked.

Treatment is multidisciplinary and is mainly symptomatic:

- It is important to keep the mouth free of ulcers by using topical steroids.
- Thalidomide and topical tacrolimus help ulceration but have no effect on ocular signs.
- Azathioprine helps decrease recurrence of ulcers.
- Major systemic involvement is treated by immunosuppression.
- Only azathioprine and ciclosporin have been evaluated in the treatment of Behçet's disease.

OTHER RHEUMATOLOGICAL DISEASES

Osteoarthritis

Osteoarthritis is a degenerative disease affecting the articular cartilage and subchondral bone. In the UK 8 million people suffer from osteoarthritis: it is the most common joint condition in people over the age of 65 years.

Risk factors

Age and sex: the chances of developing osteoarthritis increase with age. Before the age of 50 more men have osteoarthritis, while over the age of 50 more women are affected.

- Genetic background: a third of all cases have a family history. There is an association with the type 2 collagen gene (*COL2A1*) on chromosome 12.
- Lifestyle: obesity has a causal relationship and is also linked to progression of the disease.
- Trauma: work and sport may increase the stress on weight-bearing joints.

Clinical features

The main features are pain and or stiffness, especially stiffness after resting or on getting out of bed in the morning. Pain may be intermittent at first then persistent and may be associated with joint swelling. Disability is related to the site/joint affected.

Hands
- Distal interphalangeal joints and thumbs
- There are two types of disease: nodal or non-nodal. Nodal disease appears to be familial.
- Heberden's nodes appear on distal interphalangeal joints.
- Bouchard's nodes on the proximal interphalangeal joints.
- The thumb joint is also affected.

Lumbo-sacral spine
- Pain and stiffness in the back and neck result.
- If the peripheral nerves are affected paraesthesia, numbness, and weakness may result.

Hips
- Osteoarthritis of the hip is associated with severe morbidity.
- Pain may be referred to the knees or groin.
- Severely decreased mobility may necessitate hip replacement surgery.
- Stiffness may affect mobility.

Knee
- The patello-femoral and tibiofemoral joints are affected.
- The knees are the primary weight-bearing joints and tend to be very painful at night.

Feet
- The big toe is more commonly affected than the other toes.
- Hallux valgus (bending medially) and hallux rigidus (stiffening) occur.

Investigations and treatment

X-rays are the main investigation. Arthroscopy gives an idea of cartilage loss. Occasionally CT and MRI scans may be indicated.

There are a number of treatment options:

- Medication: analgesics especially NSAIDs, inter-articular steroids, glucosamine sulphate, and chondroitin sulphate
- Lifestyle: reduce weight to an acceptable level.
- Physiotherapy.
- Occupational therapy.
- Surgery may be needed for knee and hip replacement.

> **BOX 9.11** Dental relevance of osteoarthritis
> - The temporomandibular joint may be affected.
> - Oral health may be compromised by arthritis affecting the hands.
> - Patient mobility may be a problem. Patients with osteoarthritis make up a large proportion of those requiring domiciliary visits.
> - NSAIDs may affect renal function in the elderly.

Problems with steroid therapy and its dental implications

Patients presenting to dentists are frequently taking steroids or being prescribed steroids for mucosal diseases. Although often life saving, steroids have numerous side-effects and dentists should be cognisant of pitfalls, especially adrenocortical suppression, when dental patients have a major surgical procedure. Changes which might prove hazardous for dental patients are highlighted. Metabolic changes are especially hazardous, as these may give rise to other systemic diseases and complications:

- Appearance: abnormal weight distribution, cushingoid facies, buffalo hump.
- Metabolic changes: **sodium and water retention, potassium depletion, hypertension, hyperglycaemia, hyperlipidaemia**.
- **Adrenal suppression and atrophy**.
- Cataracts and raised intraocular pressure.
- Amenorrhoea and premature menopause.
- **Increased susceptibility to infection: bacterial**, e.g. **TB, fungal**, e.g. *Candida*, **viral**, e.g. **herpes**.
- Bone and muscle: **osteoporosis, aseptic bone necrosis**, myopathy.
- Gastrointestinal tract: **peptic ulcer**, dyspepsia, **pancreatitis**.
- Cutaneous changes: thinning of skin and delayed healing, striae and bruises, venous ulcers, acne, hypertrichosis.
- Central nervous system: **headache, raised intracranial pressure, euphoria, psychosis, epilepsy**.

The vasculitides

Vasculitis is a general term for a group of diseases that involve inflammation in blood vessels. Blood vessels of all sizes may be affected, from the largest vessel in the body (the aorta) to the smallest blood vessels in the skin (capillaries):

- Large vessel vasculitis: temporal arteritis, Takayashu's giant cell arteritis, Kawasaki disease.
- Small and medium size arteritis: SLE, rheumatoid arthritis, systemic sclerosis, polymyositis, dermatomyositis.
- Small vessel vasculitis: idiopathic cutaneous vasculitis, tumours, serum sickness, drug allergy, Henoch–Schonlein purpura.
- Thromboangiitis obliterans (Buerger's disease).

- Systemic vasculitis: Wegener's granulomatosis (midline granuloma oral lesions, chest, kidney cANCA positive), polyarteritis nodosa, Churg–Strauss syndrome (oesinophilic flares in asthma), Behçet's disease (orogenital ulceration, skin, joint, ocular, and nervous system involvement).

Polyarteritis nodosa

Polyarteritis nodosa is a rare disease affecting 2.4 people per million in UK. It usually presents in men aged between 20 and 50 years but can present at any age. The aetiology is unknown but a minority of cases seem to be associated with active hepatitis B virus (HBV) infection. The incidence worldwide is related to the incidence of HBV.

Polyarteritis nodosa is a vasculitis of medium sized vessels. Fibinoid necrosis of the media of the medium and small arteries occurs with infiltration of oesinophils and polymorphs. Healing by fibrosis causes small aneurysms. Subsequent thrombosis results in ischaemic lesions.

Clinical features of polyarteritis nodosa are as follows:

- General features: weight loss, fever, and malaise.
- Cardiovascular features: hypertension occurs in all cases; angina and myocardial infarction; cardiomyopathy; pericarditis.
- Renal features: progressive renal failure.
- Respiratory features: late-onset asthma.
- Nervous system: poly- or mononeuritis multiplex.
- Cutaneous features: subcutaneous nodules, nail-bed arteritis.

Investigations are:

- Full blood count, which may indicate the presence of anaemia or leucocytosis with marked eosinophilia.
- Raised erythrocyte sedimentation rate and C-reactive protein.
- Hepatitis B viral screen, which may be positive.
- Antineutrophil cytoplasmic antibodies (ANCA) negative
- Tissue biopsy shows vasculitic lesions.

Treatment of polyarteritis nodosa:

- HBV-associated polyarteritis should be treated with antivirals and low-dose immunosuppression.
- Steroids have increased survival to >70%.

BOX 9.12 Dental implications of polyarteritis nodosa

- Steroids and their associated problems.
- Hepatitis B infection and cross-infection control and liver metabolism of drugs.
- Delayed healing due to vasculitis.
- Antihypertensive drugs.

- In non-HBV-associated disease try to induce remission, because disease does not recur once remission has been induced.

Kawasaki disease

Kawasaki disease is a medium vessel vasculitis. Described by Tomisaku Kawasaki in 1967 as a 'mucocutaneous lymph syndrome'. It affects children aged between 6 months and 8 years and is more common in boys (male : female ratio 3 : 2). Children of Japanese or Korean descent have a higher incidence of the disease but it can affect all racial and ethnic groups.

Kawasaki disease is thought to be caused by an infection. The bacterial components cross react with host tissue resulting in an autoimmune reaction. No firm evidence has been found of person to person spread. Both staphylococcal and streptococcal bacteria may be implicated: bacterial superantigens may stimulate and activate T cells to produce inflammatory cytokines.

Five of the following **clinical features** must be present for a diagnosis of Kawasaki disease:

- Fever lasting more than 5 days.
- Dry, red, fissured lips.
- Erythema of the oropharyngeal mucosa.
- Red 'strawberry' tongue.
- Conjunctival congestion.
- Macular truncal rash.
- Cervical lymphadenopathy.
- Red palms and soles.
- Oedema.
- Desquamation of fingers during convalescence.

Complications may include:

- Coronary artery thrombosis, narrowing and aneurysms.
- Myocarditis, pericarditis, and mitral valve prolapse.

There are no specific tests for Kawasaki disease. Some patients are ANCA positive and aneurysms may be seen on echocardiography. *Staphylococcus aureus* and streptococcus toxin may be detected in some patients.

Treatment is with high-dose intravenous immunoglobulin, which reduces the incidence of development of aneurysms. Aspirin at 100 mg/kg/day can be given until the child is afebrile, then continue at lower dose for 6 weeks.

BOX 9.13 Dental implications of Kawasaki disease

- The patient may present to the dentist with oral changes.
- Oral changes together with swollen cervical nodes should increase the index of suspicion.
- Cardiac complications may increase the risk for bacterial endocarditis.

Wegener's granulomatosis

Wegener's granulomatosis is a small vessel necrotizing granulomatous vasculitis. It is a rare disease affecting about 10 per million population per year in the UK; all racial groups equally affected.

Wegener's granulomatosis is an autoimmune disease of unknown aetiology. Drugs such as hydralazine, penicillamine and propylthiouracil may precipitate disease in genetically susceptible people. Infections such as *Staphylococcus aureus* are associated with relapse.

Wegener's granulomatosis has many **clinical features**:

- General features: weight loss, malaise; fever and night sweats; myalgia and arthralgia; polyarthritis.
- Respiratory system: upper respiratory tract symptoms occur in more than 90% of patients; sinusitis, nasal discharge, and ulceration (the septum may be perforated with otitis media, resulting in painless deafness); shortness of breath with a chronic non-productive cough; pleurisy; haemoptysis due to lung haemorrhage—this may be life-threatening.
- Renal: haematuria and proteinuria due to proliferative glomerulonephritis occurs in almost 80% of patients.
- Eye: proptosis due to retino-bulbar pseudotumour caused by granuloma.

Investigations:

- Kidney biopsy shows small vessel vasculitis.
- The lung and nasopharyngeal tissue show non-specific inflammation.
- PR3-ANCA is specific for proteinase 3. PR3-ANCA levels correlate with disease and are both sensitive and specific.
- Circulating ANCA can be used for monitoring disease.
- Chest X-ray shows diffuse pulmonary shadowing secondary to pulmonary haemorrhage.

Treatment should take place early to prevent permanent damage. Cytotoxic drugs and steroids leads to remission in 70–80% of cases Five-year survival is 80%. Morbidity results from pulmonary haemorrhage and opportunistic infection.

Polymyalgia rheumatica

Polymyalgia rheumatica is a clinical syndrome of limb girdle pain and stiffness and constitutional symptoms. It was described by William Bruce in Scotland in

---

BOX 9.14 Dental implications of Wegener's granulomatosis

- Wegener's may present in the mouth as ulceration.
- There are the usual problems associated with steroid use.
- Cytotoxic drugs may cause mucositis.

1888. It is a chronic debilitating disease twice as common in women as men, and commonest in Whites. It usually affects adults over the age of 50 years with a prevalence of around 1 in 200. Fifteen per cent of cases of polymyalgia have giant cell arteritis (GCA).

Polymyalgia rheumatica has an immunological aetiology. There appears to be a gentic association with HLA-DR4.

Clinical features include:

- Bilateral symmetrical shoulder and pelvic girdle pain and/or stiffness.
- Muscle stiffness, which may prevent the patient getting out of bed.
- Muscle stiffness is associated with non-specific symptoms of profound fatigue and low-grade fever.
- Weight loss.
- Depression, which is usually secondary to pain and limitation of physical activity.

An erythroycyte sedimentation rate (ESR) of over 40 is a good diagnostic criterion. C-reactive protein is also high. **Treatment** is with high-dose oral steroids such as prednisolone (15–20 mg/day). ESR and CRP levels are no guide to steroid dose.

Giant cell arteritis

Giant cell arteritis is a syndrome of focal arteritis resulting in blood vessel ischaemia; it is associated with the signs and symptoms of polymyalgia rheumatica. Polymyalgia rheumatica and giant cell arteritis are considered opposite ends of the same disease spectrum. Incidence of giant cell arteritis is 1 in 50 000 per year. It is more common in females (females : male ratio 4 : 1).

Clinical features:

- Sudden onset of a unilateral throbbing headache localized to the temporal area (temporal arteritis). The pain is associated with scalp tenderness and may disturb sleep.
- The pain may occur in the occipital region (vertebrobasilar arteritis).
- Other symptoms associated with vertebrobasilar arteritis are ataxia, vertigo, and hearing loss.
- Visual symptoms may result in sudden, painless, partial or complete loss of vision.
- Facial pain may occur with chewing or speaking.
- Fifty per cent of patients may have symptoms of polymyalgia rheumatica.
- General features: fever; weight loss; weakness and malaise; arthralgia and myalgia; headache.

Investigations:

- Biopsy before or within 24 h of starting steroids.
- ESR and C-reactive protein.

> **BOX 9.15** Dental implications of polymyalgia rheumatica and giant cell arteritis
>
> • Patients may present with severe facial pain.
> • The pain may mimic pain of dental origin.
> • The pain may be mistaken for temporomandibular joint pain or prodromal symptoms of herpes zoster.

Treatment:

• If the patient has visual loss administer 500–1000 mg methylprednisolone intravenously daily for 3–4 days.
• High-dose prednisolone (40–60 mg/day).

The spondyloarthropathies

The spondyloarthropathies are a group of disease which present with arthropathy alone or arthropathy associated with underlying systemic disease. The spondyloarthropathies have a strong genetic association with HLA-B27 and tend to occur within families. Infectious agents may act as triggers.

The spondyloarthropathies have the following characterisitics:

• HLA-B27 association.
• Autoantibodies are not present.
• Arthritis affects vertebral joints and the sacrum.
• The insertion of tendons and ligaments is affected.
• There is a large clinical overlap.
• Systemic involvement is usually with the eye, skin, and vascular (aorta and aortic valve) tissues.

Ankylosing spondylitis

Ankylosing spondylitis is a multisystem disease of young adults (age of onset usually less than 40 years). Males are more frequently affected than females (3 : 1). The presence of ankylosing spondylitis generally parallels the distribution of the *HLA-B27* gene. Prevalence is higher in Whites and certain native Americans (Inuit, Haida, and Pima) than in other non-White ethnic groups, with a peak incidence in the north of Norway.

Unknown environmental factors are thought to trigger disease in susceptible people. Women may have coexistent chronic inflammatory bowel disease, whereas men tend to have psoriatic arthropathy. There is a strong family history of ankylosing spondylitis in affected individuals.

Clinical features of ankylosing spondylitis are:

• Insidious onset of pain and fatigue which may be associated with morning stiffness.

- Early onset of pain in the lumbar spine followed later by increasing pain in the dorsolumbar spine.
- Limitation of movement of the lumbar spine in three planes.
- Patients develop kyphosis.

Extra-articular manifestations:

- General features: fever; malaise and fatigue; weight loss; raised ESR; anaemia.
- Specific features: iritis in 40%; lung fibrosis giving rise to dyspnoea and cough productive of sputum; respiratory failure; ulcerative colitis or Crohn's disease; aortic incompetence, cardiac conduction effects and cardiomegaly (these are usually seen as a late complication after 12–15 years); psoriasis; Achilles tendinitis.

Investigations may find:

- Severe sacroiliitis, which may be unilateral or bilateral, on X-ray.
- X-ray may show severe ossification of the vertebral discs and epiphyseal and sacroiliac joints.
- ESR may or may not be raised.
- Autoantibodies are negative.
- HLA-B27 is usually positive.

Treatment consists of supervised exercise and analgesia.

Reiter's syndrome

Reiter's syndrome is a post-infective arthritis which affects young men and women equally. It is diagnosed after an episode of oligoarthritis of the lower limb in association with cervicitis or urethritis. The preceding infection is often a sexually transmitted disease or bacillary dysentery. HLA-B27 association increases the risk of developing Reiter's syndrome by 40.

The **clinical features** of Reiter's syndrome are:

- A combination of urethritis, cervicitis and diarrhoea, conjunctivitis, and arthritis.
- The eye is frequently affected and presents as painful and red. This is due to conjunctivitis and less commonly iritis.
- Mucocutaneous lesions such as ulcers.
- Keratoderma blenorrhagicum, a pustular psoriasis, occurs on the soles of the feet.
- Circinate balanitis is also a psoriaform rash.
- There may be on-going low-grade gut infection

Treatment is by physiotherapy and exercise. Non-steroidal anti-inflammatory drugs are usually used for analgesia. Sixty per cent of patients recover within 6 months, but 50% will have further episodes. The fifteen per cent who develop chronic disease may benefit from steroids, sulphasalzine, and methotrexate.

> **BOX 9.16** Dental implications of ankylosing spondylitis
> - Patients may present with oral ulcers.
> - If a patient presents with oral lesions and a red eye urgent ophthalmological referral is required.
> - Patients with chronic disease may be on steroids or methotrexate.
> - Methotrexate may increase the frequency of oral ulcers.

Lyme disease

Lyme disease is a disease endemic in mammals in Europe and North America. It is caused by a spirochaete bacterium *Borrelia burgdorferi* transmitted to humans by tick (*Ixodes*) bites. (see Chapter 6.)

Gout

Gout is a spectrum of diseases due to hyperuricaemia and deposition of uric acid crystals in the tissues. It occurs predominantly in adult men:

- Primary gout: due to an inborn error of metabolism or familial hyperuricaemia
- Secondary gout: myeloproliferative disease, e.g. myeloid leukaemia, polycythemia rubra vera, and myelofibrosis; drug induced, e.g. diuretics, salicylates, phenylbutazone; due to chronic renal failure.

Gout has the following **clinical features**:

- The affected joint becomes hot, red, shiny, and very tender.
- The big toe is affected in 50% of cases.
- Attacks may be recurrent and can become polyarticular and asymmetrical.
- Gouty tophi on ears and joints.
- Complications include: renal disease, hypertension, and secondary pyogenic infection.

Investigations will find:

- Serum urate raised.
- ESR raised.
- White blood count commonly raised.
- Joint aspirate shows refractile crystals under the microscope.
- X-ray in the late stages show irregular punched out bony erosions.

Treatment:

- In the acute stages give analgesia (NSAIDs) for pain. Start allopurinol as soon as the pain is relieved.
- In chronic disease give allopurinol. This blocks the metabolic pathway of purine synthesis by inhibiting xanthine oxidase creating xanthine and hypoxanthine which are more soluble than uric acid. The dose is 300 mg/day reduced to 200 mg or 100 mg/day in patients with reduced renal function.

10 The respiratory system

The function of the respiratory system is to take in oxygen and remove carbon dioxide from the body. The physiological mechanisms that control ventilation, tissue perfusion, and gas exchange are multifaceted. Ventilation is controlled by chemosensory receptors in the carotid, the aorta and spinal cord which detect carbon dioxide tension and hypoxia.

Oxygen exchange takes place in the tissues and in the lungs. Loss of respiratory function and consequent respiratory disease is a cause of considerable morbidity and mortality, especially in children and the elderly.

COMMON CLINICAL FEATURES ON GENERAL EXAMINATION

Cyanosis is a blue discoloration of the mucosae or skin. It occurs in severe oxygen deficiency, due to excess of desaturated haemoglobin, i.e. >5 g/dl of haemoglobin in capillaries or abnormal haemoglobin in blood. The presence of cyanosis is a common sign of hypoxaemia:

- peripheral cyanosis—fingers and toes;
- central cyanosis—lips, mucous membranes, tongue.

Peripheral cyanosis is due to stenotic valve disease (reduced cardiac output) or cold (local vasoconstriction).
Central cyanosis is due to:

- Pneumonia.
- Chronic bronchitis (deficient oxygenation of blood in the lungs resulting in poor ventilation).
- Poliomyelitis, motor neuron disease (reduced lung ventilation).
- Fibrosing alveolitis (reduced oxygen transfer across alveolar capillary membrane).

Coughing is caused by irritation of the airways or increase of fluid secretions in the lung tissue. It is caused by forced expiration against a closed glottis. To overcome the closure forced expiration may reach speeds of up to 120 miles per hour. Cough may be dry or productive. A productive cough is the coughing up of sputum from the lungs.

Chest pain may arise from the skin of the chest wall, muscles, ribs, or cartilage, as well as the pleura. Pleuritic pain characteristically arises on movement and coughing. Pain is also felt on inspiration. This leads to the patient taking shallow breaths increasing the difficulty of clearing mucous in the airways.

Haemoptysis is the coughing up of blood and may be a sign of serious disease. Common causes of haemoptysis are:

- carcinoma of the lung
- pulmonary tuberculosis
- acute pneumonia
- bronchiectasis
- lung abscess
- left ventricular failure
- mitral stenosis
- pulmonary infarct

Less common causes are:

- polyarteritis nodosa
- Wegener's granulomatosis
- Goodpasture's syndrome
- aspergillosis.

Clubbing is increased curvature of the nails in both longitudinal and lateral directions with loss of the normal angle (approximately 140°) between the nail and cuticle. There is obliteration of the nail angle. Causes of clubbing are detailed in Chapter 2.

Other features: wheeze may be audible without a stethoscope and indicates airway obstruction. **Cervical nodes** may be pathologically enlarged in tuberculosis or bronchial carcinoma. **Accessory muscles** may be used in chronic obstructive pulmonary disease.

EXAMINATION OF THE CHEST

Initial inspection: respiratory rate and movements. The normal respiratory rate in a healthy adult is between 12–18 breaths a minute:

- **Dyspnoea** is the subjective awareness of the need for increased respiration (difficulty in breathing).
- **Orthopnoea**: patient experiences difficulty in breathing when lying down.
- **Tachypnoea**: a fast respiratory rate.
- **Apnoea**: the patient is not breathing at all.

Shape of the chest:
The shape of the chest gives clues to underlying pathology:

- barrel shape of hyperinflated chest;
- deformities pectus excavatum, kyphosis, scoliosis;
- operation scars.

Palpation and percussion of the chest are not required of the dentist in general practice. Familiarity with the technique will give the hospital-based

---

BOX 10.1 Causes of acute breathlessness

- Anxiety.
- Hyperventilation.
- Asthma.
- Metabolic acidosis.
- Chronic obstructive pulmonary disease (COPD).
- Pneumothorax.
- Anaphylaxis.
- Pulmonary embolism.
- Pleural effusion.
- Trauma.

---

dentist vital clues as to pre- and post-operative health of patients requiring an anaesthetic.

Palpation:

- Position of the mediastinum.
- Upper part—palpate the trachea in the suprasternal notch between the tips of two fingers.
- Lower part—localize the apex beat.
- Measure the cricosternal distance between lower border of the cricoid cartilage and the sternal notch (normally two to three fingers).
- Expansion: this is normally 5 cm in men.

Percussion: compare the percussion note at several levels on both sides and at the front and the back of the chest:

- The percussion note is decreased in areas of consolidation: pleural thickening, pulmonary fibrosis, pleural effusion.
- The percussion note is increased in areas of pneumothorax and emphysema.

Auscultation: listen with the diaphragm. Instruct the patient to breathe through the mouth and listen to both sides and at the front and the back of the chest.

- Normal sounds (vesicular) are low-pitched rustling sounds. The inspiratory phase is louder and twice as long as the expiration. This is followed by a pause.
- Bronchial breathing: this is higher pitched and with blowing breath sounds which are similar to the sounds heard over the trachea. Inspiration and expiration are of equal length with a small gap between them.
- Added sounds (adventitious):
  - Wheezes (also called rhonchi): indicate narrowed airways and are more prominent in expiration. Found in asthma and chronic bronchitis, bronchial stenosis (unilateral, unaffected by coughing), and retained secretion (diffuse, cleared by coughing).

- Crackles (rales or crepitations) are caused by opening of the airways on inspiration with sudden equalization of pressure along their length. Causes are pulmonary oedema, fibrosing alveolitis, pneumonia, chronic bronchitis, and emphysema.
- Pleural rub: infection, neoplasia, pulmonary infarction (bronchial carcinoma, tuberculosis, sarcoidosis, asthma, pulmonary embolism).

BRONCHIAL CARCINOMA

Bronchial carcinoma is the commonest malignant tumour in the Western world. It is the third commonest cause of death in the UK with 35 000 deaths and 40 000 new cases each year. It is more common in males (male : female ratio 3.5 : 1), but the mortality is rising in females and is now 1 in 8, second only to carcinoma of breast. Twenty per cent of smokers will develop lung cancer. The prognosis is poor because symptoms only occur when the tumour is approximately 3 cm in size and 80% of the way through its natural history. The staging of bronchial carcinoma is shown in Table 10.1.

Aetiology

Cigarette smoking is a direct cause in over 90% of all lung cancers. Risk is related to:

- The number of cigarettes consumed in year.
- The environment (e.g. passive smoking).

Table 10.1　Staging of bronchial carcinoma

Stage	Description
Stage I	
T_1	Tumour less than 3 cm
T_2	Tumour >3 cm or invades pleura or lobar collapse at the hilum
Stage II	
T_1, T_2, N	Nodal metastases in ipsilateral hilum
Stage IIIa	
Any T_3, any T_2 and N_2	Metastases in the ipsilateral mediastinum or subcarinal nodes
Stage IIIb	
Any T and N_3	Metastases in contralateral hilar or mediastinum and/or supraclavicular nodes
T_4 any N	Invades mediastinum, vertebrae, or carina, or causes malignant effusion
Stage IV	
Any T any N and M	Distant metastases

Abbreviations: T, tumour; N, nodes; M, metastases.

- Occupation, e.g. asbestos, silicosis, aluminium industry.
- Other diseases: radiation for other tumours; alveolitis of autoimmune disease, e.g. systemic sclerosis; cryptogenic fibrosing alveolitis.

Pathology

Most bronchial carcinomas arise in the central airways in the segmental or lobar bronchi. There are a number of tissue lesions:

- Small cell (oat cell): 15–20% of cases, grows rapidly and metastasizes early.
- Large cell and anaplastic: 7% of cases, very fast growing.
- Adenocarcinoma: 10–15% of cases, slow growing, may be peripheral, metastasizes at an intermediate time.
- Squamous cell: 60% of cases, slow growing, metastasizes late.

Clinical features

Five per cent of cases are asymptomatic and are diagnosed on a routine chest X-ray. The symptoms may be due directly to effects of the tumour, to the spread of the tumour, or due to metastasis or non-metastatic effects, e.g. biochemical or endocrine effects.

Symptoms
- Cough, which is dry and productive.
- Chest pain over the site of the tumour (22% of cases).
- Cough together with pain (15% of cases).
- Haemoptysis (7% of cases).
- Breathlessness, which may be insidious.

Signs
There may be no physical signs. Important signs are:

- Inspiratory monomorphic wheeze.
- Decrease in breathing sounds.
- Pleural effusion.
- Tenderness over rib.
- Finger clubbing.
- Palpable supraclavicular nodes.

BOX 10.2 Causes of haemoptysis

Haemoptysis may be caused by respiratory and cardiovascular causes. Oral bleeding may sometimes cause confusion.

- **Respiratory causes**: bronchial carcinoma, bronchitis, bronchiectasis, cystic fibrosis, lung abscess, pulmonary tuberculosis, pulmonary infarct, pneumonia.
- **Cardiovascular causes**: mitral stenosis, acute left ventricular failure.
- **Less common causes**: polyarteritis nodosa, foreign body, Wegener's granulomatosis, Goodpasture's syndrome, bleeding diathesis.

However, physicians should be wary of patients with persistent or recurrent chest infections who may have an occult lung tumour.

Clinical features associated with spread
Intrathoracic (direct):

- Pleural effusion.
- Pericarditis.
- Superior vena cava obstruction.
- Horner's syndrome associated with Pancoast's syndrome.
- Rib metastases.
- Pain: rib erosion or brachial plexus via Pancoast's tumour.
- Hoarseness due to recurrent laryngeal nerve palsy.
- Dysphagia due to compression of the oesophagus by enlarged lymph nodes or direct invasion by tumour.

Both Horner's syndrome and superior vena cava obstruction indicate inoperability.
   Extrahepatic (metastatic):

- liver (often silent)
- adrenal
- brain
- bone.

Non-metastatic extrapulmonary manifestions
The so-called paraneoplastic syndromes associated with lung cancer (especially the endocrine and neurological types) are most commonly associated with small cell lung cancer:

- Vascular manifestations: non-bacterial endocarditis; thrombophlebitis migrans.
- Neurological manifestations: encephalopathy; neuropathy; Eaton–Lambert myasthenic syndrome.
- Skeletal manifestations: nail clubbing; hypertrophic pulmonary osteoarthropathy.
- Endocrine manifestations: ectopic antidiuretic hormone (ADH); ectopic adrenocorticotrophic hormone (ACTH); raised calcium usually associated with squamous cell Ca due to secretion of parathyroid hormone-related protein (PTHrP) and multiple bony metastases; painful gynaecomastia.
- Haematological manifestations: disseminated intravascular coagulation; anaemia.

Investigations

Management must take into account the patient's general state of health and whether the patient is operable or needs chemotherapy. To do this a tissue diagnosis must be made. To establish histological diagnosis and stage the tumour the following investigations should be carried out:

- Sputum: three specimens for cytology will give a diagnosis in 70% of all bronchial carcinomas.
- Bronchoscopy: bronchial washings and biopsy will give a diagnosis in 60–70% of all bronchial carcinomas.
- Percutaneous needle biopsy.
- Excisional biopsy (if surgery appropriate).

Treatment

Surgery

Surgery should be considered in patients with limited disease and:

- Age less than 75 years.
- Adequate respiratory reserves, e.g. FEV greater than 1 litre.
- Tumour size larger than 2 cm from main carina on bronchoscopy.
- No evidence of mediastinal, chest wall, or distant metastasis on chest X-ray, CT of chest, liver, and adrenal glands, CT of head, or isotope bone scan.

It should be noted that of patients who have surgery:

- 20–25% of patients with non-small-cell lung cancer (NSCLC) are operable.
- Of those undergoing apparently curative surgery the 5-year survival rate is only 25% owing to undetected disseminated disease in the others.
- The morbidity and mortality from the operative procedure may be high.

Chemotherapy

Chemotherapy is the first line of treatment for small-cell lung cancer (SCLC) and can result in remission in up to 50% and a response in 80%. Chemotherapeutic agents used include cyclophosphamide, doxorubicin, vincristine, cisplatin, ifosfamide, etoposide, carboplatin, methotrexate, and epirubicin. Various

---

BOX 10.3 Dental management of patient with bronchial carcinoma

- Impaired respiratory function may prove hazardous in patients who have had either lung removal or lobectomy.
- Local anaesthetic is usually safe.
- Lung metastases may present in the bone of the mandible or maxilla.
- Always examine the posterior cervical triangle for the presentation of Pancoast's tumour.
- Radiotherapy to the lungs may cause xerostomia if the salivary glands are in the radiation field.
- Chemotherapy may affect the bone marrow causing immunosuppression and delayed healing or prolonged bleeding, as well as mucositis.
- Pigmentation of the oral soft tissues is a rare but early sign of disease.

combinations are used in well-established protocols and yield better results than single-agent therapy.

Radiotherapy

Consider chest radiotherapy if disease is limited with complete remission following chemotherapy to prevent local relapse. Prophylactic cranial radiation may reduce the risk of brain metastases.

Palliative care

Specialized palliative nursing care within a multidisciplinary team is needed. Radiotherapy is useful for SVC obstruction and bone pain and endobronchial laser therapy for obstruction in the proximal airways.

Smoking and health

Every year in the UK 120 000 people die from a smoking-related disease. Thirty per cent of all deaths are caused directly or indirectly by smoking.

The Health Survey for England, 2001, found that:

- In 2001 1% 11-year-olds and 15% of 15-year-olds were regular smokers.
- In 2001 33% of men and 30% of women were regular smokers.
- The daily consumption of cigarettes has increased from 14 per day for men and 6.8 per day for women in 1949 to 15 per day for men and 13 per day for women in 2001.

Smoking is a major cause of systemic morbidity:

- It causes changes in lung tissue and function and has a causal relation with chronic obstructive pulmonary disease, asthma, and increased episodes of infective pneumonia.
- It is associated with ischaemic heart disease, hypertension, and cerebrovascular accidents.
- It is associated with peripheral vascular disease. It is the main causal factor for the increase in Buerger's disease.
- Peptic ulceration.
- Premature births and low birth weight.
- Increases likelihood of early death.
- Dementia.
- Associated with increased morbidity from deep-vein thrombosis.
- Passive smoking occurs in 42% of UK households.
- Passive smoking is associated with asthma, cot deaths, middle ear disease, coronary artery disease, and lung cancer.
- Smoking decreases male and female fertility.
- Smoking increases the propensity to develop depression.
- Smoking increases the risk of carriage of meningococcal disease.
- Smoking has a causal relationship with several cancers in addition to lung cancer: oropharynx, oesophagus, breast, pancreas, kidney, bladder.

TUBERCULOSIS

Tuberculosis (TB) is a chronic granulomatous infection caused by *Mycobacterium tuberculosis* and is the world's leading cause of death from infection responsible for 3 million deaths per year and one-fifth of adult mortality in developing countries. It is estimated that one-third of the world's population is infected, with three-quarters of these being less than 50 years of age.

The number of reported cases in the UK was 6572 in 2000 and 6838 in 2001, with 50% occurring in the London area. Sixty-five per cent of cases are of pulmonary tuberculosis. Thirty per cent of reported cases arise outside the UK.

Dye *et al.* for the WHO Global Surveillance and Monitoring Project (Dye C *et al.* (1999) Global burden of tuberculosis: estimated incidence, prevalence, and mortality by country. *J. Am. Med. Assoc.* **282**: 677–86) reported 7.96 million new cases of TB in 1997. In the same year an estimated 1.87 million people died of TB. The global prevalence of TB infection in 1997 was 32%, i.e. 1.86 billion people. Globally, eighty per cent of all cases of TB were found in Southeast Asia, sub-Saharan Africa, and eastern Europe. There is a high rates of co-infection of tuberculosis and HIV in African countries.

TB is a re-emergent problem with case rates rising in Austria, Denmark, Ireland, Italy, Netherlands, Norway, Switzerland, UK, and the USA. Additionally, TB is of increasing concern owing to rising prevalence of multi-drug resistant forms of the disease (MDRTB). The increase in TB is due to:

- Co-infection of TB with HIV is 5–10% (people infected with HIV and TB have an **annual** risk of 10% of developing active TB compared with a **lifetime** risk of 10% in people infected with TB alone).
- Increase in the number of homeless and intravenous drug abusers in large cities in the west.
- Increased immigration from and travel to developing countries, e.g. countries of the former Soviet Union, the Indian subcontinent, and Africa.
- Poor treatment completion rates in industrialized countries.
- Loss to follow-up is a significant problem, and poor treatment compliance results in increased cross-infection and drug resistance.
- Increased air travel may have led to spread form areas where TB infection is common.

Pulmonary TB is caused by infection with *Mycobacterium tuberculosis*, an atypical or opportunistic mycobacterium. Generalized (systemic) tuberculosis can also be caused by infection with *Mycobacterium bovis* found in cattle.

The mortality rate in MDRTB outbreaks which have occurred in hospitals in the USA is 43–93%. The time from diagnosis to death is 4–6 weeks. Factors contributing to outbreaks are:

- Delay in diagnosis, initiation of therapy or recognition of drug resistance.
- Inadequate ventilation of houses and isolation of smear-positive infected individual also play a part.
- Inadequate nutrition, immunosuppression.

Assessment of risk for TB

People most at risk of TB infection include:

- The homeless and those living in densely overcrowded conditions.
- Health workers and contacts of smear-positive patients.
- Immunocompromised people, e.g. AIDS patients, patients on immunosuppressive drugs, transplant patients, alcoholics.
- Children and young adults.
- People from the Asian subcontinent and Africa.

The **probability** of infection for a given individual depends on:

- concentration of infected droplets
- duration of exposure.

The **characteristics** of a TB patient that enhance risk of transmission are:

- Disease in lungs, airways, or larynx.
- Cough.
- Acid-fast bacilli in sputum.
- Failure to cover mouth when sneezing or coughing.
- Cavitation on chest radiograph.
- Inappropriate or short treatment.
- Procedures that induce coughing or aerosolization.

Environmental factors that increase risk of transmission:

- Small enclosed spaces.
- Inadequate ventilation.
- Recirculation of infectious droplets.
- Crowding, which increases close contact.

Risk of hospital transmission is increased in personnel carrying out the following procedures:

- bronchoscopy
- endotracheal intubation
- suctioning
- open abscess irrigation
- autopsy
- sputum induction
- aerosol treatments that induce coughing.

Spread of TB

Mycobacterium tuberculosis is carried in airborne particles or droplet nuclei which are generated in those who have pulmonary or laryngeal lesions by sneezing, coughing, speaking, or singing. Particles are estimated to be 1–5 μm in size.

Groups with a higher risk of active disease from latent TB infection are:

- Those with a recent TB infection (less than 2 years previously).
- Children less than 4 years old.
- Those with fibrotic lesions on chest X-ray.
- Medical, nursing, dental, and laboratory personnel.
- Those with a medical history of: HIV; gastrectomy or jejuno-ileal bypass; 10% fall in body weight; chronic renal failure with dialysis; diabetes mellitus; immunosuppressive therapy; some malignancies; silicosis.

Pathogenesis

Primary infection is 'focused' in the lung and caseous regional lymph node lesions. These heal then calcify, causing complications of primary infection. Infection can spread via the bloodstream ('haematogenous' spread) to the lungs, bones, joints, and kidneys. Acute miliary tuberculosis is acute dissemination of infection throughout body. Progressive pulmonary tuberculosis may occur after primary infection or may occur after reactivation of latent infection.

Post-primary tuberculosis is reactivation of the original infection. The characteristic lesion is tuberculous cavities in the lung formed by caseating and liquefied material discharging from the bronchus. Pleural infection may result in pleural effusion.

Clinical features

Systemic features of TB include:

- Progressive weight loss and anòrexia.
- Malaise, night sweats, and pyrexia, mainly in the evenings.

Local features include:

- Lung involvement is demonstrated by a persistent dry cough. This may be accompanied by haemoptysis.
- Oral lesions—tuberculous ulcers—may be seen in the oral capacity. They appear after coughing up of infected material. These ulcers are deep and painful. On careful examination the deep ulcer can be seem to be teeming with mycobacteria.
- Cervical nodes: tuberculosis causes a hard solitary lesion to appear in the neck. The node is a classic caseating granulomatous lesion.
- Lupus vulgaris: a tuberculosed ulcer appears on the face. This is usually a large, painless ulcerating lesion. If a local lesion is found careful examination of the patient must be made to exclude widespread systemic disease.

Complications
- Pleural effusion.
- Pneumothorax.

- Emphysema.
- Enteritis.
- Kidney disease.
- Milliary spread.
- TB meningitis.
- Cor pulmonale.
- In a late stage a mycetoma (deep fungal infection) may form in the healed open cavity.

Investigations

- Radiological assessment.
- Chest X-ray may show upper lobe calcification, cavitation calcification. In exceptional circumstances, military or nodular pattern may be seen.
- Sputum or swabs from lesion are stained with Ziehl–Neelson stain or examined using the auramine–phenol fluorescent test. Multiple samples should be examined.
- The sputum or swab can be cultured on Lowenstein–Jensen medium, but may take 4–6 weeks.
- A diagnosis can be made in 24–48 h and the organism typed by using polymerase chain reaction.
- CT scan of the thorax may give more information on the extent of the disease.
- Bronchoscopy in suspected cases with negative sputum.
- Sample of pleural effusion shows straw-coloured fluid with a high protein content.
- Tuberculin testing may be helpful in primary diagnoses but both Mantaux and Heaf tests are more valuable in secondary disease.

The **Heaf test** is carried out in patients suspected of having TB or their contacts. Purified protein derivative (PPD) is injected intradermally and read after 48–72 h. A positive test result is graded as follows:

- Grade 1: discrete papules at three or more puncture points (may be faint).
- Grade 2: coalescence of papules to form an indurated ring.
- Grade 3: raised papules and induration of the surrounding area (5–10 mm).
- Grade 4: induration including central necrosis (>10 mm).
- People who have had a previous BCG vaccination may give a grade 3 or 4 reaction. However, these grades may also indicate current infection.
- Patients with atypical infection may be grade 1 positive.

Treatment

Drugs which form first-line treatment are shown in Table 10.2. (Note that streptomycin is not a first line drug. Streptomycin causes vestibular toxicity.) Sputum-positive TB is usually treated in hospital for 14 days until the sputum

Table 10.2 First-line drugs for treatment of TB

Drug	Action	Side-effects
Rifampicin	Bactericidal	Turns urine and sputum orange
		Alteration of liver function. Liver enzyme inducer—care with P-450 drugs used in dentistry, e.g. erythromycin, flucaonazole, metronidazole, warfarin, steroids
		Erythematous skin eruption
		Vasculitis
Isoniazid	Antimycobacterial	Hypersensitivity reactions
		Polyneuropathy which may affect the cranial nerves
		Inability to concentrate
		Low toxicity
		Hepatitis
Pyrazinamide	Bactericidal	Rashes
		Hepatitis (problems with drugs in dentistry, as above)
		Gout
		Hypersensitivity
Ethambutol	Bacteriostatic	Optic neuritis, which may be irreversible, may occur
		Renal function may be affected
		Hypersensitivity

BOX 10.4 Prevention of TB and the role of the dental surgeon

Prevention of TB depends on several measures including control-of-infection procedures:

- BCG intradermal injection may give 75–80% protection for 15 years in a UK based population.
- Dentists should maintain a high index of suspicion.
- Remember TB is spread by aerosol. Dental premises need to be well ventilated.
- Tuberculous ulcers in the mouth have mycobacteria in the base which stick to rubber gloves.
- Patients most at risk are the very young, the elderly, and the immunosuppressed. Dental staff are also at risk.
- Sputum and ulcer microscopy and direct smear examination are the best methods of detecting TB.
- Tuberculous cervical lymphadenopathy is the second commonest form of TB after pulmonary disease.

BOX 10.5 Further dental implications of tuberculosis

- Dental treatment of patients with known smear-positive pulmonary TB should be postponed until patients are given the all-clear by a physician.
- Patients with TB may also be infected with HIV.
- Rifampicin used in the treatment of TB causes red secretions, including staining of the saliva.
- TB organisms may survive for up to 2 weeks on dental equipment and work surfaces.
- Cross-infection between dental staff and patients may occur.

BOX 10.6 A risk assessment of dental surgery procedures for TB

- Assess the hazard of TB.
- Assess which patients or staff may come to harm.
- Assess how patients or staff may come to harm.
- Evaluate the risks associated with TB.
- Record findings.
- Review assessment with a view to modifying practices in the light of the TB hazard.

BOX 10.7 Modification of premises for TB prevention

- Local exhaust ventilation.
- General ventilation: HEPA filters (>99.97% of 0.3 μm droplets removed).
- UV germicidal irradiation 253 nm (UV-C 100–290 nm).
- Personal respiratory protective equipment: paper masks give very little protection. Plastic masks prevent inhalation of air-borne material.

---

is clear. Treatment failure is usually due to non-compliance, resistance, or inadequate therapy. Patients with HIV are more prone to TB and the disease is widely disseminated. Care must be taken with medication in HIV patients as rifampicin interacts with protease inhibitors and other antiretroviral drugs.

Contact tracing is very important in TB prophylaxis. The BCG (Bacille Calmette-Guérin) vaccine has variable success, but should never be given to immunosuppressed patients.

Atypical TB is frequently drug resistant.

Infection control procedures

There are law on infection control which may affect the dental surgeon. The following regulations have implications for the practicing dentist:

Health and Safety at Work Act 1974

This places a duty on all dentists to ensure the welfare, health, and safety of all their employees in the workplace and that all practices, information, instruction, and training are provided to ensure a safe working environment.

The 1992 Management of Health and Safety at Work Regulations
This requires assessment of the work environment as well as work practices.

*1992 General Dental Services NHS Regulation (as amended) and NHS
(Service Committees Tribunal amendment) Regulations 1996*
This regulates the suitability of premises and all equipment. If a lack of infection control has been deemed to take place, the local health authority may act through the NHS Tribunal or the General Dental Council directly to suspend a practitioner. **All dental premises are subject to inspection at any time by the Health and Safety inspectors**.

SARCOIDOSIS

Sarcoidosis is a granulomatous disorder of unknown aetiology. It is more common in Afro-Caribbeans and in the Irish and more women than men are affected. It usually occurs in people between the ages of 20 and 40.

The pathological features of sarcoidosis are non-caseating granulomas and infiltration of T cells around the granulomas.

Clinical features

Patients may be totally asymptomatic and the finding incidental or may be severely compromised by the disease:

- Bilateral hilar lymphadenopathy may be found incidentally on X-ray examination.
- Shortness of breath with or without a cough. This may vary from mild disease to incapacitating cough and distress due to shortness of breath.
- Systemic clinical manifestations: malaise, anorexia, weigh loss, salivary gland enlargement, jaundice due to liver involvement, erythema nodosum accompanied by tender red nodules over shins, joint pains and fever. Cerebral involvement ranges from mild headaches to disorientation. Renal involvement gives signs of renal failure.

Investigations and treatment

- Chest X-ray—even in asymptomatic patients bilateral hilar lymphadenopathy may persist for years. Serial chest X-rays are important in assessing the need for therapeutic intervention.
- Sputum for acid-fast bacilli is negative on culture and microscopy.
- Serum calcium and serum angiotensin converting enzyme both tend to be elevated in patients with active disease.
- Pulmonary function tests may show the restrictive nature of pulmonary involvement. Sequential measurement for disease activity is essential.
- Gallium scan isotope uptake is most frequent in the lungs, lachrymal, and submandibular glands.

> **BOX 10.8 Dental relevance of sarcoidosis**
>
> - The salivary glands are frequently involved. Patients present with bilateral or uni-lateral swellings of either the parotid or submandibular glands. Biopsy of the glands will slow typical non-caseating granuloma. Pain and fever may accompany swelling of the glands (Heerfordt's syndrome).
> - Care is necessary with patients undergoing general anaesthetic procedures. The first indication of disease may be during the pre-operative assessment chest X-ray, or unexplained hypoxia during a surgical procedure.
> - Seventy-five per cent of all patients with sarcoidosis have hepatic involvement from mildly abnormal liver function tests to frank and severe jaundice.
> - The abnormal liver function may impair metabolism, e.g. metronidazole, picana-zoles, erythromycin, precipitate hepato-renal syndrome, and increase perioperat-ive bleeding.
> - Renal involvement may precipitate both renal failure and hypertension.
> - Medication may include antihypertensive drugs as well as corticosteroid therapy.
> - Corticosteroid therapy affects both immunosuppression and delays wound heal-ing and may precipitate adrenocortical failure postoperatively.

- The Heaf test is usually negative. Kveim tests are no longer performed.
- Slit-lamp examination of eyes.
- Lashley cup collection of saliva or whole saliva.

   Treatment depends on whether the patient is symptomatic or not:

- Asymptomatic patients: review at 1, 2, 6, and 12 weeks.
- Symptomatic patients: the mainstay of treatment is corticosteroids. How-ever, specific treatment for major organ involvement may also be necessary.

ASTHMA

Asthma is caused by a reversible airway obstruction which resolves spontan-eously or with treatment.

   Asthma is increasing in incidence, with 10% of children in the UK having asthma. In adults males and females are affected equally, but in children boys are more often affected than girls. Asthma is most common in the first decade of life. The next peak in incidence is in the third and fourth decades.

Aetiology

Intrinsic asthma:

- Atopy: an increased sensitivity to common environmental agents associated with raised IgE levels. Related to a gene on the short arm of chromosome 11 which is also implicated in hay fever and atopic eczema.
- Bronchial hyperactivity.

Extrinsic asthma:

- Asthma brought on by specific allergens, e.g. house dust mite, pollen, cats, dogs.

  Factors which may provoke asthmatic attack include:

- exercise or cold air
- night or early morning
- allergens, e.g. house dust mite, cat and dogs, pollen
- stress and emotion
- respiratory infection, e.g. viral
- drugs e.g. beta blockers, aspirin
- diet, e.g. tartrazine and other allergens
- occupational exposure.

Pathogenesis

Asthma is characterized by a triad of oedema, bronchoconstriction, and increased mucus secretions. These changes are mediated by mast cells—histamine, prostaglandin D2, leucotrienes—and lymphocytes—IL5 activates eosinophils which release major basic proteins which cause shedding of the lung epithelium.

Clinical features

The natural history is characteristic:

- Patients may have a history of atopy.
- Breathlessness.
- Wheeze (expiratory polyphonic).
- Cough (often nocturnal) may be the only symptom.

Not all symptoms may be present, and asthma can mimic recurrent chest infections. Provoking factors may also help in making a diagnosis.

Examination may be normal. A widespread expiratory wheeze may be heard, which may be provoked if not present on examination.

Investigations and management

- Sputum and peak expiratory flow rate (PEFR).
- Chest X-ray excludes pneumothorax and hyperinflation.
- Arterial blood gases will be measured in hospital in patients who are having an acute attack: in a life-threatening attack there will be a normal or high $Paco_2 > 5$ kPa, $Pao_2 < 8$ kPa and a low pH of less than 7.35.
- Lung function tests show an obstructive pattern: PEFR shows a $>15\%$ improvement with bronchodilators; peak flow charts are useful in management.
- Skin tests may identify extrinsic causes.
- Other tests: allergen provocation test may identify causes; exercise test; methacholine bronchial provocation test.

BOX 10.9 Dental relevance of asthma

- Oral candidosis is common with inhaled steroids, patients should be told to rinse after using their inhaler.
- Hoarseness may occur due to myopathy of the vocal cords secondary to inhaled steroids.
- Beta agonists may cause tremor, cramps, and headaches.
- Anxiety in dental patients may precipitate an asthmatic attack: reassure patients and reduce anxiety.
- Patients may be asked to use a bronchodilator before treatment.
- Dental procedures should be carried out under local anaesthesia where possible.
- Prolonged use of steroids may cause delayed healing and adrenocortical suppression.
- Analgesics such as aspirin and NSAIDs used for dental pain relief may precipitate an asthmatic attack.

BOX 10.10 Clinical features in a patient having an asthma attack in the dental surgery

Severe attack:

- Inability to complete sentences in one breath.
- Respiratory rate greater than 25 per minute.
- Pulse greater than 110 beats per minute.
- Peak expiratory flow less than 50% of predicted or best value.

Life-threatening features:

- Peak expiratory flow less than 33% of predicted or best value.
- Silent chest.
- Feeble respiratory effort.
- Cyanosis.
- Bradycardia or hypotension.
- Exhaustion or confusion or loss of consciousness.

BOX 10.11 Initial management of an acute asthmatic attack in the dental surgery

- Stay calm and reassure the patient.
- Stop all dental treatment.
- Sit the patient upright.
- Administer 100% oxygen.
- Administer the patient's own inhaler or oxygen with 5 mg of nebulized salbutamol.

The British Thoracic Society guidelines on therapy for prevention of asthma attacks are:

- sodium cromoglicate (β2 adrenoceptor agonist)
- beclomethasone (systemic corticosteroid)
- in severe asthma immunosuppressive drugs—methotrexate and cyclosporin—may even be used.

CHRONIC OBSTRUCTIVE PULMONARY DISEASE (COPD)

Is a collection of heterogeneous conditions including bronchitis, emphysema, and chronic persistent asthma, which result in progressive pulmonary airway obstruction. It is often called the English disease and is associated with cigarette smoking, pollution, and cold wet weather.

Chronic bronchitis has:

- A cough productive of sputum on most days for 3 months of 2 successive years.
- Obstruction caused by narrowing the airway lumen with mucosal thickening and excess mucus.

Emphysema has:

- Dilation of the air spaces by destruction of their walls.
- Obstruction by decreasing the lungs' elastic recoil which holds airways open in expiration.

Clinical features

Symptoms are cough, sputum, dyspnoea, and wheeze. **Signs** are hyperinflation, hypertrophied accessory muscles, wheezes, crepitations, cyanosis, quiet breath sounds, and cor pulmonale.

'Pink puffers' and 'blue bloaters'
Pink puffers:

- increased alveolar ventilation
- normal or low P_{CO_2}
- normal P_{O_2}
- breathless but not cyanosed
- may progress to type I respiratory failure.

Blue bloaters:

- decreased alveolar ventilation
- raised P_{CO_2}
- low P_{O_2}
- cyanotic, and if cor pulmonale develops 'blue bloaters' rely on hypoxic drive.

Investigations

- Chest X-ray shows hyperinflation more than six anterior ribs above the diagram, bullae, and a flat hemidiaphragm.
- Lung function tests: obstruction with air-trapping FEV1/FVC $\ll 70\%$ (ratio of the forced expiratory volume in the first 1 s to the forced vital capacity of the lungs).
- Residual volume (RV) high.

- Total lung capacity (TLC) high.
- Full blood count: secondary polycythaemia (i.e. increase in red blood cells and Hb without an increase in red cell mass).

Treatment

The aim of treatment is to reduce symptoms and improve the quality of life. The most important measure is cessation of smoking. Symptomatic relief is provided by bronchodilators. The use of bronchodilators depends on the severity of disease:

1. Salbutamol.

- Mild disease: beta agonist or an anticholinergic drug. 2. ipratropium.
- Moderate disease: beta agonist combined with an anticholinergic drug.
- Severe disease: combination of beta agonist, anticholinergic via nebulizer, and theophylline. Continuous oxygen via an oxygen concentrator may prolong survival.

RESPIRATORY FAILURE

There are two types of respiratory failure:

- Type 1 respiratory failure. Arterial $Pao_2 < 8$ kPa + $Paco_2 < 6.5$ kPa. Due to a failure of the lungs to exchange gas (pneumonia, asthma, pulmonary embolism, pulmonary fibrosis).

BOX 10.12 Dental relevance of COPD

- Dental treatment should be carried out using local anaesthesia in patients with COPD.
- Patients may have bouts of uncontrollable coughing making long dental procedures difficult.
- Treat patients in the upright position. They become increasingly breathless when supine and may have heart failure.
- Avoid rubber dams, they cause further airway obstruction.
- Avoid general anaesthetic.
- If general anaesthetic is required keep the surgical procedure as short as possible, admit preoperatively, make sure patients stop smoking, and introduce intensive pre-operative physiotherapy. Monitor blood gases.
- In the hospital setting opiates are contraindicated, use pethidine for analgesia. Monitor arterial blood gases.

BOX 10.13 Dental aspects of management of patients with respiratory failure

- General anaesthetic is contraindicated.
- Avoid sedatives.
- Both the above will worsen respiratory failure.

- Type 2 respiratory failure. Arterial $Pao_2 < 8$ kPa $+ Paco_2 > 6.5$ kPa. Type 2 respiratory failure is due to a number of conditions: fatigue of the respiratory muscles (e.g. polyneuritis); damage to the respiratory centre (e.g. trauma to the head or cerebrovascular accident); disturbance of central control of respiration (e.g. exacerbation of COPD).

Clinical features

- Low oxygen levels (hypoxaemia) cause cyanosis, confusion, restlessness, and coma.
- High carbon dioxide levels (hypercapnia) cause bounding pulse, flapping tremor of hands, warm peripheries, and drowsiness.

Treatment

Treat the underlying condition. Give supplemental oxygen by mask or nasal cannula (note: patients with COPD cannot tolerate high concentrations of oxygen).

PULMONARY EMBOLISM

Pulmonary embolism (the process by which a solid, liquid, or gas enters and lodges within blood or lymphatic vessels during life) occurs when a thrombus that has formed in the deep venous circulation breaks away from its site of origin and travels to the lungs, via the right side of the heart. Lodging in the pulmonary arteries it obstructs the blood flow through the lungs causing hypoxia and possibly death. (A thrombus is a solid mass formed in the circulation from the constituents of the blood. If platelets and fibrin are dominant the thrombus is pale and if many red cells dominate the thrombus is dark red.). Thrombosis is caused by:

- changes in the coagulation mechanism of the blood,
- changes in the endothelium,
- changes in blood flow

known as **Virchow's triad**.

The risk of fatal pulmonary embolism in high-risk patients in hospital is 5%. Deep vein thrombosis (DVT) occurs in 33% of patients in intensive therapy units, in 8–15% of patients after major surgery, and in 40–80% after knee replacement. DVT may spread in calf veins and extend proximally into pelvic veins. Fragments of pelvic vein clot may break off to form pulmonary embolism. For every 1000 post-operative patients pulmonary embolism cause two deaths per year. Most patients who are going to die from a pulmonary embolism do so in the first 30 min. Thirty to 60% of patients who suffer a DVT develop post-phlebitic limb syndrome.

Pulmonary embolism is more common over the age of 40, but can occur in young women taking the combined oral contraceptive pill and during pregnancy. Women are more often affected than men due to the above factors.

Predisposing factors for pulmonary embolism:

- Age over 40.
- Severe obesity.
- Immobility, e.g. more than 4 days' bed rest.
- Pregnancy and the puerperium.
- High-dose oestrogens.
- Previous deep vein thrombosis or pulmonary embolus.
- Thrombophilia, e.g. in systemic lupus erythematosus or lupus anticoagulant.
- The following diseases or surgical procedures: trauma or surgery, malignancy, heart failure, recent myocardial infarct, paralysis of the lower limbs, severe infection, nephritic syndrome, polycythaemia, Behçet's disease.

Clinical signs

A **small embolus** may be asymptomatic except for a few basal crackles. A **large embolus** has the following signs:

- The patient is short of breath.
- The patient looks unwell and may have cyanosis.
- Sudden death.
- Right ventricular heave, gallop rhythm, tachycardia.
- There is a prominent A wave in the jugulo-venous pressure.
- The second heart sound may be loud because of pulmonary hypertension.

In **all emboli**:

- A pleural rub may be heard.
- There is pyrexia if infarction is present.
- Haemoptysis.

Investigations

The following investigations should be performed:

- Full blood count.
- Arterial blood gases.
- Chest X-ray.
- ECG.
- Ventilation/perfusion scan.
- Pulmonary angiography (for large emboli).
- Microscopy (at post-mortem).

Management

Prevention
- Be aware of risk.
- Use compression stockings.

- Use intermittent pneumatic compression.
- Use subcutaneous low-molecular-weight heparin.
- Give warfarin.

Treatment
The following treatments are used:

- intravenous/subcutaneous heparin
- intravenous fluids
- thrombolysis
- embolectomy
- warfarin.

The exact treatment mode depends on the size of the embolus:

- Small: patient may asymptomatic. Short-term anticoagulant or aspirin.
- Medium size embolus: start with subcutaneous low-molecular-weight heparin and intravenous fluids. Consider thrombolysis, then warfarinize. Long-term anticoagulants.
- Large embolus: Urgent, medical emergency. Embolectomy and thrombolysis. Patients frequently do badly.

PNEUMONIA

Pneumonia results from inflammation of the lungs. It is the most common form of infection of the lower respiratory tract. Pneumonia may be either primary or secondary. Primary infection usually occurs in the community, whereas secondary infection occurs in patients who have underlying lung pathology. The aetiology depends on the infecting organism and initial state of health of the patient.

Pneumonia affects 2–2.6 per 1000 adults per year in the UK. This figure is higher in the elderly and infirm.

Infective pneumonia can be caused by bacterial (see Table 10.3), viral (respiratory syncytial virus, influenza, mumps, Varicella zoster; these usually result in a secondary bacterial infection), or fungal (Candida, Histoplasmosis, *Pneumocystis carinii* in immunosuppressed patients, toxoplasmosis) infection. In addition allergens, chemicals, and physical agents can all cause non-infective pneumonia.

Clinical features

Symptoms of pneumonia are

- Non-specific symptoms: fever, sweats, confusion.
- Respiratory symptoms: cough, with or without sputum, shortness of breath, haemoptysis.

Table 10.3 Causes of bacterial pneumonia

Bacterium	Percentage of cases
Streptococcus pneumoniae	35–40%
Haemophilus influenzae	10–15%
Mycoplasma pneumoniae	7–10%
Legionella pneumophila	5%
Chlamydia psittaci	3%
Staphylococcus aureus including MRSA	5%
Mycobacterium tuberculosis	0.5–1%
Klebsiella pneumoniae	1%

MRSA, methicillin-resistant *Staphylococcus aureus*.

Table 10.4 Clinical and laboratory features of severe pneumonia

Clinical features	Respiratory rate >30
	Mental confusion
	Diastolic blood pressure <60 mmHg
	Atrial fibrillation
	Multilobar involvement
Laboratory features	White cell count $<4 \times 10^9$
	Bacteraemia
	Urea >7 mmol/l
	Albumin <35 g/dl

Lobar pneumococcal pneumonia can give rise to the following complications:

- Non-specific symptoms: septicaemia, Herpes labialis, arrhythmias, deep vein thrombosis, cardiac failure.
- Respiratory symptoms: pleurisy with effusion, empyema, delayed resolution.

Investigations

- Sputum for microscopy, culture, and sensitivity.
- White cell count and blood cultures.
- Urea and electrolytes, liver function tests.
- Chest X-ray and blood gases.

Table 10.4 shows the clinical and laboratory features of severe pneumonia.

Treatment

Treatment depends on the infecting organism; local protocols should be followed. Common forms of community acquired pneumonia require empirical treatment before culture and sensitivity results are available—use amoxicillin or erythromycin/clarithromycin. In severe cases the advice of a microbiologist must be taken.

CYSTIC FIBROSIS

Cystic fibrosis is a multisystem disorder caused by defective sodium and chloride transport across the lung epithelium. The airways are obstructed by tenacious secretions and patients are at risk of repeated chest infections.

Cystic fibrosis is a common autosomal recessive disorder which mainly affects Whites of northern European ancestry. It leads to early death from respiratory failure, but recent treatment advances have improved morbidity and length of life. The gene for cystic fibrosis (*CFTR*) is located on the long arm of chromosome 7, encoding for the cystic fibrosis transmembrane conductance regulator. A mutation in the *CFTR* gene results in defective transport of sodium and chloride ions and highly viscous secretions. Cystic fibrosis occurs in 1 in 2500 live births and the carrier frequency is 1 in 25.

Clinical features

Cystic fibrosis has numerous clinical features:

- repeated lower respiratory tract infections
- bronchiectasis
- nasal polyps
- finger clubbing
- abnormal sweat secretion
- pancreatic insufficiency
- diabetes mellitus
- steatorrhoea
- jaundice due to liver disease
- portal hypertension
- gallstones
- fractures from osteoporosis
- infertility
- arthritis
- risk of pneumothorax.

Investigations

- A sweat test shows >60 mmol/l sodium and chloride.
- Patients can be screened for polymorphisms of the defective gene.
- Chest X-ray shows varying degrees of bronchiectasis.

Management

- Physiotherapy with patients participating in home self-directed activity.
- Antibiotics, which may need to be given prophylactically. Patients often require courses of antibiotics for pseudomonal and staphylococcal chest infections.

- Bronchodilators for symptomatic relief.
- Pneumococcal and influenza vaccine as prophylaxis.
- Nutritional pancreatic supplements.
- In the later stages patients may require supplemental oxygen and heart or lung transplantation.

GENERAL PROBLEMS FACED BY RESPIRATORY PATIENTS REQUIRING DENTAL CARE

- All patients with respiratory disease have the right to good oral health.
- The main symptom of respiratory disease is breathlessness.
- Patients with chronic breathlessness, as in chronic obstructive pulmonary disease, often do not present for care because of difficulty with mobility which is restricted because of breathlessness.
- At the dental surgery breathlessness may be exacerbated by anxiety and hyperventilation.
- Patients have difficulty lying flat and need to be treated in the upright position.
- Dental procedures by necessity partially occlude the airway and increase dyspnoea. For this reason many patients cannot tolerate the use of a rubber dam.
- Patients with respiratory disease tend to be smokers, which causes staining as well as predisposing to periodontal disease and poor wound healing.
- Steroid medication in inhalers and taken systemically predisposes these patients to oral candidosis.

BOX 10.14 Procedure for dealing with a respiratory patient who becomes acutely breathless

- The main cause is usually anxiety together with pain of dental origin.
- Make sure there is no obstruction to the airway.
- Reassure the patient by acting and speaking in a calm manner.
- Sit patient upright in the dental chair.
- Use the patient's own inhaler and ask the patient to take two puffs.
- Give the patient 30% oxygen via a mask.
- Stay calm and count the respiratory rate.
- If there is no improvement in 5 min give 5 mg of nebulized salbutamol.

BOX 10.15 Dental relevance of diseases of the respiratory system

- Patients have a right to good oral health.
- Patients frequently do not attend dental appointments because of recurrent chest infections.
- Patients have recurrent lower respiratory tract infections and may be on long-term antibiotics.
- Patients may also have: chronic sinusitis, nasal polyps, liver disease, diabetes.
- Patients become increasingly short of breath as the disease progresses.

- Steroids and hypoxaemia also predispose to poor wound healing and the development of a dry socket after extraction.
- Antibiotics used for recurrent chest infections interact with the patient's therapeutic regime. Examples are: erythromycin and ciprofloxin which interact with aminophylline; erythromycin which interacts with antifungals.
- Some drugs suppress the respiratory system and should be used with caution: e.g. benzodiazepines.
- Do not give any sedative premedication: dihydrocodeine, pethidine, morphine, or potent analgesics.

11 Psychiatry

THE MENTAL STATE

Psychosocial disorders are an essential component of human disease. It is extremely important when dealing with patients to be able to establish good rapport and recognize any abnormal psychosocial problems. When examining the mental state, the aim is to build up a comprehensive picture of the patient's life, aspects of which are:

- social: occupation, age, sex, family, marriage, etc.
- physical: medical illnesses, heredity
- psychological: cognitive, e.g. thinking, perceiving, remembering, IQ; affective, e.g. emotion, conative, e.g. motivation.

Formal testing includes orientation in time and place, memory, concentration, intelligence, general knowledge, attention and concentration, and insight. When taking a history and assessing the patient note:

- General behaviour: observe the patient closely during the interview, at daily living if possible and interaction with other patients and staff.
- Speech: note both form (how the patient talks, e.g. fluid, stuttering, staccato) and content (if the content is appropriate or not), if spontaneous, and note topics of conversation covered.
- Mood: observe the patient's mood with reference to the content of speech. Note if the patient's observed mood is the same or discrepant with their subjective account of their mood.
- Delusions and hallucinations: note the patient's beliefs, whether are they appropriate, and if the patient has any hallucinations. Record the type of hallucination, whether visual, olfactory, tactile, or auditory

The neurotic state

People with neuroses form the largest group of patients consulting psychiatrists. They usually have insight into their problems. Types of neuroses include anxiety disorders, obsessive disorders, and phobic disorders.

The psychotic state

Psychoses are major psychiatric illnesses. The patient has no insight into their problem. The major forms are manic depressive psychoses and schizophrenias.

Definitions and terminology

The **Mental Health Act 1959, Section 4**, defines a psychopathic disorder as a persistent disorder/disability of the mind (whether or not including subnormality of intelligence) which results in abnormally aggressive or socially irresponsible conduct on the part of the patient and requires or is susceptible to medical treatment.

The **Mental Heath Act 1983, Section 1** gives a definition of mental disorder divided into four categories: severe mental impairment, mental impairment, psychopathic disorder, and mental illness. These are detailed below:

Mental disorder

The Mental Heath Act 1983, Section 1 defines mental disorder as: 'Mental illness, arrested or incomplete development of mind, psychopathic disorder and any other disorder or disability of mind.' The four subcategories of mental disorder are:.

- **Severe mental impairment:** Defined by the Act as 'A state of arrested or incomplete development of mind which includes severe impairment of intelligence and social functioning and is associated with abnormally aggressive or seriously irresponsible conduct on the part of the person concerned.'
- **Mental impairment:** Defined by the Act as 'A state of arrested or incomplete development of mind (not amounting to severe mental impairment) which includes significant impairment of intelligence and social functioning and is associated with abnormally aggressive or seriously irresponsible conduct on the part of the person concerned.'
- **Psychopathic disorder:** Defined by the Act as 'A persistent disorder or disability of mind (whether or not including significant impairment of intelligence) which results in abnormally aggressive or seriously irresponsible conduct on the part of the person concerned.'
- **Mental illness:** This is not defined under the Act. It leaves this as a matter for 'medical judgement'. However, this is the most common form of mental disorder.

The Department of Health provides a guide to mental illness where the patient has one or more of the following characteristics:

- more than temporary impairment of intellectual functions;
- more than temporary alteration of mood (including delusional ideation);
- delusional beliefs, persecutory, jealous, or grandiose;
- abnormal perceptions associated with delusional misinterpretation of events;
- thinking disordered to such a degree to warrant the detention of the patient.

ANXIETY AND ANXIETY DISORDERS

Anxiety is a normal response to stressful events. **Fear** is defined as a state of acute anxiety linked to the presence of a particular object, person, or stimulus, which subsequently leads to avoidance behaviour. **Anxiety disorder** is defined as an unpleasant emotional state with autonomic symptoms. In anxiety disorder there is the development of significant physical and psychological symptoms, in the absence of stress, which impairs the patient's day to day functioning.

There are a number of types of anxiety disorder:

- panic attacks
- phobias
- obsessive and compulsive disorder
- generalized anxiety.

Panic attacks

Three per cent of the population are affected by panic attacks, which generally occur in early adulthood. Panic attacks are severe and frightening attacks of anxiety of sudden abrupt onset. The attacks are accompanied by feelings of impending doom as well as autonomic symptoms of palpitations, shortness of breath, and dizzy spells, with or without collapse. An attack usually lasts a few minutes.

Panic attacks are seen in patients with chronic medical disorders, or patients who have been investigated for unexplained symptoms. The attacks are, however, associated with but not caused by any of the above. Patients suffering from panic attacks may have been under severe stress in their personal or working environment.

Treatment is by cognitive therapy with or without the use of drugs.

Phobias

Eight per cent of the population are affected by a phobia. Phobias are characterized by a fear of a place, object, or situation. The phobic situation precipitates sudden severe anxiety. Treatment is usually by supervised exposure using cognitive therapy.

Common phobias are:

- Agoraphobia: fear of open spaces. Usually occurs in middle-aged females. The patient can become housebound.
- Social phobia: a fear of being evaluated by others. Usually begins in the teens. Patients avoid social situations and show symptoms of anxiety and fear when exposed socially.
- Discrete phobias of an object or situation: These start in childhood, and are usually irrational fears of, for example, flying, spiders, or snakes. The patient tries to avoid any situation in which the object of the fear could be encountered.

Compulsive/obsessive disorder

These are repeated acts, thoughts, or speech present for at least 2 weeks:

- **Compulsion** is the insistent urge to perform or repeat an act which the patient consciously repudiates.

> **BOX 11.1** Dental relevance of anxiety disorders
> - The dental management of patients with anxiety disorders may become very difficult.
> - A previously simple problem assumes a significance out of all proportion to its importance.
> - Careful assessment of both the patient's oro-dental problem as well as their mental state may preclude complicated treatment which may never be perceived as satisfactory. Patients must be reassured, as any indication of pathology will elicit exaggerated morbid or obsessive thoughts and increase underlying anxiety or reinforce obsessive behaviour or phobia.

- **Obsession** is a constantly recurring thought of which the patient tries to rid their mind and is also recognized as being their own.

Obsessive thoughts or compulsive acts are unpleasantly repetitive and distressing and interfere with daily activity.

Treatment is by serotonin inhibitors, e.g. clomipramine, fluoxetine, sertraline, and fluvoxamine, and behavioural or psychosocial therapy.

SCHIZOPHRENIA

In the UK the incidence of schizophrenia is 0.1 or 0.2 per 1000 and the prevalence 3 per 1000. The incidence of schizophrenia is higher than average in people of Afro-Caribbean and African origin living in the UK. More males than females develop schizophrenia (male : female ratio 1.42 : 1).

Schizophrenia is a multifactorial, multidisease process which comprises a number of severe mental disorders. Components are: thought disorder, withdrawal from reality, disorders of perception (hallucinations and illusions), disorders of affect, and disorders of behaviour. There are four types of schizophrenia: simple, catatonic, hebephrenic, and paranoid.

Schizophrenia is a disorder of neurological development involving lateral ventricle enlargement, reduced size of the temporal lobes, widening of the cortical sulci, and dopamine transmission abnormalities. There is a genetic component to the development of the disease, with twin studies showing concordance rates of 35–40% in monozygotic twins and 10–15% in dizygotic twins. First-degree relatives of schizophrenics have an increased risk of being affected. People born in late winter or early spring have an increased risk of developing schizophrenia. It is also increased in first-generation immigrants.

Clinical features

First-rank symptoms (Schneider)
- Auditory hallucinations: audible thoughts; third person commenting on subject's actions; third person directing, talking, or arguing with the subject.

- Somatic passivity—belief that feeling, thoughts etc. are imposed and not the patient's own.
- Thought broadcast.
- Thought withdrawal or insertion.
- External control of feelings or actions.
- Delusional perception.

It is important to remember that first-rank symptoms may occur in hypothyroidism, drug-induced psychosis (e.g. alcoholism, amphetamines, LSD, cocaine), temporal lobe epilepsy, and cerebral infection, trauma, or tumours.

Clinical presentations
- Thought disorder occurs in up to 20% patients.
- Patients may make up new words (neologisms) or use known words in new ways (parapluralism).
- Speech may be totally incomprehensible.
- Hallucinations: these are usually auditory; but may be visual or olfactory sensations which occur without external stimuli. The hallucinations tend to be a prominent feature and each episode may be prolonged.
- Mood: the patient's mood may be exhibited by a flat affect (flat emotional response). Similarly they may experience delusional feelings.
- Delusions: these are false beliefs that are held and are not in keeping with the patient's social or cultural background, and despite all the evidence and rational arguments are still firmly held by the patient. Paranoid delusions are very common. They may be bizarre and vary from hypochondriacal and persecutory delusions to the religious, grandiose, or maniacal.
- Passivity: this is delusional in that the patient believes that the thoughts, emotions, and sensations experienced are not personal but are imposed by an outside force.

Treatment

There are two main forms of treatment: antipsychotic drugs and social management.

Drugs
Drugs are the mainstay treatment. They are used to control both psychotic symptoms and behaviour. It is important to remember that antipsychotic drugs may have oral side-effects:

- Chlorpromazine has side-effects postural hypotension and extrapyramidal effects including dry mouth and lichenoid reactions.
- Clozapine has fewer extrapyramidal effects but hypersalivation is common. Patients may also become neutropenic, resulting in oral ulceration. They are at increased risk of seizures.

> **BOX 11.2** Dental relevance of schizophrenia
>
> - The oral side-effects of some antipsychotic medication may mean that patients with schizophrenia will have a high requirement for dental care.
> - Practice point: if a patient becomes acutely unwell in the dental surgery let the patient know that you want to help. Remain calm and non-judgemental. This may help to decrease the patient's agitation. Leave the surgery door open and position yourself so that you have a clear exit route. If you think the consultation may end in violence call for help. If you feel insecure or frightened, leave quickly and return only when you have sufficient support.

Social management

Social management will take place after acute drug management, during recovery. It may include occupational and behavioural therapy with the help of a multidisciplinary team.

PSYCHIATRY IN GENERAL DENTISTRY

Dentists should be aware of psychiatric problems in patients presenting for dental care. These may not always be apparent but will have a major influence on both symptoms and outcome of treatment. Problems occur throughout all age groups from childhood and adolescence, to adults as well as the elderly.

Childhood psychiatric problems

Childhood psychiatric problems include disorders of emotion, affect, behaviour, and somatization. They become a problem when they interfere with natural development. They tend to be exaggeration of natural development and are usually dealt with by a reduction of stressful situations and behavioural therapy. Children attending a dental surgery may have unexplained oro-dental problems. These children tend to have associated **emotional disorders**, have high family and personal expectations, and have a close family member with a medical problem.

Depression

Depression becomes increasingly common by mid-adolescence, with up to 4–5% of girls being affected. The symptoms are the same as in adults. Patients usually respond to a reduction in stress, the removal of adverse situations, and cognitive therapy.

Behavioural problems

Behavioural problems may have both social and environmental roots and may occur in as many as 10% of 9–10-year-olds in urban areas.

Hypkerkinetic disorders are associated with overactive behaviour in a child, associated with marked inattentiveness, and may be associated with learning difficulties. Children may have high caries rates and find it difficult to follow oral health guidance. They may be unable to attend an appointment with the dentist for coating with fluoride varnish or gel. The incidence varies depending on country and treatment centre. In the United States a figure of 8% or more is given. Methylphenidate may be prescribed for those children in whom a definitive diagnosis is reached.

Enuresis and **encoporesis** may present as behavioural problems in children over the age of 5. These should always indicate referral to the general medical practitioner for assessment as there may be an underlying physical problem which should be excluded before a behavioural diagnosis is made.

Child abuse

Child abuse may be identified by a careful and observant general dental practitioner. This may present itself as: **non-accidental injury**. The head and face are the most common site for signs of bruises. The lesions all tend to be of different ages. Fractures of the skull and jaw are also commonly found. The injuries tend to multiple and are often complicated. The site and type of injury are variable and associated with an inappropriate history. There may be signs of bruises and burns on the arms and legs. These children may be inappropriately fearful and display 'frozen watchfulness'.

Neglect and emotional abuse is very difficult to define as well as identify, especially in a dental setting where visits are short and infrequent. These children may be brought to see a general dental practitioner only in extreme circumstances. The child might appear to be 'failing to thrive' or be unable to interact in a social context. Any suspicions aroused should be conveyed to the general medical practitioner who will alert the social services.

Sexual abuse in children is usually not evident to the dentist. However, unexplained and uncharacteristic oral lesions which may be of venereal origin must entertain a high index of suspicion.

Transcultural psychiatric problems

It is important to be aware that psychotic disorders are present in all cultures and that cultural factors will affect the presentation of all oro-dental problems. It is equally important for the dentist to recognize their own cultural limitations in understanding their patients. When dealing with immigrant populations consider the following points.

Somatization

Somatization is the presentation of oro-dental problems combined with other symptoms for which no organic cause is found. Somatization is often exacerbated by anxiety or depression, which both have prominent autonomic physical symptoms and are expressed in terms of these. Commonly the cultural expression of the patient's mental problems and distress is expressed in terms of atypical facial pain or toothache. It is important to elicit patient responses to questions such as: 'What do you think is causing the pain?'; 'Do you think something serious may be wrong?'; 'What do you worry about most when you have the pain?'. It is important to provide satisfactory answers to queries and to reassure patients. Do not become involved in prolonged unnecessary investigations.

Psychotic disorders

It has been shown that there is an increased incidence of schizophrenia in second-generation Afro-Caribbean immigrants.

Post-traumatic stress syndrome

Refugees may be subject to terrifying experiences of war, personal violence, and torture of family and friends. These traumatizing psychological experiences remain with them throughout their lives, no matter what the apparent assimilation into their new culture.

Patients experience nightmares, flashbacks, and intrusive memories and thoughts. They often do not complain or share these problems, and may present with dysfunctional behaviour in the working environment, and in their social interaction, and are usually unable to maintain stable relationships. The effect on their dental management includes:

- non-attendance;
- late presentation for dental treatment;
- the frequent display of exaggerated startle responses to dental stimuli;
- dental treatment may precipitate flashback and reliving of traumatic experiences.

Psychiatric problems in the elderly

These may result from organic neurological states which result in acute and or chronic confusion or functional neurological states.

Organic neurological states

Acute confusional states

Acute confusional states are due to acute but widespread problems with cerebral function which result in an organic brain syndrome. The causes include hypothyroidism and hypoglycaemia and/or renal and or hepatic failure, infection and hypoxia or vascular disorders. A common underestimated cause is drugs, with the elderly frequently being prescribed cocktails of drugs requiring

---

BOX 11.3 Causes of acute confusional states

- Alcohol.
- Drugs.
- Metabolic: hypoglycaemia, hypothyroidism.
- Hypoxia: cerebrovascular accident, myocardial infarction, pulmonary embolism.
- Organ failure: renal, hepatic, cardiac.

complicated regimes. These acute confusional states do not present in a dental setting and usually last less than 7 days.

Chronic confusional states

Dementia is an acquired syndrome which may be a primary neurodegenerative disease which results in a progressive decline in intellect, behaviour, and personality. However, an indistinguishable clinical syndrome occurs secondary to repeated cerebral trauma, space-occupying lesions, and metabolic and vascular disorders including chronic cerebral infections.

Alzheimer's disease is responsible for over 70% of the causes of dementia. There is a high incidence of depression in these patients, as well as aggressive behavioural patterns including physical and verbal aggression and uncooperativeness. Some patients may be on antidepressants, as well as tacrine, a centrally active non-competitive reversible acetylcholinesterase inhibitor, which results in cognitive benefit but with considerable side-effects. Patients present with abnormal liver function tests as well as gastrointestinal effects of nausea and vomiting.

Patients with **vascular dementia** have a higher incidence of depression. In addition they display excessive emotional lability. Patients may also be hypertensive. Unlike in Alzheimer's disease these patients retain insight late into the disease process. These patients are very difficult to manage dentally with ever-increasing deterioration of living skills. They increasingly neglect their oral hygiene and are unable to tolerate a course of therapy. They often become abusive or aggressive during treatment; frequently forgetting where they are or why they are at the dentist's. They also develop spatial disorientation, resulting in wandering behaviour.

Functional neurological states

Functional disorders are not uncommon in the elderly and are frequently overlooked. These include affective disorders (depression, anxiety disorder, mania), adjustment disorders (bereavement), and schizophrenia-like syndrome. The incidence is the same or slightly increased compared with the general adult population. The risk of suicide in this group is high.

The dental management of these patients may be complicated by:

• Exaggerated reactions to oral conditions.
• Depression and anxiety disorders presenting as atypical facial pain, recurrent denture problems, and sore mouths with no apparent cause being found.
• Oral symptoms such as hypo- or hypersalivation associated with medication, e.g. hypersalivation with methyldopa and clomipramine and hyposalivation with anticholinergic drugs, tricyclics, and major tranquilizers.
• Mucosal ulceration secondary to drugs.
• Lichenoid reaction secondary to drugs.
• Mucosal infection secondary to dry mouth, dentures, and age-related immunosuppression.

Medication used in clinical psychiatry

Drugs used as medication in clinical psychiatry are in common use. They should be carefully monitored in the dental setting as they interact with or potentiate side-effects of other drugs, with consequent oral morbidity.

Antidepressants

There are a very large number of different antidepressant drugs in use:

- **Tricyclic antidepressants:** patients may have cognitive impairment, dry mouth, hypotension, cardiac arrhythmias, or blurred vision.
- **Selective serotonin re-uptake inhibitors (SSRIs):** side-effects include anxiety, headache, dry mouth, loss of appetite. SSRIs inhibit hepatic P-450 enzyme (potentiate warfarin, metronidazole, erythromycin).
- **Monoamine-oxidase inhibitors (MAOIs):** interact with sympathomimetic drugs (e.g. adrenaline), opiates and SSRIs.
- **Lithium:** side-effects include dysarthria, ataxia, tremor, goitre, thirst (rarely diabetes insipidus), increased white cell count, altered taste, increased acne and psoriasis, increased thyroid-stimulating hormone, increased intraoral ulceration.
- **Carbamazepine** (usually used for facial pain): side-effects of ataxia and drowsiness, reduced white cell count, hyponatraemia, erythematous rash, anorexia and nausea, conduction disturbances, increased thyroid-stimulating hormone.

Antipsychotic drugs

Side-effects of antipsychotic drugs include: tardive dyskinesia, e.g. choreoathetoid movements of the tongue, lips, and jaw; increased creatinine phosphokinase; sedation; postural hypotension; weight gain; and increased salivation.

Benzodiazepines

Benzodiazepines induce dependence and withdrawal syndrome and are both respiratory and cardiac depressants.

SUBSTANCE ABUSE

Almost any substance, either natural or synthetic, can be used to alter the mental state. Commonly used substance with widespread public acceptance are tobacco and alcohol. In some societies other substances are routinely used, e.g. paan in the Asian subcontinent, cannabis in Rastafarians and some Afro-American societies and qat in Yemeni, Ethiopian, and Sudanese populations. These substances are accommodated by longstanding social acceptance in the above groups.

Prescribed drugs such as amphetamines, benzodiazepines, especially tamazepan, and narcotic analgesics have all been used as substances of abuse.

Other substances include volatile substances, e.g. varnish, glue, petrol, cigarette lighter fuel, propane and butane as well as amyl nitrate.

Cannabis

Cannabis comes from the plant *Cannabis sativa* and contains tetrahydro-cannabinols which affect the central nervous systems (CNS). The drug is usually smoked, incorporated into foodstuffs and ingested, or drank as an infusion. It is rarely injected intravenously.

Clinical features

These depend on whether intoxication is acute or there has been chronic abuse:

- **Acute intoxication** results in euphoria with drowsiness. Colours and sounds may be distorted. Some patients become very withdrawn. Visual and auditory hallucinations may occur. There are also direct effects on the circulation, with resultant tachycardia, hypotension, and conjunctival suffusion. There is an increase in the white blood count, especially the neutrophil count. Very occasionally the blood sugar is lowered.
- **Chronic abuse**: the individual may become apathetic and withdrawn, with depression and a lack of desire to achieve. Continued use may result in depersonalization. In some cases chronic abusers become aggressive. Persistent cardiac effects include sinus tachycardia, hyper- or hypotension, and angina.

  Few **oral effects** are seen except with chronic abuse, when aphthous ulceration may occur.

  Most patients do not require any **treatment**. It is not advisable to administer any medication or dental treatment to an intoxicated patient. Disruptive patients may require intramuscular injections of haloperidol (2.5–5 mg), or chlorpromazine (50–100 mg).

Ecstasy

3,4-methylenedioxymethamphetamine (MDMA) is commonly known as 'ecstasy'. MDMA was originally used as an appetite suppressant but has become one of the commonest drugs of abuse in Europe. In the UK a third of children under the age of 13 have been exposed to ecstasy. It is taken orally either as a capsule or tablet.

Clinical effects

The clinical effects of ecstasy are characterized in the acute phase by tachycardia, hypertension, sweating and dilated pupils. These effects are exacerbated by exertion and dehydration, resulting in hyperthermia, rhabdomyolysis, acute renal failure, and intravascular coagulation. Fulminant hyperthermia has also been seen which may result in death.

Oral effects include trismus which may be severe. Repeated trismus may result in long-term temporomandibular dysfunction. Facial pain may also be a resultant effect.

Treatment
Treatment includes rehydration with intravenous fluids. In severe cases dantrolene, 1 mg/kg body weight, is given.

Amphetamines

Amphetamines are central nervous system stimulants. Metamphetamine is the most potent form. Most metamphetamine available are home made (alled crank, crystal, ice, glass, or speed). They are usually ingested, 'snorted', or injected.

Clinical features
The clinical features include:

- A state of self-confidence and heightened awareness coupled with extrovert euphoric behaviour with loss of the desire to eat or sleep.
- The heart rate, respiratory rate, and blood pressure all increase. Arrhythmias may be experienced.
- Inability to urinate.
- The mouth becomes dry and there is difficulty in swallowing.
- Speech becomes rapid then slurred.
- In a few cases paranoid delusions, agitation and violent behaviour may occur.
- Rarely patients experience hyperthermia, cardiac arrhythmias, and rhabdomy-olysis all of which have an increased associated mortality.
- Orofacial effects: typically fissured ulceration; vascular infarcts may be seen anywhere in the head and neck area.

Treatment
Chlorpromazine (50–100 g intramuscularly) is used in acute cases. Both gastric lavage and activated charcoal have been used.

Cocaine

Cocaine is an extract from the coca plant. It has a local anaesthetic and vaso-constrictor action. Cocaine may be snorted, smoked, ingested, injected, or inhaled.

Clinical features
Clinical features are similar to those of amphetamines, with abusers feeling and acting invincible. Features include sinus tachycardia, hypertension, sweat-ing, euphoria and/or agitation. Hallucinations may also occur. Prolonged con-vulsions may lead to hyperthermia and rhabdomyolysis. Severe intoxication may result in ventricular arrhythmias with consequent cardiac arrest. Chronic

intranasal ingestion results in perforation of the nasal septum and thinning of the cribiform plate.

Oral effects: ulceration of the buccal mucosa or buccal sulcus where cocaine is held in the mouth; perforation of the nasopalantine bone resulting in communication between the mouth and nose; facial dystonia; rarely, perforation between the nose and mouth has been reported.

Treatment

In acute intoxication diazepam (5–10 mg intramuscularly or intravenously) may be used. Cardiovascular problems may be controlled symptomatically.

Opioids

Opioids include heroin, morphine, methadone, pethidine, and codeine.

Clinical features

Clinical features of opiod use include: depression or alteration of consciousness; respiratory depression, including depressed cough reflex (in acute respiratory depression every effort should be made to take a chest X-ray, as sudden onset of pulmonary oedema may have fatal consequences); cardiovascular depression with bradycardia and hypotension. Skin wounds occur which may be infected but give clues to injection sites, especially in the groin, anticubital fossae, hands, and feet. However, any site where a blood vessel is felt to be accessible may be used (e.g. neck veins).

Oral and facial signs: central cyanosis apparent to the tongue and lips. The pupils may be pinpoint. The facial muscles are relaxed and hypotonic.

Treatment

Acute cases of cardiorespiratory arrest should be given naloxone, 1–2 mg intra-muscularly in an adult. The patient should be transferred to hospital with oxygen support. If no help arrives within 30–40 min the dose should be repeated.

Lysergic acid diethylamide (LSD)

The mode of action of LSD is unknown. Theories about the mode of action include: a vascular effect as the muscles in the blood vessels contract and relax causing redistribution of blood flow; increased permeability of the blood–brain barrier; antagonism of the activity of serotonin. This drug is usually taken orally or snorted.

Clinical features

The acute phase includes agitation and excitement or aggression. The pupils are dilated with tremor of the limbs and hand. Respiratory depression as well as CNS depression may occur when large doses have been taken. Fifteen to 20% of users experience repeated 'flashbacks' and re-enactment of the visual hallucinations;

agitation and aggression may occur without further ingestion of the drug. Morbidity is related to accidents during hallucinations.

Orofacial features: perioral erythematous spots and rashes may occur; breath may smell of solvent; oral ulceration; lichenoid reactions.

Treatment

Sedation and supportive measures are used in those are severely affected.

Volatile substance abuse

This is a common practice, usually in boys aged 13–15 years, some of whom progress to alcohol or other drugs of abuse. Substances abused include chlorinated hydrocarbons, e.g. paints, varnishes, lacquers, acetone (nail varnish remover), butane and propane (cigarette lighter fluid), petrol, amyl nitrite. These are usually inhaled using either a bag containing the solvent or a cloth. Sometimes petrol or acetone is mixed with Coca-Cola or other drinks and consumed.

Clinical features

Clinical features are both medical and psychological. The medical effects may cause CNS and cardiovascular stimulation followed by depression. Morbidity depends on the toxicity of the substance abused. Fatalities are high.

Specific problems:

- Amyl nitrites also cause methaemoglobinaemia.
- Petrol may cause an acute encephalopathy.
- Toluene causes cerebellar atrophy.
- In all cases fatal arrhythmias and renal failure may occur with continued use.

Orofacial features: perioral erythematous spots and rashes may occur; breath may smell of solvent; oral ulceration; lichenoid reaction.

Qat

Qat is grown in Northern Yemen and Ethiopia and is widely used as a stimulant by Yemenis, Sudanese and Ethiopians. The largest immigrant groups using the drug are settled around Sheffield and the Manchester area. Qat is legally imported into the UK but is a prohibited drug in most other countries.

Qat is chewed, kept in the buccal sulcus and the stimulant juice swallowed. Occasionally qat is pre-soaked to release the active ingredients. It is often chewed alongside use of the 'hubble bubble' containing flavoured tobacco.

Clinical effects

Qat is a stimulant and produces a euphoric state. The side-effects include abdominal pain and constipation.

Orofacial effects: plasma cell gingivitis; ulceration (typical linear ulcers in the buccal sulcus); severe lichenoid reactions.

12 Liver disease

The liver plays a major role in the general metabolism of the body. Any acute or chronic liver disease will result in abnormalities of biochemical function. Derangement of liver function has consequences for the provision of dental care of patients. Both metabolism and detoxification of drugs are dependent on effective enzyme systems, while tooth extraction and wound healing are dependent on production of clotting factors and protein metabolism.

Viral infection of the liver may put dental personnel at risk of cross-infection. All dental personnel should be vaccinated against hepatitis B.

FUNCTIONS OF THE LIVER

- Metabolism of amino acids, proteins, and lipids. Amino acids are synthesized directly from dietary protein. Unwanted amino acids are degraded or catabolized to urea and excreted. The enzyme processes involved are transamination and oxidative deamination. Amino acids play a part in the citric acid cycle to function in the intermediary metabolism of lipids and carbohydrates.
- The liver synthesizes all proteins needed for general cellar function. The most important of these being albumin, which is produced in the largest quantities. Other proteins include blood clotting factors, fibrinogen, prothrombin (factor II), factors V, VII, IX, and X. Factors II, VII, IX, and X are vitamin K respondent and thus also dependent on normal intestinal fat absorption. In response to tissue damage the liver synthesizes acute phase proteins, e.g. fibrinogen, C-reactive protein, and transferrin. Serum α and β globulins are synthesized by the liver (γ globulins are produced by plasma cells).
- Metabolism of carbohydrates. The liver plays an important part in glucose metabolism. The liver controls the level of glucose by storage of glucose as glycogen and regulating the uptake of glucose. Stored glycogen is converted into glucose by glycogenolysis when required. Glucose is also produced from non-carbohydrate stores. It is important to note that hepatic stores are depleted after 24 h of fasting. In these cases the use of glucagon to treat acute hypoglycaemia is ineffective. This is an important point for the practising dentist to remember, i.e. the use glucagon in diabetic hypoglycaemia is ineffective in a starving patient.
- The liver is actively involved in the production of lipids, especially triglycerides which are excreted into the blood.
- Cholesterol and bile acid synthesis are mainly carried out by the liver.
- The liver metabolizes and detoxifies drugs, hormones, and vitamins.

- In the liver biochemical oxidation or energy production occurs via aerobic respiration, during which energy is transferred to ATP and flavin nucleotides which are used for biochemical work.
- Nitrogen metabolism in the liver produces ammonia which is rapidly converted to urea, a non-toxic end product (recall the Krebs cycle); it is one of the intermediate steps during which arginine is converted to ornithine.

HEPATITIS

Hepatitis A

Hepatitis A is an infection is caused by a small non-enveloped symmetrical virus of the Picornaviridae group. It is endemic in large parts of the developing world, where most children (95%) have asymptomatic infection by the age of 5 years. There may be large outbreaks of infection: the largest recently recorded outbreak, in 1988, saw 300 000 cases due to infected clams in Shanghai, China.

The disease is transmitted by the faeco-oral route. Faecal contamination may be waterborne, via contaminated food, or by person to person contact. The incubation period is 2–6 weeks.

Clinical features
The illness starts with a prodromal period of a week when the patient suffers from malaise, is anorectic, and has nausea and vomiting associated with a low-grade fever.

- This is followed by dark urine, pale faeces, and jaundice indicating cholestasis; this lasts for 2–3 weeks.
- The stool then returns to a normal colour and the patient's symptoms slowly disappear.

Complications include prolonged cholestasis for up to 18 weeks and relapse within 1–3 months.

Investigations and treatment
Liver function tests show a large increase in bilirubin and an increase in alanine transferase related to the severity of the disease.

- Urobilinogen is present in the urine.
- Antibodies to hepatitis A virus (HAV): IgM to HAV may last 3–6 months.
- IgG to HAV indicates past exposure to HAV and immunity to the virus.

There is no specific **treatment** for hepatitis A and supportive treatment is given. Resolution is complete and chronic infection does not occur.

Hepatitis B

Hepatitis B is caused by a double-stranded DNA virus belonging to the Hepadna virus group. Hepatitis B is endemic, with 350 million people affected worldwide.

The disease is transmitted parenterally. Activities which carry a risk of infection are blood transfusion, unprotected sexual intercourse, intravenous drug abuse with used needles, and dental or surgical procedures using non-sterile instruments.

Once infected a poorer outcome is dependent on increasing age, male sex, the presence of hypogammaglobulinaemia, and the genetic background HLA-DRB1 : 1302. The incubation period is 3–6 months.

Clinical features
- Patients may be asymptomatic.
- Acute symptomatic patients present with a serum sickness-like illness of arthralgia, fever, and urticaria which lasts about a week, followed by jaundice, malaise, fatigue, arthralgia, and right hypochondrial pain.
- In less than 1% of patients severe liver failure ensues, which may result in death.
- Co-infection of hepatitis B virus (HBV) and hepatitis D or delta virus (HDV) results in an acute self-limiting infection.
- Chronic infection results in cirrhoses which cause portal hypertension. The resultant varices may bleed.
- Ascites may result in liver failure.
- Cirrhoses may ultimately result in hepatocellular carcinoma.

Investigations
- Liver function tests show greatly raised bilirubin, raised alanine transaminase (ALT), and raised alkaline phosphatase (ALP).
- In clinical disease there is a series of stages: in the initial stage infection is positive for hepatitis Be antigen (HBe), followed by HBe-negative infection.
- In some areas HDV may co-infect patients with HBV. HDV requires the presence of HBV for its expression and replication (see below).

Treatment
Treatment is symptomatic. In progressive disease the best therapy is interferon. However, fewer than 50% of cases respond to therapy and there are side-effects associated with treatment. The interferons used are α, β, and γ. Interferon α is the most promising, with 40% of treated patients clearing HBV DNA and HBV e antigen (HBV eAg). The antiviral nucleoside agents famciclovir and lamivudine are under trial at present. Liver transplant is also an option in patients with early hepatocellular carcinoma and cirrhoses.

Hepatitis D

HDV is an RNA virus with no envelope and is a nuleocapsid antigen. HDV can only replicate in patients infected with HBV. To do this HDV uses the HBV envelope. Co-infection with HBV and HDV may occur in the acute or chronic phase of HBV infection. In acute HBV infection co-infection leads to an acute self-limiting infection which accounts for over 95% of HBV and HDV infection.

Co-infection rarely occurs in the chronic stage of HBV infection and results in a more severe hepatitis.

Hepatitis C

The hepatitis C virus (HCV) is enveloped single-stranded RNA virus. It is a member of the Flaviviridae family. Worldwide, 170 million people are infected with HBC.

Transmission of HBC occurs when blood or body fluids from an infected person enter the body of a person who is not infected. Routes of transmission include infected blood products, blood transfusion, intravenous drug abuse with used needles, dentistry and other healthcare procedures, acupuncture, tattooing, and ear piercing.

Clinical features

There is an incubation period of 6–12 weeks. In **acute disease** patients may be asymptomatic or have very mild disease. Fewer than 25% of patients are jaundiced. In chronic disease most patients run an asymptomatic course but after 10 years they either develop rapidly progressive or benign slowly progressive cirrhosis.

Infection may cause systemic disease: autoimmune hepatitis, cryoglobulinaemia, porphyria cutanea tarda, lymphocytic sialodenitis, or membranous glomerulonephritis.

Investigations and treatment

Anti-HCV antibody is present within 1–2 weeks of infection. There is an increase in bilirubin and alanine transferase

Treatment is with inteferon α but relapse occurs in 50% of cases. There is no vaccination available but patients must be vaccinated against HAV and HBV.

Hepatitis E

The hepatitis E virus is a single-stranded non-enveloped calcivirus which was discovered in 1983. It is endemic in Asia, Africa, the Middle East, and Central America. In these areas 40% of adults are affected and 5% of children under 10 are hepatitis E positive. Transmission follows the faeco-oral route, and may be zoonotic or person to person. The incubation period is 2 weeks to 20 months.

Clinical features

Hepatitis E is an acute self-limiting disease which has clinical features resembling those of hepatitis A. In pregnant women there can be a mortality of 25% due to fulminant hepatitis in the third trimester. There is no chronic liver disease.

IgM antibody to HEV in the serum provides a definitive disgnosis. Supportive treatment only is necessary as the disease is self-limiting.

> **BOX 12.1 Risk factors for gallstones**
> - 'Fair, fat, female, and over forty'.
> - Age 30–50.
> - Female.
> - Obesity.
> - Pregnancy.
> - Hormone replacement therapy and the combined oral contraceptive pill.
> - Drugs, e.g. clofibrate, octreotide, and parenteral nutrition.
> - Systemic problems, e.g. diabetes mellitus, cirrhosis, and surgery.
> - Cirrhosis and haemodialysis are risk factors for pigment stones. These are more common in East Asians.

GALLSTONES

Two types of gallstone occur: cholesterol stones (80% of cases) and pigment stones. Pigment stones are opaque and contain unconjugated bilirubin, bile salts, calcium, and cholesterol. The incidence of gallstones is 5–8 per 1000 population. The prevalence is highest in those over 55 years of age, when the male to female ratio is 1 : 1.

Clinical features

Seventy per cent of people with gallstones are asymptomatic. Biliary colic ('gallstone attack') may occur. This is the sudden onset of severe pain in the right hypochondrium which radiates to the back accompanied by nausea and vomiting. Other features also occur but these are secondary to the associated complications.

The following **complications** can occur:

- Acute cholecystitis (inflammation of the gall bladder) is associated with fever, biliary colic and positive Murphy's sign (tenderness over the gall bladder).
- Blocked common bile duct. This is usually caused by a stone and presents with biliary colic and jaundice.
- Acute cholangitis (infection of the biliary tract) presents with biliary colic and jaundice.
- Acute pancreatitis presents with severe abdominal pain which radiates into back. Patients complain of tenderness on rebound when palpating the abdomen.
- Acute pancreatitis may also result in collapse due to hypotension.

Investigations

The following investigations may be done:

- Abdominal ultrasound.
- Plain abdominal X-ray; this will show fewer than 25% of stones.

- An oral cholecystogram will identify the radiolucent stones.
- CT scan.

Treatment

Treatment is only necessary if patient is symptomatic.

- **Medical treatment**: Lithotripsy for radiolucent stones. Solvents, e.g. methyl tert-butyl, applied directly to the stone via a percutaneous transhepatic catheter. This procedure can cause severe pain and there is a risk of recurrence. Bile acids are also used. These give early symptomatic relief by decreasing gallbladder contraction.
- **Surgical treatment:** 50 000 cholecystectomies occur per year in the UK. Laparoscopic cholecystectomy is more commonly performed than open surgery. The main problem is damage to the common bile duct.

HEPATIC TUMOURS

Primary tumours of the liver are uncommon except for hepatocellar carcinoma.

Hepatocelluar carcinoma

Hepatocelluar carcinoma is the commonest primary liver tumour and accounts for over 85% of cases. There are 3 cases per 100 000 population in Western Europe and 30 per 100 000 in Africa and Southeast Asia.

The known risk factors for hepatocelluar carcinoma are:

- male sex
- cirrhosis
- HBV infection
- HCV infection
- exposure to aflatoxin (a naturally occurring mycotoxin produced by two types of *Aspergillus* fungus, and sometimes found in grains and peanuts which have been badly stored).

Clinical features
Symptoms:

- nausea
- vomiting
- abdominal pain
- jaundice.

Signs:

- fever
- weight loss
- ascites
- hepatomegaly.

Investigations
- Liver function tests are abnormal.
- There is raised alpha-fetoprotein.
- Ultrasound and CT scan.
- Biopsy should not be performed as there is a risk of bleeding and spontaneous rupture.

Treatment
- Surgical resection is the only hope of cure. However, only 15% of cases are curable.
- The tumour may be localized by local alcohol injection.
- Targeted chemotherapy using epirubicin attached to lipoidal may also be used to localize the tumour, with better results.
- Secondary tumours are common: the liver is the second most common site for metastases after the lymph nodes. Tumours that frequently metastasize to the liver are colorectal tumours, carcinoid, and neuroendocrine tumours. Less frequently, bone, breast, and kidney tumours metastasize to the liver.

AUTOIMMUNE HEPATITIS

Autoimmune hepatitis was previously known as chronic active hepatitis. It is a chronic disease of unknown aetiology and is characterized by a history of other autoimmune diseases, high serum levels of immunoglobulins, and serum autoantibodies. The disease is most common in females between the ages of 20 and 40 years.

Clinical features

Onset may be insidious or acute. The most common presentation is the slow development of anorexia, weight loss, and abdominal pain with later onset of jaundice. Physical signs include palmar erythema and spider naevi for some time before jaundice develops. Patients with disease of rapid onset have all the above features plus hepatomegaly. Fifty to 60% of patients will develop other features:

- arthralgia, skin rashes
- lymphadenopathy
- low platelet count
- haemolytic anaemia
- ulcerative colitis.

Investigations and treatment

Liver biopsy shows piecemeal cellular necrosis and periportal inflammation with fibrosis causing rosettes of cells. There is very little regeneration. Progression to cirrhosis usually occurs. Liver function tests may show a moderate rise in bilirubin and alkaline phosphatase. IgG levels and autoantibodies are raised. Three distinct patterns of raised autoantibodies occur: antinuclear and anti-smooth muscle antibodies; antiliver–kidney and microsomal antibodies; anti-soluble liver antigen/liver pancreas antibodies. Lupiod cells are found in 10–15% of patients.

Treatment is with corticosteroids and or azathioprine. End-stage disease is treated with liver transplantation.

PRIMARY BILIARY CIRRHOSIS

Primary biliary cirrhosis is a chronic liver disease which is common in northern Europe and America and rare in Asia and Africa. The aetiology is unknown, but there is an association with other autoimmune diseases. It is a chronic progressive disease and is seen mainly in females between the ages of 30 and 50 years.

Clinical features

Asymptomatic patients may have abnormal liver function with circulating antimitochondrial antibodies (AMA) found on routine screening.

Symptomatic patients:

- Complain of pruritus, anorexia, and lethargy.
- Signs of chronic liver disease become apparent.
- Dentists may notice increasing facial pigmentation, xanthalasmata, and clubbing in patients.
- There are usually no spider naevi.
- Hepatomegaly is present in more than half of patients.
- Liver decompensation (jaundice, ascites, and portal hypertension with variceal hemorrhage) follows. The natural pattern of disease from diagnosis to death is 7–10 years.

A number of autoimmune diseases are associated with primary biliary cirrhosis. It is frequently associated with primary Sjögren's syndrome. Less common associations are with thyroid disease, fibrosing alveolitis, and Raynaud's syndrome.

Investigations and treatment

Liver biopsy shows granulomatous cholangitis and inflammation. Cirrhosis is present later. Liver function test shows cholestasis, raised bilirubin, raised alkaline phosphatase, and γ-glutamyl transferase. Serum IgM is increased and antinuclear antibodies to nuclear pore protein (gp120) and AMA are present.

Treatment is usually symptomatic. Ursodeoxycholic acid may improve time to transplant and slow progression but it is not clear if survival is increased.

Immunosuppressives have little effect but liver transplantation has good results with survival of over 80% over 5 years.

HAEMOCHROMATOSIS

Haemochromatosis is the excessive uptake of iron into the body, resulting in iron overload. Iron is used for electron transfer as well as oxygen exchange, but in excess it causes tissue damage and fibrosis. It is a common disease with an incidence of 1 in 200–300 with 1–10 being carriers.

Two mutations, C282Y and H63D account for almost all cases with over 90% of cases of hereditary haemochromatosis associated with a mutation of the *HFE* gene. A homozygous substitution of tyrosine for cysteine (C282Y) at amino acid position 282 of the HFE protein occurs. C282Y is found exclusively in CeHs. Rarer causes are abnormalities associated with ferroportin and the transferrin receptor-2.

In the UK 1 in 300 population are homozygous and 1 in 10 population are heterozygotes. Not all homozygotes have iron overload, which is determined by iron and alcohol intake. In addition to hereditary haemochromotosis (known as primary haemochromatosis) there are a number of other causes of iron overload:

- prolonged iron therapy
- excess iron with repeated blood transfusions
- excess iron with chronic haemodialysis
- portocaval anastomosis for liver disease
- misdiagnosed anaemia in thalassaemia
- Bantu siderosis resulting from beer brewed in iron pots
- excess alcohol intake
- porphyria cutanea tarda.

Clinical features

Haemochromatosis often presents between the ages of 40 and 50 years. Men usually present earlier as women lose iron through menstrual bleeding and pregnancy. Juvenile haemochromatosis presents in the second decade.

Haemochromatosis is asymptomatic in the early stages. Liver disease results from iron loading of the hepatocytes; fibrosis occurs and this leads in turn to cirrhosis. In the late stages hepatocellular carcinoma may develop. Other changes include:

- Diabetes mellitus Type 2 may develop.
- Skin and mucosa become pigmented.
- Cardiac arrhythmias, followed later by cardiac failure.
- Arthritis.
- Loss of libido.
- Abdominal pain.

Investigations and treatment

Specific tests for haemochromatosis are:

- Serum ferritin greater than 300 mg/l in men or 200 mg/l in women.
- Liver function tests are abnormal.
- Liver biopsy.
- MRI scan.
- Genetic testing.

Other less specific tests that may be done are blood sugar and ECG.

Treatment is by phlebotomy once a week until serum ferritin is below 50 mg/l. Other symptoms should be treated as they occur, e.g. arthritis, diabetes, rhythm abnormalities, or liver failure. Once treatment is commenced many symptoms improve. Screening of relatives is very important.

WILSON'S DISEASE

Wilson's disease is a disorder of abnormal copper deposition. Copper is deposited in the liver until saturation occurs. It is then excreted into the blood and deposited in the tissue spaces causing clinical problems.

Wilson's disease is a genetic disorder associated with a mutation in the gene *ATP7B* on chromosome 13. It is an uncommon autosomal recessive disorder with a prevalence of 30 per million. It should be considered as a disgnosis in any young child or teenager presenting with abnormal liver function.

Clinical features

Hepatic features include:

- raised aminotransferases
- hepatomegaly
- hepatitis
- in rare cases fulminant hepatic failure.

Neurological features:

- clumsiness
- slow writhing choreoathetoid movements
- tremor
- rigidity may resemble Parkinson's disease
- handwriting very small
- epileptic seizures
- deposition of copper in the eyes to give Kayser–Fleischer rings.

Psychiatric features:

- severe depression
- neurotic disorders

- emotional lability
- aggression.

Less common symptoms:

- pancreatitis
- gallstones
- cardiac arrhythmias
- hypothyroidism.

Investigations and treatment

The following investigations will assist in diagnosis of Wilson's disease:

- serum copper
- urinary copper (raised 24 h)
- increased hepatic copper
- abnormal liver function
- low serum caeruloplasmin
- Kayser–Fleischer rings seen by slit lamp examination
- liver biopsy may show fibrosis, cirrhosis, hepatocellular necrosis, and steatosis.

The following **treatment** can be given:

- Lifelong low copper diet and cessation of all alcohol intake.
- Penicillamine acts as a chelator of copper; trientine has fewer side-effects.
- Zinc to deplete body copper stores.
- Vitamin E as adjunct therapy.
- Liver transplantation in severe cases or fulminant hepatic failure.

ALCOHOL AND THE LIVER

The **recommended safe limits** for alcohol intake are 21 units (a unit being half a pint of beer, a glass of wine, or a single measure of spirits) a week for women and 28 units for men. Men who drink more than 52 units and women who drink more than 35 units have an increased risk of liver disease. The risk is further increased by binge drinking. The increase in alcoholic liver disease is related to increased drinking at a younger age and increased drinking by women:

- Alcohol intake is directly related to death from chronic liver disease.
- Alcohol is primarily oxidized in the liver and its breakdown product, acetaldehyde, causes toxic liver damage.
- Fifty per cent of oriental people lack aldehyde dehydrogenase, causing flushing due to accumulation of acetaldehyde.

Clinical features

The **CAGE questionnaire** is useful in patients who deny alcohol problem but in whom one is suspicious of alcohol excess. One point is given for every 'yes' answer, and two or more points suggest an alcohol problem:

- Have you ever
- Felt a need to **C**ut down?
- Been **A**nnoyed at the suggestion of a drinking problem?
- Felt **G**uilty about a drinking problem?
- Had to have a drink (**E**ye opener) in the morning?

Symptoms of alcohol excess unrelated to the liver are psychological, nausea, and diarrhoea.

Patients with mild/moderate alcoholic hepatitis may be asymptomatic in early stages or have tender hepatomegaly or jaundice. Patients with severe alcoholic hepatitis have jaundice, ascites, hepatic encephalopathy, haemochromatosis.

Extrahepatic disease related to alcohol excess includes:

- parotid enlargement
- alcoholic cardiomyopathy
- testicular atrophy
- Dupuytren's contracture
- hepatocellular carcinoma
- chronic pancreatitis
- diabetes Type 2 (a consequence of cirrhosis and increases the risk of cirrhosis)
- duodenal ulceration
- peripheral sensory neuropathy
- cerebral atrophy
- cerebellar atrophy
- Wernicke's encephalopathy
- Korsakoff's dementia.

Investigations and treatment

Full blood count may show leucocytosis, macrocytosis, and low platelet count. Prothrombin time may be prolonged. Liver function tests show raised enzymes especially γ-glutamyl transferase; aspartate transaminase (AST) is greater then alanine transaminase (ALT). Other tests:

- increased serum IgA
- abdominal ultrasound to exclude biliary obstruction and portal hypertension
- liver biopsy.

In an emergency **treatment** with oral pentoxifylline improves survival in acute cases. For alcoholic withdrawal treat with chlodiazepoxide.

In the short term treatment with corticosteroids may be given in severe alcoholic hepatitis without infection. The mainstay of long term treatment is abstinence. Acamprosate and naltrexone may reduce alcohol dependence. Liver transplantation may be used.

Complications of alcohol abuse and liver damage include:

- ascites
- hepatic encephalopathy
- septicaemia
- hepatorenal failure
- chronic liver disease.

ACUTE LIVER FAILURE

Acute liver failure occurs in the absence of pre-existing liver disease. Table 12.1 shows the main causes of acute liver failure.

There are three forms of acute liver all presenting with encephalopathy after the onset of jaundice and mild tender hepatomegaly:

- **Hyperacute liver failure:** onset is within 7 days. Causes include paracetamol overdose and hepatitis A and B infection. There is a prolonged international normalized ratio (INR), a high incidence of cerebral oedema, early regeneration, and reasonable prospects for survival.
- **Acute liver failure:** has an onset with 8–28 days. The aetiology is mixed, but with similar characteristics to hyperacute failure. Prospects for survival are poor.
- **Subacute liver failure:** onset is within 5–12 weeks. Coagulation is not greatly prolonged. There is a low incidence of cerebral oedema. Prospects for survival are very poor and infection may contraindicate transplantation.

Investigations and treatment

- Full blood count.
- Prothrombin time or INR. This will give an indication of acute liver disease.
- Liver function tests.
- Urea and electrolytes.
- Ultrasound to exclude pre-existing disease in acute cases, e.g. splenomegaly and varices and Budd–Chiari syndrome.

Table 12.1 Causes of acute liver failure

Cause	Percentage of cases
Paracetamol	70
NANBNC	8
Drug toxicity	2
Hepatitis A	2
Hepatitis B	2

NANBNC, non-A, non-B, non-C hepatitis.

> **BOX 12.2** Liver transplantation
>
> Types of liver transplants
> - Standard cadaveric.
> - Auxillary.
> - Living related.
> - Two-step procedure.
>
> Outcome of liver transplantation
> - Standard: 74% 1-year and 55% 10-year survival, but may be up to 90% 1-year survival.
> - Auxillary: 72% 3.5-year survival.
> - Living related: 90% 5-year survival.

> **BOX 12.3** Causes of death in patients with acute liver failure
> - Infection.
> - Cardiovascular and neurological collapse.
> - Multi-organ failure.
> - Failure to obtain donor.
> - Post-transplant death.

- Exclude coexisting liver disease.
- Hepatitis A IgM.
- Hepatitis B core IgM.
- Serum copper and caeruloplasmin and ophthalmology for Kayser–Fleischer rings in Wilson's disease.

Treatment needs to be in specialist unit with a multidisciplinary team, with recognition of multisystem problems. Transplantation may be considered.

DRUGS IN DENTISTRY AND LIVER DISEASE

Several drugs used in dentistry may cause transient or permanent liver damage. Liver damage may affect metabolism of drugs, resulting in unexpected side-effects from commonly used drugs.

Effects of common drugs

Alcohol

Alcohol is the most common cause of liver damage. Initial damage results in a fatty liver which progresses to alcoholic hepatitis and finally cirrhosis. Patients may progress to hepatocellular carcinoma. Alcoholic damage may

> **BOX 12.4** Dental relevance of drug interactions in hepatic disease
>
> Patients with established hepatic disease have an increased risk of adverse drug reactions during routine treatment. A careful medical history may list any of these:
>
> - Oral hypoglycaemics increase the risk of hypoglycaemic events.
> - NSAIDs increase the risk of gastrointestinal bleeding.
> - Cimetidine may increase the risk of confusional episodes.
> - Angiotensin converting enzyme inhibitors increase the risk of hypotensive episodes.
> - Need to decrease the dose of warfarin as previous therapeutic doses increases the risk of post-extraction bleeding.
> - Gentamicin has an increased risk of causing renal toxicity.

also increase the progression of HCV to chronic disease. Alcohol induces both cytochrome P-450 and alcohol dehydrogenase. Many drugs used in dentistry are metabolized via the P-450 enzyme pathway.

Analgesics

- Paracetamol: an overdose of paracetamol causes acute hepatitis. The risk of liver toxicity is increased in alcoholic patients, the elderly, the malnourished, or those taking enzyme-inducing drugs. Fulminant liver failure and death may occur. Administration of N-acetyl cysteine in paracetamol overdose helps to prevent liver damage.
- NSAIDs: piroxicam and diclofenac can cause acute hepatitis and cholestasis. Aspirin in continued large doses can cause acute hepatitis and granulomatous changes.

Anaesthetics

Halothane can cause hepatitis, especially after repeated administration. Liver damage may present with fever and raised alanine transaminase at day 7 after anaesthetic administration.

Antibiotics

Erythromycin, penicillin, flucloxacillin, amoxicillin and cephalosporins (first generation) may all cause cholestasis and mild hepatitis.

Immunosuppressive drugs

Azathioprine causes hepatitis and cholestasis. The rise of liver enzymes on routine testing may be the first indication of liver damage. Methotrexate may cause slow insidious damage. Corticosteroids after prolonged use may cause microvesicular damage and fatty change. Ciclosporin and cyclophosphamide cause acute cholestasis and hepatitis. Colchicine used in oral medicine for the treatment of ulceration may cause cholestasis and hepatitis.

> **BOX 12.5 Dental relevance of jaundice**
>
> **Practice point**: The dentist may be faced by a patient in acute pain who needs urgent treatment but who is jaundiced. In this case elective work will not be able to be deferred until a diagnosis is made. The patient has a right to good oral care.
>
> **Problems to avoid are:**
> - Patient cooperation may be compromised because of drug or alcohol abuse.
> - Universal precautions for cross-infection control should be strictly applied because of the risk of underlying viral infection.
> - It is safe to use local anaesthetic.
> - There is an increased risk of post-extraction bleeding. This may be secondary to failure to produce vitamin K-dependent clotting factors.
> - Drugs which are metabolized or excreted by the liver may have a prolonged half-life. Examples are paracetamol, NSAIDs, halothane, metronidazole, erythromycin, and sedatives.
> - Post-extraction healing may be compromised in patients because of reduction of protein synthesis.
> - Reduce the dose of oral or inhalation sedation because of potentiation of the metabolic half-life of these drugs.
> - Intravenous sedation and general anaesthetics should be avoided.
> - In the hospital environment, dentists working with inpatients should be careful with the use of halothane which is hepatotoxic, and may precipitate hepatorenal syndrome.

Recreational drugs

Cocaine causes ischaemic liver damage and ecstasy causes acute hepatitis. Contaminants of these drugs may be responsible for HBV, HDV, and HCV infection, further compromising liver function.

JAUNDICE

Describes a yellow discoloration of the skin and mucous membranes. It is due to an increase in bilirubin levels in the plasma. Bilirubin levels in jaundice are usually two to three times the normal level of <18 mmol/l.

Clinical signs and causes

In pale skinned individuals the sclera of the eyes, the mucous membranes, and the skin are good indicators. In Asian and Black patients apply pressure on the palmar creases. This will show yellow against the pigmented skin.

The **causes** of jaundice are:

- Pre-hepatic: haemolysis due to red cell destruction. This may result from autoimmune causes, abnormal haemoglobin, or red cell membrane abnormalities.
- Hepatic: viral hepatitis, e.g. HAV, HBV, HCV, HDV, and HEV, and Epstein–Barr virus (EBV) and cytomagalovirus (CMV); drug-induced hepatitis, e.g. alcohol,

paracetamol, NSAIDs, isoniazid for TB, cephalosporins, and metronidizole; cirrhosis caused by alcohol, chronic hepatitis, or autoimmune-induced cirrhosis.
- Post-hepatic: biliary obstruction by stones or carcinoma; pancreatic carcinoma; carcinoma, both primary and secondary, may cause pre-hepatic, hepatic, or post-hepatic jaundice.

Investigations

- Liver function tests: bilirubin will indicate the degree of jaundice; alanine transaminase is raised in hepatic jaundice due to necrosis and inflammation; alkaline phosphatase is raised in obstructive jaundice.
- Clotting studies to include the prothrombin time and INR. Clotting factors II, VII, IX, and X, the vitamin K-dependent factors.
- Hepatitis serology for HBV, HCV, HAV, EBV and CMV.
- Full blood count indicates haemoglobin or red cell abnormality.
- Serum albumin, which is produced in the liver and decreases with loss of the ability of the liver to synthesize proteins.
- Abdominal ultrasound may be helpful in the diagnosis of carcinoma, biliary disease and obstruction, and cirrhosis.

13 Haematology

Blood is a complex fluid containing multiple cellular elements derived from bone marrow and thymus proteins, including clotting factors, derived from liver, and antibodies derived from plasma cells.

Haemopoiesis occurs in the liver in the fetus and in the bone marrow in both children and adults. The spleen or liver also produce haemotopoietic cells under conditions of stress.

Haemopoietic stem cells are pluripotent, giving rise to erythroid cells (red cells), myeloid cells (white cells), and megakaryocytes, as well as T and B lymphocytes. The high rate of cell turnover required in the bone marrow to manufacture cellular elements for the blood at a rate that matches their loss produces a large demand for nutritional elements such as vitamin B_{12}, folate, iron, and growth factors such as stem cell factor (SCF), interleukin-3 (IL-3), granulocyte–macrophage colony stimulating factor (GM-CSF), monocyte colony stimulating factor, IL-5, erythropoietin, and thrombopoietin. Deficiency of these elements will affect blood and other rapidly dividing tissues such as the oral mucosa.

BOX 13.1 Haemopoietic growth factors

- Steel factor—important for cell migration.
- Interleukin-3 (IL-3)—multipotent growth factor.
- Granulocyte–macrophage colony-stimulating factor (GM-CSF)—stimulates production neutrophils, oesinophils, monocytes and granulocytes.
- Granulocyte colony-stimulating factor (G-CSF)—stimulates production of granulocytes.
- Monocyte colony-stimulating factor (M-CSF)—monocyte growth factor.
- Interleukin-5 (IL-5)—oesinophilic growth factor.
- Erythropoietin—induces red blood cell (RBC) proliferation.
- Thrombopoietin—stimulates megakaryocyte proliferation.
- Vitamin B_{12} and folic acid—required for DNA synthesis.

BOX 13.2 Problems of haemopoiesis relevant to the dentist

- Diseases affecting haemopoiesis will also affect the oral mucosa (both are high-turnover tissues).
- Changes in the number of blood components may lead to oral changes.
- Blood clotting factor problems may lead to increased bleeding in the mouth.

THE RED BLOOD CELL

The function of red blood cells (RBC) is to carry haemoglobin (Hb), the prime role of which is the delivery of oxygen to the tissues. Haemoglobin is a tetramer of two α and two non-α globin chains. It has both haem groups and a globin fraction, which comprises four peptide chains.

Haemoglobin chains differ in the adult and the fetus:

- Adult HbA: two α and two β chains ($\alpha_2\beta_2$).
- Adult HbA$_2$: two α and two δ chains ($\alpha_2\delta_2$).
- Fetal Hb (HbF): two α and two γ chains ($\alpha_2\gamma_2$).

Fetal Hb is replaced by adult Hb within the first 6 months of life.

Production of RBCs is controlled mainly by erythropoietin which is produced in the kidney in response to reduction of blood oxygen content:

- Adults produce 25×10^{10} RBCs per day, i.e. 40–50 ml of blood.
- The average lifespan of a RBC is 120 days, with 1% of total RBCs lost each day.
- RBCs develop from reticulocytes which are released from the bone marrow; they are larger than mature RBCs.
- Low levels of iron, vitamin B$_{12}$, and folate all affect the development of erythrocytes.
- A number of factors affect the development of RBCs: increased sudden blood loss; increase in the number of reticulocytes in circulation; insufficient iron, resulting in small pale cells; insufficient vitamin B$_{12}$ or folate results in large cells which may retain nuclei.

Red blood cell disorders

Red blood disorders include the haemoglobinopathies (haemoglobin disorders), the thalassaemias, RBC membrane defects, anaemia, and polycythaemia.

Sickle cell disorders

Sickle cell (SC) disease is due to homozygosity for HbS (sickle cell haemoglobin), containing a mutation of the normal β chain. Homozygoity for HbS (i.e. HbSS, >50% abnormal Hb) results in a severe clinical syndrome. Sickle cell trait (heterozygous for HbS, e.g. HbAS, <50% abnormal Hb). These patients only have clinical problems in severe hypoxia. Patients with HbC (SC disease) have near normal Hb levels and a milder clinical disease but are at high risk of retinopathy.

Clinical features

- Painful sickling crises which are precipitated by infection, dehydration, and exposure to low temperatures. Particular care should be taken with dental procedures which may precipitate a crisis.

> **BOX 13.3** Dental implications of sickle cell disease
> - Check racial background and check sickling test on any at-risk patient before a general anaesthetic.
> - Treat infections promptly with antibiotics.
> - High index of suspicion of aseptic bone necrosis, especially in the premaxilla area.
> - Care in giving routine blood transfusion because of danger of increased vaso-occlusive complications.

- Human parvovirus B19 causes a rapid fall in Hb with absence of reticulocytes resulting in aplastic crises.
- Infection may cause high morbidity and mortality.
- Salmonella osteomyelitis may present in a dental setting.
- Pneumococcal vaccine should be given to prevent pneumonia which may be fatal.
- Renal damage occurs due to constant sickling of red blood cells damaging the kidney.
- Aseptic bone necrosis and ulceration of the skin may occur in the head, neck, and orodental tissues.
- Gallstones result from excess bilirubin.
- Infarction may be responsible for priapism, pulmonary hypertension, cirrhosis, and cerebrovascular accidents.

Thalassaemia

There are two types of thalassaemia: α thalassaemia and β thalassaemia. α Thalassaemia occurs almost exclusively in the Middle Eastern and Asian populations. There is a deficiency of α chains of haemoglobin. β Thalassaemia occurs in almost all races, with a predominance in the Mediterranean and the Middle and Far East.

α Thalassaemia

There are four clinical types of α thalassaemia related to α-globin gene deletions (a healthy individual has two normal α-globin genes on each chromosome 16 (i.e. four in total):

- A silent carrier occurs with no haematological abnormality: usually due to single gene deletions.
- Thalassaemia trait: patients have hypochromic, microcytic anaemia resulting from the deletion of two α-globin genes.
- HbH disease: this results from the deletion of three α-globin genes
- Hb Bart's (hydrops fetalis) result in death *in utero* or shortly after birth due to deletion of all four α-globin genes.

> ### BOX 13.4 Dental implications of thalassaemia
>
> - Bony abnormalities including bossing of the skull and other deformities: X-ray has typical appearance and other bones become increasingly brittle.
> - Anaemia with hypochromic microcytic pattern associated with problems with general anaesthesia.
> - Regular transfusions can lead to iron overload resulting in cardiac failure.
> - Patients are prone to recurrent infections.
> - Splenectomy increases risk of infection, especially from pneumococcal bacteria.
> - The patient might be immunosuppressed because of bone marrow transplantation.

β Thalassaemia

The clinical disease depends on the base pair mutations in the β chain of the globin molecule. In thalassaemia major (Cooley's anaemia) patients are severely affected clinically. This results from being homozygous or doubly heterozygous for β-globin mutations. These patients now live to adulthood because of effective therapeutic treatment.

RBC membrane defects

Hereditary spherocytosis, elliptocytosis, and **stomatocytosis** are all RBC membrane defects. Only hereditary spherocytosis is common. It affects 1 in 5000 of the population. It is caused by a deficiency of spectrin, ankyrin, and skeletal proteins:

- The RBC membrane is very permeable, causing the cells to become spherical. They have a decreased lifespan.
- The main clinical problem is haemolytic anaemia.
- Treatment is by splenectomy which results in an effective cure.

Anaemia

Anaemia is due to the decrease in the amount of haemoglobin. It has several causes:

- Failure to make RBCs.
- RBCs are abnormal, e.g. abnormal membrane, enzymes, Hb structure, Hb chains, or nucleus.
- Decreased RBC lifespan.
- Increased RBC loss.

Iron deficiency anaemia

The total body iron stores in an adult are 3–4 g. Haemoglobin contains 75% of total body iron, the remainder being stored as ferritin or haemosiderin in the liver and macrophages, in cytochrome oxidase and in the tongue. Loss of iron occurs via the oral and gastrointestinal mucosa at a rate of 1 mg/day. Each ml of RBC contains 1 mg of iron. Iron is used in the synthesis of haemoglobin in

---

BOX 13.5 Terminology used in haematology associated with anaemia

- Normochromic: normal colour.
- Normocytic: normal size.
- Hypochromic: decreased colour.
- Microcytic: small.
- Macrocytic: large.
- Megaloblastic: large with immature nucleus.
- Reticulocyte: a RBC released early.

BOX 13.6 Effect of iron deficiency on the oral mucosa

- As the body runs out of iron the oral mucosa will suffer before the bone marrow.
- The body rations iron, preserving what is available for blood formation at the expense of other tissues.
- Iron is stored in the tongue in filiform papillae; this is considered a non-essential store.
- As iron deficiency worsens the oral mucosa may initially show few or no signs. Thereafter they may present with burning mouth but normal looking mucosa.
- Later there is atrophy of the filiform papillae. Other clinical signs are worsening of recurrent oral ulceration.
- After prolonged iron deficiency Plummer–Vinson syndrome may occur. This is dysphagia due to oesophageal web formation, pale smooth tongue, and koilynychia.

---

developing RBCs and also plays a vital role in many cellular enzyme systems, e.g. cytochrome systems.

Aetiology: Iron deficiency is not a disease in its own right, but merely a sign of disease:

- In young women menstrual loss is a probable cause. Menorrhagia is a common cause of chronic bleeding.
- Dietary deficiency must be excluded in all age groups.
- In older patients there is the possibility of occult bowel loss due to from hiatus hernia, carcinoma of the bowel, or diverticular disease.
- Coeliac disease, Crohn's disease and post-gastrectomy can all cause problems with absorption of iron.

Investigations:

- The routine clinical test for iron deficiency is serum ferritin assessment. However, the gold standard investigation is bone marrow examination.
- The serum ferritin may be decreased long before clinical signs of anaemia develop.
- Ferritin is an 'acute phase' protein and may be raised in inflammatory conditions such as systemic lupus erythematosus and chronic infections, despite iron deficiency.

- The RBCs in iron deficiency anaemia are small (microcytic) (mean cell volume (MCV) < 80 fl) and pale (hypochromic). They vary in shape (poikilocytosis) and size (anisocytosis). Note that there is a similar picture in patients with thalassaemia who are at risk of iron overload. These patients have an inappropriately low MCV for the stated Hb level.

Vitamin B$_{12}$ deficiency

Vitamin B$_{12}$ is involved in the transfer of single carbon units in the synthesis of DNA, therefore deficiency leads to abnormal cell growth and maturation. Vitamin B$_{12}$ (cobalamin) is found in small amounts in all animal tissues but is absent from foods of vegetable origin. It is absorbed in the terminal ileum after binding to intrinsic factor, a glycoprotein secreted by gastric parietal cells. It is transported by the carrier protein transcobalamin and stored in the liver. Total body stores are about 3 mg. A daily intake of 1 to 3 μg is needed to maintain the 3 mg store. There are a number of causes of deficiency of B$_{12}$:

- Vegan diet (vegetarians who eat milk and eggs are likely to obtain sufficient from dietary sources).
- Partial gastrectomy resulting in decreased secretion of intrinsic factor (IF).
- Autoantibodies to IF in Addisonian pernicious anaemia.
- Competition for B$_{12}$ by fish tapeworm (*Diphilobothram latum*) or bacteria in blind loops of the intestine.
- Resection of the terminal ileum.

The main effect of B$_{12}$ deficiency is on the bone marrow. This leads to the production of large RBCs (macrocytes), some of which may be primitive with nuclei (megaloblasts), neutrophils with hypersegmented nuclei, and abnormal platelets. In the mouth the classical effect is a glossitis with a 'beefsteak' like tongue. Worsening of recurrent oral ulcerations and mucosal dysplasia are also recognized.

Clinical features: in addition to signs of anaemia there is:

- Glossitis and angular cheilitis.
- Smooth sore tongue due to epithelial atrophy.
- Mild jaundice due to premature destruction of RBCs.
- Sensory peripheral neuropathy.
- Subacute combined degeneration of the spinal cord.

Investigations:

- Full blood count shows macrocytic RBCs.
- Red cell B$_{12}$ and folate will be reduced.
- The Schilling test (tests vitamin B$_{12}$ absorption).
- Examine bone marrow for megaloblasts.

Management:

- Treat the cause and treat the underlying disease.
- Pernicious anaemia is the most common cause of B$_{12}$ deficiency in the UK.

BOX 13.7 Differentiated diagnosis of macrocytosis without megaloblasts

- Haemolytic anaemia.
- Hypothyroidism.
- Alcohol excess.
- Liver disease.
- Drugs, e.g. azathioprime, metronidizole.

Points to note

A commonly made mistake: macrocytic **does not mean** megaloblastic. The degree of macrocytosis gives a clue to the likely aetiology:

- MCV $<$ 110: alcohol, liver disease, thyroid, or azathioprine.
- MCV $>$ 110: B_{12} and folate deficiency or myelodysplasia.

- Absorption problems also occur in Crohn's disease and post-gastrectomy.
- Treat with B_{12} replacement therapy—oral if the deficiency is dietary or by injection if there is an absorption problem.

Pernicious anaemia

Pernicious anaemia is due to poor intestinal absorption of vitamin B12, which is caused by faulty production of intrinsic factor by the gastric mucosa.

It affects 1 in 8000 people over the age of 60 years, but occurs at a younger age ($<$55 years) in patients with a family history.

It is more common in:

- women than men
- fair haired and skinned people
- people who develop grey hair early
- patients with gastric atrophy

Furthermore:

- there is an association with other autoimmune diseases, especially hypothyroidism (2.4%)
- there is also an increased risk of tumour development (both gastric and carcinoid)

Clinical features are the same as other causes of B12 deficiency.

Investigations:

- Serum B12
- Blood film shows low WBC, low platelets and low Hb
- Parietal and Intrinsic factor antibodies
- Bone marrow shows megaloblasts, later a pancytopenia may develop
- Schilling test
- Treatment is by injection of B12 (1000 mcg of hydroxyhydrocobalamin) intramuscularly once every 3 months

The initial treatment is with high doses of vitamin B12, to restore normal B12 stores. Thereafter, once every 3 months, an injection is required for the rest of the patient's life to prevent relapse.

Folic acid deficiency

Like B_{12}, folate is used for single carbon unit transfer in DNA synthesis. Folic acid stores are only sufficient for 3.5 to 4 months, resulting in severe deficiency in patients whose diet consists mainly of ready-prepared meals devoid of vegetables. The main effect of folic acid deficiency is on the bone marrow. Deficiency leads to the production of large RBCs (macrocytes), some of which may be primitive with nuclei (megaloblasts). Neutrophils have hypersegmented nuclei and platelets are abnormal. There are a number of causes of folate deficiency:

- haemolytic anaemia
- fast-growing tumours
- pregnancy
- malabsorption
- a diet of convenience food and lacking in vegetables
- drugs: antiepileptics, antimalarials, and oral contraceptives.

Clinical features: deficiency of folate causes a similar picture to B_{12} deficiency. Signs in addition to those of anaemia are:

- mild jaundice due to unconjugated bilirubin in destroyed immature cells
- smooth tongue and glossitis
- angular cheilitis.

Causes of folate deficiency include dietary deficiency, malabsorption, phenytoin, and increased bodily demands.

Investigation requires measurement of the red cell folate level (serum folate does not assess anything other than recent intake). **Treatment** is by oral folate therapy. (Note: giving folate therapy without excluding B_{12} deficiency may lead to spinal cord degeneration.)

Polycythaemia

Polycythaemia is an increase in red blood cell count, packed cell volume (PCV), or haemoglobin level. There are two types of polycythaemia:

- Absolute: primary—polycythaemia rubra vera—and secondary to pathology from renal, endocrine, cardiac and respiratory courses.
- Relative: reduction in plasma volume with normal red cell mass.

Primary polycythaemia (polycythaemia rubra vera)

Polycythaemia rubra vera may be regarded as a myeloproliferative disorder that results from an abnormal proliferation of red cell precursors derived from a haemopoietic progenitor cell. There is a consequent increase in the production of RBCs, white blood cells (WBCs), and platelets.

Clinical features:

- Patients complain of persistent, severe pruritus especially after bathing.
- The spleen is enlarged.
- Cardiovascular presentation includes angina or intermittent claudication.
- Central nervous system symptoms include headaches, dizziness, and visual and hearing disturbances.
- Patients appear plethoric with a cyanotic tinge.
- There is a tendency to bleed caused by abnormal platelet aggregation.
- Peptic ulceration.

Investigations show:

- Increase in haemoglobin levels and PCV.
- Absolute increase in red cell mass.
- Increase in white cell and/or platelet count.
- Increase in uric acid.
- Increase in leucocyte alkaline phosphatase.
- Bone marrow examination shows active marrow but erythropoiesis is normoblastic.

Early complications of polycythaemia rubra vera are death secondary to bleeding and cardiac emergencies. Later complications include thrombocythaemia, leukaemia, and myelofibrosis.

Secondary polycythaemia

In secondary polycythaemia there is an increase in the RBCs but not WBCs or platelets, and the spleen is not enlarged. Secondary polycythaemia has numerous causes:

- renal disease (tumours, post transplant)
- respiratory (altitude, chronic lung disease, Pickwickian syndrome)
- cardiac (congenital cyanotic heart disease)
- endocrine (Cushing's disease, phaeochromocytoma)
- tumours (cerebellar haemangioma, uterine fibroids, hepatoma).

BOX 13.8 Dental implications of polycythaemia

- Operative risk—thrombosis.
- Keep patient well oxygenated during surgical procedures.
- Prophylactic measures needed for DVT.
- In primary polycythaemia patients are at an increased risk of bleeding.
- Chronic myeloid leukaemia may present with gingival infiltration.
- Watch blood pressure in Addison's and Cushing's patients; they may need perioperative steroids.

Relative polycythaemia

There are two types of relative polycythaemia:

- Caused by diminished plasma volume, e.g. severe dehydration, Addison's or Cushing's disease.
- Caused by obesity in middle-aged males with a red cell mass at the upper limit of normal and a plasma volume at the lower limit of normal. This results from changes in venous capacity secondary to age-related changes in the autonomic nervous system.

Laboratory investigations should look for cerebrovascular disease and coronary artery disease.

THE WHITE BLOOD CELLS

The function of white blood cells is as part of the immune system. White blood cells (WBCs) are classified as:

- neutrophils
- lymphocytes
- monocytes
- basophils
- oesinophils.

Neutrophils and **monocytes** phagocytose and kill micro-organisms by degranulation using enzymes and the oxidative free radicals. **Monocytes** and **macrophages** are also directly involved in killing intracellular micro-organisms, especially those responsible for chronic infective states such as mycobacterial infection. Macrophages are also capable of specialized immune functions such as antigen presentation. **Lymphocytes** are divided into **T cells** and **B cells**. T cells are involved in the cellular immune response whereas B cells are involved in the humoral immune response. Oesinophils are involved in allergic reactions.

Leukaemia

Leukaemia results from malignant clonal proliferation of one of the bone marrow cell lines. There are two main groups of leukaemias, acute and chronic, classified according to the type of cell proliferation.

Leukaemic cells result from a multifactoral environment and host factors. Random or chance damage to DNA during cell division may result from radiation, alkylating chemicals, or immunosuppressive drugs. Genetic factors are also involved, e.g. people with Down syndrome are at a higher than normal risk of developing leukaemia. Infections may also play a part in the aetiology, but no direct evidence of this exists for humans.

The disease produces its effect by direct invasion, causing bone marrow failure or accumulation of leukaemic cells. Bone marrow failure results in

Table 13.1 Clinical features of acute leukaemia

Clinical feature	Association
Anaemia	Marrow aplasia
Bruising and bleeding	Marrow aplasia
Recurrent infection	Marrow aplasia
Bone pain	Marrow cell replacement
Hyperviscosity syndrome	Large numbers of cells in circulation
Gingival hypertrophy (in AML)	Tissue deposits of leukaemic cells
Neurological involvement	More common in ALL than in AML
Lymphadenopathy	More common in ALL than AML
Splenomegaly	More common in ALL than AML
Hepatomegaly	More common in ALL than AML
Bleeding	Special feature of promyelocytic leukaemia

AML, acute myelogenous leukaemia; ALL, acute lymphoblastic leukaemia.

anaemia, leucopenia, and thrombocytopenia. Leukaemic cells may also accumulate in tissues to produce neurological problems and enlargement of the liver, spleen, and lymph nodes.

Acute leukaemia

The acute onset causes tiredness, malaise, and pyrexia (especially night sweats). In the terminal phase of the disease undifferentiated stem cells proliferate in massive amounts causing numerous symptoms.

The **clinical features** of acute leukaemia are set out in Table 13.1.

Treatment aims to destroy the rapidly dividing malignant cells and depends on the classification of the acute leukaemia. Current therapy includes chemotherapy, radiation, and bone marrow transplantation. Gene fusion therapy results in a cure rate of 90% with minimal long-term side-effects. Prognosis has improved markedly over the last 15–30 years. Several factors affect the prognosis, including the treatment selected and the total WBC count at presentation. The best prognosis is seen in acute lymphoblastic leukaemia.

Acute lymphoblastic leukaemia

Acute lymphoblastic leukaemia (ALL) is the most common childhood leukaemia, with the peak incidence between the ages of 2 and 10 years. The cure rate varies from 60–90% depending on treatment and prognostic factors.

Acute myelogenous leukaemia

Acute myelogenous leukaemia (AML) is a heterogenous group of disorders, with the possible involvement of all cell lines (see Table 13.2). AML accounts for 80% of all adult leukaemias.

Table 13.2 Proliferating cell lines in AML

Proliferating cell line	Disease from myeloblastic progenitor
Myeloblasts (MO and M1)	Myeloblastic leukaemia
Granulocytes (M2)	Myeloid leukaemia
Promyelocyte (M3)	Promyelocytic leukaemia
Myelomonocyte (M4)	Myelomonocytic leukaemia
Monocyte (M5)	Monocytic leukaemia
Erythroblasts (M6)	Erythroblastic leukaemia
Megakarocyte (M7)	Megakaryoblastic leukaemia

BOX 13.9 Dental implications of acute leukaemia

- Oral manifestations may be severe in acute leukaemia. This may be the presenting complaint in approximately 40% of patients. However, clinical examination reveals that up to 70% of patients have oral signs at the time of diagnosis.
- Signs in head and neck area: cervical lymph node enlargement (in ALL), cranial nerve palsies (in ALL), facial or intra-oral infection, gingival hyperplasia (fragile and bleeding) (in AML), gingival or periodontal infection, gingival and mucosal bleeding.
- Spontaneous bleeding is unlikely until the platelet count drops below $30 \times 10^9/l$. However, the low platelet count combined with gingival infection causes intense bleeding during toothbrushing.
- Dental extractions may provoke haemorrhage at counts below $80 \times 10^9/l$.
- Orodental infections should be treated aggressively, as a lack of neutrophils and lymphocytes may lead to fatal overwhelming infection.

Oral infections in acute leukaemia

- Fungal—*Candida* causes a sore mouth.
- Viral—HSV, CMV, and herpes zoster cause vesicular ulceration.
- EBV causes ulcers and hairy leucoplakia,
- Bacterial—acute ulcerative necrotizing gingivitis (ANUG).

Chronic leukaemia

Chronic leukaemia may be asymptomatic for many years. There are two forms: chronic myeloid leukaemia (CML) and chronic lymphocytic leukaemia (CLL).

Chronic myeloid leukaemia

CML is seen mainly in adults. A CML variant in children runs a much more aggressive course.

CML is due to proliferation of the pleuripotent stem cells together with the Philadelphia (Ph) chromosome. The Ph chromosome results from a reciprocal translocation between one chromosome 9 and one chromosome 22 (designated t(9;22)). This results in one chromosome 9 longer than normal and one

> **BOX 13.10** Oral problems caused by treatment regimes
>
> Treatment of leukaemias also causes oral problems. Both chemotherapy and irradiation cause orodental problems:
>
> - Bone marrow failure secondary to bone marrow irradiation.
> - Salivary gland damage causes dry mouth within 1 week, with swollen painful glands and long-term gland atrophy.
> - Osteoradionecrosis secondary to irradiation damage to the blood supply.
> - Mucositis caused by the direct effect of chemotherapy and radiotherapy on the mucosae.

chromosome 22 shorter than normal; the latter is called the Philadelphia chromosome. Only 5 to 10% of patients with CML may present without the Ph chromosome.

Clinical features: the symptoms of CML may be non-specific:

- In 50% of cases, the diagnosis is made during haematological tests for another reason
- tiredness
- malaise
- weight loss
- signs of anaemia
- splenomegaly in 90% of cases
- hepatosplenomegaly in 50% of cases

The initial chronic phase lasts 2–3 years before the disease enters a blastic phase which may be either lymphoid (40%) or myeloid (60%).

Investigation and treatment

The white cell count on **diagnosis** is high, 20–400 $\times$ 10^9/l with a large increase of neutrophils, myelocytes, and blast cells. Thrombocytophilia, oesinophilia, and basophilia are also prominent.

Treatment is initially with interferon-α (IFN-α) and bone marrow transplantation. Imatinib (Gleevec) may be used when IFN-2 fails or in accelerated phase or blast crises.

Chronic lymphocytic leukaemia

CLL results from clonal proliferation of mature B lymphocytes. It accounts for 25% of all leukaemias. Patients present with a WBC count of greater than 10×10^9/l. The disease is more common in men and affects the elderly (60–80-year-olds). Unlike CML, transition to acute leukaemia is rare.

The **clinical features** of CLL include: painless lymphadenopathy; recurrent infections; and anaemia, lymphopenia, thrombocytopenia due to bone marrow failure.

Treatment should not be given in the advanced stages of the disease. The most successful treatment to date has been with alkylating agents, although splenectomy, splenic irradiation, leucophoresis, monoclonal antibodies such as Campath-1H, and methylprednisolone are also treatment options.

Lymphoma

Non-Hodgkin's lymphoma

Non-Hodgkin's lymphoma (NHL) is characterized by the finding of collections of abnormal lymphocytes within lymph nodes. Although unknown, the aetiology may be due to infection by micro-organisms (e.g. HIV, Epstein–Barr virus (EBV), *Helicobacter*), drugs, as well as autoimmune and genetic conditions, e.g. ataxia telangiectasia. NHL is seen in middle-aged to elderly people.

There are three clinical variants of NHL (see Table 13.3). Treatment is based on this classification. Patients with stage I of the intermediate stage can be cured by radiotherapy alone. High-grade lymphoma necessitates therapy directed at preventing CNS involvement.

Hodgkin's lymphoma

Hodgkin's lymphoma is rare in the UK and shows a 3 : 2 male:female preponderance. There is a large peak in incidence between 20 and 30 years with a smaller peak between the ages of 50 and 60 years.

Table 13.3 Clinical variants of NHL (based on the WHO/REAL classification)

Grade	Disease course	Per cent of patients
Low	Indolent	40
Intermediate	Aggressive	50
High	Very aggressive (risk of CNS disease)	10

BOX 13.11 Dental implications of NHL

- Patients may present with cervical lymphadenopathy or intra-oral lesions.
- Lesions may be found in minor or major salivary glands. They may be associated with gastric MALT (mucosa-associated lymphoid tissue) lymphomas.
- Lesions on the palate are more likely to spread to the CNS.
- Anticipate oral infections—treat 'trivial' infections aggressively and maintain a high standard of oral hygiene.
- Patients need to be immunosuppressed. Do not expose them to cross-infection risks.
- Extraction of teeth should necessitate a full blood count to check the platelet count.
- Treat mucositis.
- Remember that there may be an underlying systemic problem, such as HIV or Sjögren's syndrome.

Table 13.4 WHO/REAL classification of Hodgkin's lymphoma

Histological type	Phenotype of RS cells
Nodular lymphocytic predominant	CD20+, CD30+, CD75+, EMA+
Nodular sclerosing	CD15+, CD30
Mixed cellularity	CD15+, CD30+
Lymphocyte depletion	CD15+, CD30+
Lymphocyte-rich, classical Hodgkin's disease	

RS = Reed-Sternberg; EMA, epithelial membrane antigen.

EBV is implicated in the aetiology, with the virus localized to the Reed–Sternberg cells. A genetic component is also important, with a 99-fold increased risk apparent in monozygotic twins. Occupational risks include exposure to benzene and nitrous oxide used by dentists in relative analgesia.

Histological diagnosis is carried out using the WHO/REAL (1994) classification as shown in Table 13.4.

The **clinical features** of Hodgkin's lymphoma are as follows:

- Ninety per cent of patients present with painless lymphadenopathy: 80% located in the neck cervical nodes or supraclavicular fossae and 15% in the axillae.
- Nodes are rubbery and firm on inspection.
- Spread is contiguous.
- Other symptoms include: fever, weight loss, pruritus, alcohol-induced pain, recurrent infection.

Investigations and treatment

Staging is important in defining treatment regimes (see Table 13.5).

Treatment is by radiotherapy or chemotherapy. Cure rates are high but 15% of cured patients develop a second malignancy within 15 years.

Radiotherapy can have a number of adverse affects due to radiation damage of tissues:

- Damage to salivary glands—swollen parotids and xerostomia.
- Damage to bone—osteoradionecrosis.
- Damage to teeth—radiation caries.
- Mucous membranes—mucositis, recurrent infection.
- Damage to lungs—pneumonitis.
- Damage to thyroid—hypothyroidism.
- The field radiation dose may give rise to solid tumours, myeloid leukaemia, or non-Hodgkin's lymphoma.
- General adverse effects are malaise and skin burns.

Table 13.5 Cotswolds staging in Hodgkin's disease

Stage	Feature
I	Disease in single node region or structure
II	Disease in two or more regions are same side of diaphragm
III	Disease in two or more regions on both sides of diaphragm
III(1)	With or without splenic, hilar, coelic, or portal nodes
III(2)	With para-aortic, iliac, or mesenteric nodes
IV	Involvement of extranodal sites

Suffixes are added to any of the above stages (e.g. IIIE): A, no systemic symptoms present. B, systemic symptoms present. E, extranodal involvement, contiguous or proximal to known site. X, bulky disease.

BOX 13.12 Problems presented to the dental surgeon by treatment for Hodgkin's disease

- Careful treatment planning before radiotherapy or chemotherapy begins. Any carious teeth should be restored or extracted.
- Patients should be instructed about good oral hygiene.
- During cancer treatment, anaesthetic and antibacterial mouthwashes should be given. Do not carry out any extractions or endodontics. However, emergency treatment must always be given.
- After radiation or chemotherapy, treat antifungal or bacterial infections promptly.
- Treat dry mouth with sialogogues. Ensure oral comfort. Review the teeth and jaw regularly for radiation caries and osteoradionecrosis.
- Maintain a high index of suspicion for the presence of recurrent tumours in the head and neck area years after treatment.

Other lymphomas

- Maltoma: lymphoma of mucosa-associated lymphoid tissue. Affects the gut and may be linked to *Helicobactor pylori* infection. Treatment of infection may lead to regression of the lymphoma.
- Sjögren's syndrome. Risk of development of lymphoma in the major or minor salivary glands.
- Oral lymphomas occur in HIV infection.

- Burkitt's lymphoma is an Epstein–Barr related lymphoma common in Africa with predilection for sites in the jaw. There are associated chromosomal translocations.
- Adult T-cell lymphoma is related to HTLV1 infection and is common in Afro-Caribbeans in the UK.
- Cutaneous T-cell lymphoma, e.g. mycosis fungoides.

PLASMA CELLS

Multiple myeloma

Multiple myeloma is the result of a monoclonal expansion of immunoglobulin-producing plasma cells within the bone marrow cavity, at multiple sites. Extramodullary deposits may also occur. The clonal immunoglobulins may be detected in serum and urine. They produce abnormal light chains called Bence-Jones protein. The disease is more common in men of African descent after 60 years of age.

Clinical features
- Asymptomaic—paraproteins may be found on routine screening.
- Bone pain secondary to increased osteolysis.
- Osteolytic lesions may be seen in the skull, long bones, or any other part of the skeleton.
- Five to 10% of patients develop primary amyloidosis.
- Renal failure caused by excessive Bence-Jones protein, hypercalcaemia, drugs such as non-steroidal anti-inflammatories, infection, dehydration, or amyloid deposits in the kidney.
- Infections: oral fungal and bacterial infections as well as chest infections are common.
- Peripheral neuropathy may occur, e.g. carpal tunnel syndrome.
- Congestive cardiac failure.

Investigations
- Because the cells all arise from a single clone, a single localized 'M band' or paraprotein is seen on electrophoresis.
- Three per cent of the elderly have benign monoclonal gammopathy.
- In 25% of cases light chains formed in the urine are the only recognizable product.
- In 50% of cases the paraprotein is IgG and in 20% it is IgA. It is very rare to have IgM light chains.

The IgM paraprotein causes problems of hyperviscosity (Waldenström's macroglobulinaemia), agglutination of RBCs, and gangrene of the extremities at low temperatures.

> **BOX 13.13** Dental implications of multiple myeloma
> - May present with lytic lesions in the jaws or skull.
> - May present with bleeding problems.
> - Inability to metabolize drugs. Analgesics, e.g. NSAIDs, make renal failure worse.
> - May present with non-dental pain in jaws or skull.
> - Patients are prone to infections such as oral candidosis.

Treatment

There is no effective treatment at present. Median survival is 3–4 years. Treatment options include chemotherapy and interferon. Maintenance therapy includes bone marrow transplantation.

A regime for younger patients includes vincristine and adriamycin with dexamethasone followed by autologous transplantation. In older patients melphalan and prednisolone or cyclophosphamide are given.

TRANSFUSION OF BLOOD AND BLOOD PRODUCTS

In the UK blood and blood products are obtained for transfusion from unpaid donors. They supply one unit (450 ml) of blood two or three times a year. The blood is screened for HIV-1, HIV-2, hepatitis B and C viruses, and syphilis. Screening for CMV antibodies is used for blood or blood products used for bone marrow transplantation. Leucodepletion is used on all blood preparations because of the risk of new variant Creutzfeldt–Jakob disease (CJD) as there is no test at present for prion proteins.

Problems associated with transfusion of blood and blood products

- Circulatory overload.
- Pyrexia.
- Transfusion of the wrong blood or blood component—ABO incompatibility.
- Infection due to viruses, bacteria, or parasites.
- Hypersensitivity reactions: anaphylaxis due to IgA deficiency in recipient; transfusion-associated lung injury due to donor WBC antibodies; post-transfusion purpura due to platelet antigens; delayed transfusion reactions due to RBC antigens; rhesus sensitization by RBC antigens.
- Iron overload.
- Hypothermia.
- Transfusion haemolysis.
- Hyperkalaemia.
- Clotting problems.
- Intravenous additives.
- Dangers of massive transfusion may lead to deficiency of clotting factors and platelets, cardiac arrest due to excess citrate, excess potassium and cold blood.

- Haemosiderosis—there is 1 mg of iron in every millilitre of packed red cells; continued transfusions may lead to massive iron excess.
- Mechanical hazards: air embolism, catheter embolism, thrombophlebitis.

In the UK serious adverse reactions are compulsory reported (serious hazards of transfusion (SHOT)). The data are collected randomly. SHOT reports show that transfusion of incorrect blood or blood components is the major cause of transfusion reaction accounting for up to 60% of all adverse effects.

BLEEDING DISORDERS

Congenital bleeding disorders

Congenital bleeding disorders can be divided into **coagulation factor deficiencies** and **vascular defects**. Coagulation factor deficiencies include:

- haemophilia A
- haemophilia B
- von Willebrand's disease
- factor XIII deficiency (results in delayed wound healing)
- afibrinogenaemia (rare, and bleeding problems are minor).

Vascular defects include:

- hereditary haemorrhagic telangiectasia
- Ehlers–Danlos syndrome.

Platelet abnormalities are rare

Acquired bleeding disorders

Acquired bleeding disorders can be divided into **coagulation factor defects** and **platelet abnormalities**. Coagulation factor deficiencies occur:

- due to vitamin K deficiency
- post-partum bleeding
- as a result of drug reaction, e.g. penicillin
- in systemic lupus erythematosus
- with cirrhosis of the liver.

Platelet abnormalities may be due to:

- thrombocytopenia
- chronic idiopathic thrombocytopenia
- drug-induced thrombocytopenia.

Screening tests

- A full blood count will detect thrombocytopenia, anaemia, leukaemia, and disseminated intravascular coagulation (DIC). The blood film will show any abnormal morphology of the cells.

- Coagulation screening tests are shown in Table 13.6.
- Perform specific assays, bleeding time, or platelet aggregation tests as indicated (Table 13.7).

Table 13.6 Coagulation screening tests

Test	Abnormality
Bleeding time	Platelets, von Willebrand's disease
APTT	Factors XII, XI, XI, IX, VIII, V, II, I
PT	Factors X, VII, V, II, I
TCT	Factors I, fibrinogen degradation products

APTT, activated partial thromboplastin time; PT, prothrombin time; TCT, thrombin clotting time.

Table 13.7 Results of coagulation screening tests in different disorders

Disorder	PT	APPT	TCT	Platelets
Haemophilia A	UC	↑	UC	UC
Haemophilia B	UC	↑	UC	UC
Liver disease	↑↑	↑	UC, ↑	↓
Von Willebrand's disease	UC	↑	UC	N
DIC	↑	↑	↑↑	↓
Aspirin	↑	UC	UC	↓
Warfarin	↑	↑	↑	UC
Heparin	↑	↑	↑	UC
Factor VII deficiency	↑	↑	UC	UC

APTT, activated partial thromboplastin time; PT, prothrombin time; TCT, thrombin clotting time; UC, unchanged; DIC, disseminated intravascular coagulation.

BOX 13.14 Dental implications of post-extraction or post-operative bleeding

- Do not forget to take a history of the duration and type of bleeding, family history, other diseases, e.g. of the liver and kidney, as well as patient drug history.
- Remember the most common cause is local factors.
- Examine the wound for signs of trauma, infection, or bony or root fragments.
- Apply local measures, e.g. debridement or wound pressure packs; EDTA rinse if oozing continues.
- Carry out the basic screening tests as described in the text.

Note that vitamin K deficiency affects the production of factors II, VII, IX, and X. Liver disease, which affects the production of vitamin K, will also affect the production of these factors. Drugs are an important cause of bleeding: for example warfarin and heparin sulphate, aspirin and NSAIDs, new antiplatelet drugs, e.g. clopidogrel (Plavix), ticlopidine (Ticlid), and dipyridamole (Persantine).

Once the above screening tests are carried out specific assays for clotting factors, platelet function and platelet antibodies should be carried out.

HAEMOSTASIS

Trauma to the tissues commonly results in a disturbance of haemostasis resulting in the clinical picture of bruising or post-extraction bleeding. Haemostasis is further compromised by other factors such as fever, hypoxia, metabolic disturbance, drugs, or systemic disease. Haemostasis is the response of the tissue to vascular damage. It is maintained by:

- the formation of a platelet plug
- constriction of blood vessels
- local blood coagulation
- fibrin formation
- fibrinolysis.

For clots to form a series of interactions take place between platelets, blood vessels, and clotting factors. The initial event is the adhesion of platelets to the collagen of exposed endothelium. Platelets respond by releasing adenine nucleotides and serotonin from their storage granules, which cause a change in the shape of the platelets and the formation of pseudopodia. The prostaglandin pathway is also activated by the simultaneous release of arachidonic acid.

Blood vessel endothelium releases prostacyclin, which is a powerful inhibitor of platelet aggregation. The prostaglandin-, platelet-, and endothelial-derived factors maintain a state of balance between circulating platelets and the vessel wall.

Local trauma, e.g. extraction, disturbs this balance causing increased adhesion and aggregation. As platelets become more activated, surface membrane lipid activates prothrombin to produce thrombin, which in turn activates fibrin. Plasmin is also released by tissue damage; this activates fibrinolysis. Fibrinolysis becomes a problem in extensive injury where there is a large amount of tissue damage.

Coagulation

Fibrin is used to reinforce the initial platelet plug. Fibrin is produced by the clotting cascade of serine proteases that amplify the initial message to produce large amounts of fibrin at the site of injury. Simultaneous activation of the fibrinolytic system prevents production of fibrin where it is not needed. The coagulation pathways are shown in the figure.

Anticoagulant drugs act on the coagulation pathways as follows:

- Heparin: enhances the activity of antithrombin III.
- Warfarin: inhibits post-translational γ carboxylation of the N-terminal glutamic acid residues in factors II, VII, IX, and X, synthesized in the liver, which prevents them binding calcium. These are the vitamin K-dependent factors.

Clotting factor abnormalities, e.g. haemophilia, as well as inappropriate coagulation, deficiencies of natural anticoagulants, e.g. proteins C and S, and excessive activation, e.g. in DIC, all act to cause problems of bruising and bleeding.

Inherited diseases of haemostasis

Haemophilia A: factor VIII deficiency
Haemophilia A is a congenital deficiency of factor VIII. It is an X-linked recessive disorder affecting 1 in 10 000 males. Affected females are carriers and transmit the disease. Carriers have levels of factor VIII which are 50–60% of normal and may become symptomatic following major trauma. There are currently 5500 people with haemophilia A on the UK Register.

The **clinical features** of haemophilia A are dependent on amount of factor VIII activity (see Table 13.8).

A **diagnosis** of haemophilia A should be considered in males with a family history of a bleeding disorder. Coagulation tests will show an increase in the APTT and specific factor analysis will differentiate between factor VIII and IX deficiency.

The **management** of haemophilia A requires a multidisciplinary approach headed by a physician and a haematologist with a special interest in the disease. The team should include a dentist who is familiar with the special needs of those patients. Treatment is directed towards dealing with a specific problem or prophylactic therapy:

- Factor VIII replacement using either cryoprecipitate or freeze-dried factor VIII. For surgical procedures the amount of factor VIII needed depends on the procedure. Minor surgery may need a level of 30–40% whereas major surgery requires approximately 50–100%.
- Prophylactic therapy is given when anticipated bleeding situations may occur. The level is then increased to 15%.

Haemophilia A has a number of **complications**:

- Pain is a major clinical problem for haemophiliacs. Paracetamol should be used for analgesia. Ibruprofen is thought to be safe and effective.
- Anticipated problems as complication of treatment: infection; hepatitis; HIV; other as yet characterized viruses.
- Inhibitors to factor VIII: 10–15% of haemophiliacs develop these.

Haemophilia B (Christmas disease)
There are only 1100 patients with haemophilia B on the UK Register. It is inherited as an X-linked recessive trait caused by a mutation in the gene for factor IX.

Three variants have been defined with a fourth unique variant—haemophilia B Leiden:

- CRM (cross-reacting material) positive is most common: factor IX is non-functional.
- CRM negative: factor IX is quantitatively reduced in antigenicity and activity.
- CRM^R variable.
- Haemophilia B Leiden is inherited as CRM negative but becomes CRM positive with aging.

The clinical features of haemophilia B are identical to those of haemophilia A.

Diagnosis is made using specific factor IX assay and the thromboplastin generation test.

Treatment is with specific factor IX concentrate. Always check therapy using the Recommendations of the United Kingdom Haemophilia Centre Directors Organisation.

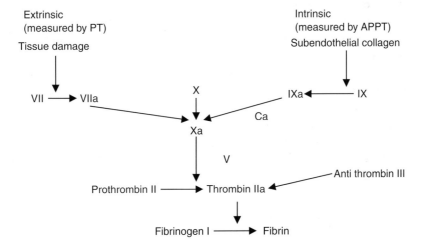

Table 13.8 Clinical features of haemophilia A

Factor VIII activity (% of normal levels)	Clinical problems
<1%	Bleeding soon after birth Spontaneous bleeding Haemarthrosis Soft tissue bleeding, e.g. mucous membranes in mouth and oropharynx
1–5%	Bleeding following trauma
>5%	Minor bleeding episodes only
>25%	Asymptomatic

Von Willebrand's disease

Von Willebrand's disease (VWD) is the most common inherited clotting disorder, affecting 125 per million population. It is inherited as an autosomal dominant or recessive trait, and is characterized by quantitative and/or qualitative abnormalities in platelet, endothelial, and plasma von Willebrand factor (VWF). This disorder is heterogenous with three main variants:

- Type I accounts for 75% of all cases. There is a quantitative deficiency of VWF.
- Type II accounts for 20% of all cases. There is functional defect of VWF. Both type I and type II VWD are inherited in an autosomal dominant fashion.
- Type III is the homozygous form of the disease and is relatively uncommon. It is responsible for major bleeding problems. Transmission of type III is autosomal recessive with no family history or as a double heterozygote with a family history of consanguinity.

Clinical features of VWD include:

- Mucocutaneous haemorrhages (the most common feature).
- Patients may present with gingival bleeding without any dental cause.
- Prolonged bleeding may be precipitated by dental extraction, surgical procedures such as tonsillectomy, post-partum haemorrhage, and menorrhagia.

The main abnormality is prolonged bleeding time. Therefore, the main aim of **treatment** is to correct the bleeding time to maintain haemostasis:

- In mild cases use desmopressin (DDVAP) (0.3 mg/kg) by slow infusion.
- Local haemostasis may be obtained by using fibrin glue, collagen, and topical thrombin.
- In the dental situation antifibrinolytic treatment such as tranexamic acid is useful.
- Highly purified VWF concentrate is now available. It is useful in major bleeds and will correct the bleeding time for up to 12 h.
- Do not use platelet inhibitory agents, e.g. aspirin.
- Do not use dextran for volume replacement.
- Do not use intramuscular injections and avoid dental blocks in these patients.

Acquired disorders of haemostasis

Acquired disorders of haemostasis are much more common than inherited disorders. They usually affect multiple factors. The same screening tests are used. The screening test will involve using a mixture of equal parts of the patient's and control plasma to distinguish the patient's deficiency from the presence of abnormal inhibitors. The commonest acquired deficiency is anticoagulant therapy. Liver disease, disorders of vitamin K metabolism, and DIC are also common.

Coumarin anticoagulants

Coumarin anticoagulants are competitive inhibitors of vitamin K and therefore decrease the availability of vitamin K in the hepatocyte. This leads to a decrease in factors II, VII, IX, X, and proteins C and S because no γ-carboxyglutamic acid

Table 13.9 Drugs interacting with warfarin

Class of drug	Increases warfarin activity	Decreases warfarin activity
Antibiotics	Ciprofloxacin	
	Cotrimoxazole	
	Erythromycin	
	Metronidazole	
	Sulphonamides	
	Trimethoprim	
Antiepileptics	Phenytoin	Carbamazepine
		Phenobarbital
		Phenytoin
Antifungals	Fluconazole	Griseofulvin
	Miconazole	
	Itraconazole	
	Metoconazole	
Hormones	Corticosteroids	
	Stanazol	
	Danazol	
	Tamoxifen	
	Thyroxine	
Cardiac drugs	Quinidine	Quinidine
	Amiodarone	
Analgesics	Phenylbutazone	Mefenamic acid
	Mefenamic acid	
Antigout medication	Allopurinol	Allopurinol
Ulcer related	Cimetidine	Sucralfate
	Omeprazole	
Others	Alcohol	Oral contraceptives
		Barbiturates
		Vitamin K

residues are added to the factors, resulting in loss of binding to the phospholipid 'skeleton' of the coagulation sequence. The overall effect can be measured by the prothrombin time (PT) and the International Normalized Ratio (INR). Many drugs interact with the commonly used coumarin anticoagulant warfarin, either increasing or decreasing its effect (see Table 13.9).

Heparin

Heparin is a glycosaminoglycan and is a heterogeneous preparation. This gives heparin a variable half-life depending on the dose and preparation administered. Patients also vary in their responses, necessitating dose adjustment. Its anticoagulant effect is due to its high-affinity binding to antithrombin. Once bound to heparin, antithrombin undergoes a conformational change that will rapidly inactivate thrombin, factor IXa and factor Xa.

Therapy is monitored using the partial thromoplastin time (APTT). Side-effects include haemorrhage, thrombocytopenia, and osteopenia.

Disorders of vitamin K metabolism

Vitamin K is a fat-soluble vitamin found in green vegetables. There may be deficiency in neonates hepatic disease malabsorption of fat from the gut. Warfarin is the most common cause of vitamin K deficiency.

Deficient Vitamin K results in loss of clotting factors II, VII, IX, and X. All neonates are routinely given Vitamin K at birth to prevent neonatal haemorrhage.

Liver disease

The liver synthesizes all the coagulation factors except factor VIII. It also has an important role in clearing the blood of active enzymes, in blood coagulation, and in fibrinolysis. There are a number of causes of bleeding in liver disease:

- In obstructive jaundice there is malabsorption of fat and vitamin K deficiency.
- In hepatocellular disease there is defective liver synthesis of multiple clotting factors.
- In portal hypertension increased fibrinolysis may contribute to a minor bleeding tendency and platelets may be sequestered in the spleen.

Screening tests, PT, PTT, TCT, fibrinogen and platelet count should be carried out. There is usually a prolongation of PT and APTT. Deficiency of vitamin K-dependent factors (II, VII, IX, and X) is reflected in moderately prolonged PT and APTT values. TCT and fibrinogen levels are usually normal (fibrinogen levels may be increased).

Renal disease

There is an increased likelihood of bleeding in renal disease. Associated clinical problems seen in ureamia are:

- Purpura,
- gingival bleeding,
- gastrointestinal bleeding.
- In severe case, intracranial bleeding and haemopericardium may occur.

Disseminated intravascular coagulation (DIC)

Disseminated intravascular coagulation is a pathological response to underlying disorders. It is characterized by widespread activation of haemostasis involving coagulation factors, platelets, physiological factors, fibrinolysis-activated endothelium, and the formation of soluble and insoluble fibrin within the circulation. Most cases present with bleeding, but in approximately 10% widespread thrombotic problems occur.

DIC has the following **clinical features**:

- The patient is very ill.
- There is bruising.
- Oozing from injection or venepuncture sites.

- Post-partum bleeding from the vagina may be catastrophic.
- Thrombotic microemboli of fingers and toes occur.

There are a number of pathological conditions which may predispose to DIC:

- Severe infections causing scepticaemia.
- Shock secondary to surgical trauma.
- Obstetrics.
- Malignancy, especially associated with metastatic disease.
- Liver disease.
- Incompatible blood transfusion.
- Fat embolism.

Management of DIC involves:

- Treatment of the underlying disorder.
- Treatment of shock.
- Screen blood for PT, PTT, fibrinogen and fibrinogen degradation products and platelets.
- Transfusion with fresh frozen plasma.
- Cryoprecipitate concentrate may be given. Aim to maintain PT and PTT within a ratio of 1.5 of control values, fibrinogen levels of greater than 1 g/l, and the haematocit greater than 0.30.

Platelets

Platelets are small granular non-nucleated cells. They are approximately 1.4 μm in size and are found at a concentration in the blood of 150–400 $\times$ 10^9/l. Platelets are rich in intracellular granules including:

- Lysosymal granules: dense granules containing calcium, ATP, ADP, and serotonin.
- Alpha granules containing platelet factor IV, factor V, beta thromboglobulin, factor VIII/VWF and fibrinogen.

The membrane contains a number of receptors involved in adhesive protein binding. A deficiency of blood platelets is termed **thrombocytopenia**, whereas an increased number of platelets is termed **thrombocytosis**.

The function of platelets is to initiate primary haemostasis by:

- **Activation:** Exposure of the sub-epithelium and collagen activates platelets. They change shape, produce pseudopodia, and expose receptor sites.
- **Adhesion:** The pseudopodia adhere to the damaged area via receptor sites which interact with high-molecular-weight multimers of factor VIII (factor VIII/VWF and fibronectin).
- **Aggregation:** Platelets aggregate using fibrinogen as an intercellular bridge. They then contract releasing more proaggregatory factors, ADP, serotonin, thromboxane A, fibrinogen, and VWF. ADP is also released from damaged red blood cells at the site of injury.

- **Clot regeneration:** The extrinsic pathway of coagulation is activated by tissue factor. Thrombin is generated which is a potent activator of the common pathway of coagulation.

Drugs and platelets

The figure shows the platelet metabolic pathways. The relative balance of the two arms of the pathway can be exploited by antiplatelet drugs at the correct dose and frequency (see Table 13.10). Too much drug, or too frequent a use of these drugs, will not be beneficial. Remember that NSAIDs such as ibuprofen and diclofenac have a reversible effect on platelet aggregation. However, platelet function is restored once the drug is cleared from the circulation.

Table 13.10 Effect of antiplatelet drugs on haemostasis

Drug[†]	Effect
Aspirin	Inhibits platelet aggregation irreversibly (lasts 7–10 days)
Clopidogrel	Inhibits platelet aggregation
Ticlopidine	Irreversible inhibition of platelet aggregation
Dipyridamole	Reversible inhibition of platelet aggregation

[†]All antiplatelet drugs affect clotting by inhibiting platelet aggregation.

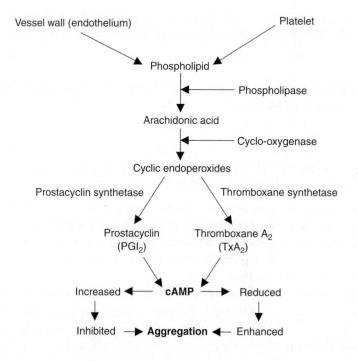

BOX 13.15 Dental implications for patients on antiplatelet medication

The dental implications for patients on antiplatelet medication depend on the drugs being used as well as the underlying disease and dental procedure:

- Antiplatelet medication includes: low-dose aspirin (75–300 mg daily), clopidogrel, triclopidine, dipyridamole.
- Patients at risk of bleeding may have liver disease, renal failure, a known clotting defect, or be undergoing radiotherapy or chemotherapy.

Dental procedures which can be carried out include:
- In dental practice NSAIDs do not pose a risk for surgical procedures.
- Extraction of up to three teeth.
- Gingival surgery.
- Non-traumatic surgical removal of a tooth.

Procedures to follow to reduce the risk of bleeding:
- Use an aspirating local anaesthetic syringe.
- Use a vasoconstrictor in local anaesthetic.
- Use a pack soaked with absorbable dressing, e.g. oxidized cellulose or collagen sponge, in the extraction site.
- Suture the socket carefully.
- Apply pressure to the extraction site with a gauze pad for 15–30 min.
- The patient should rest while local the anaesthetic wears off to give a clot time to form (2–3 h).
- Do not rinse the mouth for 24 h.
- Do not dislodge the clot.
- Avoid hot drinks and do not chew on affected side.
- Avoid NSAIDs: use paracetamol for pain relief.

Although trauma aggravated by local factors is the major cause of bleeding, oozing, and bruising of tissues, underlying systemic problems must be excluded. These disorders may be both genetic and acquired.

Disorders of platelets

Abnormal platelets either quantitatively or functionally are characterized by a long bleeding time from small puncture wounds. Clinically this presents as purpura. The dental implications of platelet disorders are important because the mouth is a common site of bleeding. Treatment using platelet transfusions may be necessary. Disorders of platelet function are summarized in Table 13.11.

Inherited platelet disorders

The inherited platelet disorders are:

- **Grey platelet syndrome**. This is characterized by Mild to moderate thrombocytopenia. It is a rare syndrome inherited as autosomal dominant trait

Table 13.11 Disorders of platelet function

Type of disorder	Inherited	Acquired
Adhesion	Von Willebrand's disease	Myeloproliferative disorder
	Bernard–Soulier syndrome	Renal failure
		Scurvy
Aggregation	Glanzmann's thrombasthenia	Myeloma
		Dextran
		Aspirin
Release	Storage pool deficiency	Penicillin
		Phenylbutazone
		Sulfinpyrazone

From chapter by F. Fortune in *Clinical Methods* published by Blackwell Scientific.

characterized by abnormal platelet activation. The alpha granules, which contain the platelet-specific factors, are abnormal. Bleeding may be moderate or severe. For severe episodes, platelet infusions may be needed. During moderate episodes DDAVP may shorten bleeding time.

- **Glanzmann's thrombasthenia**. Glanzmann's thrombosthenia is inherited as an autosomal recessive trait. Family history often reveals consanguinity. The pathology in the gene results in a deficiency of the proteins GPIIIb/IIIa resulting in an inability of fibrinogen to bind to the platelet membrane and platelet aggregation fails to occur. Symptoms occur early in childhood and the disease characterized by moderate to severe mucocutaneous haemorrhages and menorrhagia. Treatment is by HLA-matched platelet transfusions.
- **Von Willebrand's disease**. This heterogeneous condition is characterized by both qualitative and quantitative abnormalities in platelets together with endothelial and plasma VWF. The platelet abnormality results in an adhesion defect.
- **Bernard–Soulier syndrome**. There is a deficiency of platelet surface glycoproteins. It is rare and transmitted in an autosomal and incompletely recessive trait. The main symptoms are mucocutaneous bleeding and menorrhagia.

Acquired platelet disorder: autoimmune haemolytic disease
In autoimmune haemolytic disease there are antibodies to platelets. The antibodies may be warm IgG at 37 °C or cold IgM at 4 °C. Although both cold and warm antibodies are usually primary they may also be secondary:

- The cold antibodies may be secondary to infection, most commonly EBV or mycoplasma infection.

- The warm antibodies are secondary to systemic lupus erythematosus, lymphoma, or drugs.

The **clinical features** of autoimmune haemolytic disease are:

- anaemia
- mild jaundice
- mild splenomegaly.
- Additional features are: clinical features of the underlying problem. In cold haemagglutinin disease (CHAD) there is acrocyanosis, which is a purple discoloration of the ears, nose, and digits.

Treatment involves treatment of the underlying condition. In primary disease:

- plasma exchange
- immunoglobulin infusion
- folic acid.

In warm antibody disease:

- immunosuppression with steroids or azathioprine
- splenectomy.

In cold antibody disease:
- splenomegaly and immunosuppression are unhelpful.
  Other causes of acquired platelet disorder are **drugs**:

- aspirin—thromboxane A_2 inhibitor,
- dipyridamole—phosphodiesterase inhibitor,
- ticlopidine—prostacyclin analogue,
- clopidrogel—affects PIIIb/IIIa,

renal failure, which affects platelet aggregation, and **cardiopulmonary bypass**, which causes platelet fragmentation.

14 Endocrine disorders and disorders of bone metabolism

THE PITUITARY GLAND

The pituitary gland produces hormones which regulate the function of the endocrine organs such as the thyroid gland, the adrenal cortex, the breast, and the gonads, as well as targeting non-endocrine organs and tissues. Each pituitary hormone is regulated by hypothalamic-derived substances as well as regulated in a negative-feedback loop by substances produced by its target organs. Negative feedback occurs at both hypothalamic and pituitary levels.

The **hormones secreted by the pituitary** are as follows:

- Anterior pituitary: follicle-stimulating hormone (FSH), luteinizing hormone (LH), adrenocorticotrophic hormone (ACTH), thyroid-stimulating hormone (TSH), growth hormone (GH), prolactin.
- Posterior pituitary: antidiuretic hormone (ADH), oxytocin.

The **hypothalamic trophic hormones** are: CRH (corticotrophin releasing hormone), thyrotrophin-releasing hormone (TRH), somatotrophin, growth hormone-releasing hormone (GHRH), corticotrophin-releasing hormone (CRH).

Because of the position of the pituitary space-occupying lesions have a major effect. Space-occupying lesions found in the pituitary include:

- Secreting adenomas: found in Cushing's disease (basophil adenoma), acromegaly (eosinophil adenoma), and prolactinoma.
- Non-secreting adenomas: granulomas, e.g. in TB, sarcoidosis, Wegener's granulomatosis; lymphomas; metastatic carcinoma; craniopharyngioma.

Clinical features of these may be due to the direct effect of excess secretion (hypersecretion) or undersecretion (hyposecretion) (see Tables 14.1 and 14.2) or local effects of a space-occupying lesion, such as headache or bitemporal hemianopia.

Acromegaly

Acromegaly is a result of prolonged increased levels of circulating growth hormone (GH) in adults. High levels of growth hormone in children before fusion of the epiphyseal plates results in acromegalic gigantism.

Acromegaly is uncommon, with approximately five cases per million population per year, and the prevalence rate 30–40 per million. The most common cause is a benign oesiniphilic adenoma secreting growth hormone. Other causes are a benign adenoma secreting growth hormone and prolactin, pituitary

Table 14.1 Effects of pituitary hypersecretion

Hormone	Effect
TRH	Hyperthyroid
ACTH	Cushing's disease
Growth hormone	Gigantism
	Acromegaly
	Diabetes
Prolactin	Galactorrhoea
	Amenorrhoea
	Sterility
Gonadotrophins	Modification of sexual function

Table 14.2 Effects of pituitary hyposecretion

Hormone	Effect
TRH	Hypothyroidism
Growth hormone	Dwarfism
ACTH	Features of Addison's disease
Prolactin	Failure of lactation
Gonadotrophic hormones	Amenorrhoea
	Sterility
	Impotence

carcinoma, or an association with multiple endocrine neoplasia type I (affecting the parathyroid and pancreas).

Clinical features

Acromegaly has a very long list of clinical features:

- **General features**: acne, hirsuitism, and excessive sweating.
- **Facial features**: general coarse features with soft tissue thickening, broad nose, prominent supraorbital ridges, and enlarged sinuses.
- **Intraoral features**: bimandibular prognathism; increased separation of teeth especially where there have been extractions; macroglossia and increased salivation.
- **Hands and feet**: large spade-like hands and feet; carpal tunnel syndrome due to compression of the median nerve.
- **Cardiovascular features**: hypertension, coronary artery disease (from hypertension and diabetes), and cardiomyopathy.
- **Metabolic features**: type 2 diabetes secondary to insulin resistance; menstrual problems in women (amenorrhoea and galactorrhoea); men have hypogonadism, low libido, and impotence.

- **Direct effects of tumour**: headache; visual field defects (classically bitemporal hemianopia); squinting due to compression of cranial nerves III, IV, and IV; hypopituitarism affecting secretion of anterior pituitary hormones (hormones affected are LH, TSH, and ACTH).
- **Arthritis** affects the spine and weight-bearing joints.

Investigations
- Check levels of growth hormone.
- Insulin-like growth factor (IGF-1) is increased. Its production in the liver is stimulated by GH. It is a more reliable indicator than GH as the levels do not fluctuate during the day.
- The glucose tolerance test measures both glucose and growth hormone.
- In acromegaly growth hormone stays elevated whereas in healthy individuals the levels are undetectable.
- X-ray of the skull shows enlargement of the supraorbital ridges, mandible and maxilla, and sella turcica.
- X-ray of the hands and feet shows tufting of the terminal phalanges and thickening of the heel pad.
- Chest X-ray may show left ventricular enlargement.

Treatment
The metabolic abnormalities need to be reversed with symptomatic relief and systemic effects. Growth hormone should be reduced to <5 mU/l.

- **Medical treatment**: somatostatin analogue octreotide or lanreotide; dopamine agonist such as cabergoline (no longer widely used); GH receptor agonists reduce IGF-1 levels very effectively.
- **Surgical treatment**: the transphenoidal approach is the treatment of choice and is used as first-line treatment in most centres. It gives good results in experienced hands.

BOX 14.1 Dental relevance of acromegaly

- Both hard and soft tissues are affected, resulting in facial changes. The dentist may be the first to notice the results of excess growth hormone.
- Patients may have a class III malocclusion or spacing of teeth.
- Extractions may be difficult because of bony ankylosis.
- Macroglossia makes routine procedures difficult.
- Dental management may be complicated by diabetes mellitus, hypertension, cardiac rhythm abnormalities, and cardiomyopathy.
- Remember patients become progressively hypopituitary and are at risk of collapse.
- Practical procedures may be hampered by visual field defects.
- Patients develop arthritis early and the occipito-axial and temporomandibular joint may be affected.

- **Radiotherapy**: used if surgery does not reduce levels to <5 mU/l. Yttrium implants or external irradiation is used.

Treatment should be instituted early as life expectancy can be halved. With or without treatment patients progressively develop hypopituitarism.

Diabetes insipidus

Diabetes insipidus is a rare disease characterized by the passage of large amounts of urine—usually more than 3 l per 24 h with an osmolality of less than 300 mOsmol/kg. This is due to a lack of antidiuretic hormone (ADH, also known as vasopressin).

Vasopressin is produced in the hypothalamus in the magnocellular neurons of the supraoptic nucleus and stored in the posterior pituitary. It is released into the circulation in response to changes in blood osmolality. It acts on the distal renal nephron and concentrates the urine. Loss of body water will increase osmolality which in turn will stimulate vasopressin release as well as stimulate thirst.

Diabetes insipidus has a number of possible causes:

- familial idiopathic diabetes insipidus is the commonest form;
- malformations, e.g. Laurence–Moon–Biedl syndrome;
- autoantibodies to magnocelluar neurons;
- craniopharyngioma;
- secondary tumours;
- in rare cases surgery or irradiation to the pituitary;
- head injury;
- infections such as meningitis;
- granulomas such as tuberculosis, oesinophilic granuloma, or sarcoidosis;
- drugs, e.g. lithium carbonate.

The mechanism for polyuria is:

- Nephrogenic: i.e. reduced renal response to vasopressin. This is usually inherited.
- Hypothalamic: i.e. the inability to regulate vasopressin.
- Primary polydipsia: i.e. where patient drinks excessive amounts of water persistently.

The main **clinical features** are polyuria and polydipsia. In psychogenic polydipsia thirst is the main clinical feature.

Polyuria itself can have a number of causes in addition to diabetes insipidus:

- chronic renal failure
- hypercalceamia
- hyperkalaemia
- diabetes mellitus.

Investigations

- Urine volume should be >3 l per 24 h with low osmolality (300 mOsmol/kg).
- Exclude common causes of polyuria by performing blood sugar and serum potassium and calcium tests.
- Desmopressin fluid deprivation test: Make sure the patient is well hydrated before test. Measure urine volume and osmolality then restrict fluid for 8 h weighing the patient every 2 h. Weight loss should be no more than 5% of starting weight. Inject 2 μg desmopressin intramuscularly and obtain blood and urine for osmolality and urine volume at 12 and 24 h after commencing the test. In diabetes insipidus the blood osmolality rises but not the urine osmolality.
- Pituitary and hypothalamic MRI may establish causal factors.

Treatment

For nephrogenic diabetes insipidus:

- Correct the metabolic disturbance and ensure adequate fluid intake.
- Urine output may be reduced by a combination of indomethacin and thiazide diuretic.

For hypothalamic/cranial diabetes insipidus:

- Ensure adequate fluid intake.
- Treat those with high volume output >4 l per 24 h with desmopressin orally or intranasally (watch for hypernatraemia).

For primary polydipsia:

- Treat the underlying disorder which may be psychogenic.
- Restrict the patient's water intake.

THE PARATHYROID GLAND

Ninety-five per cent of individuals have four parathyroid glands. They are small and embedded in the thyroid gland. The upper pair is derived from the fourth pharyngeal pouch and is situated in the upper posterior surface, whereas the lower pair is derived from the third pharyngeal pouch, situated close to the lower pole of the thyroid. Occasionally the lower pair is situated in the mediastinum. The diseases affecting the gland are mainly due to hyper- and hypo-function and tumours. Its major function is that of calcium metabolism.

Hypoparathyroidism

Common causes of hypoparathyroidism are:

- post-thyroid surgery (thyroidectomy)
- idiopathic/autoimmune causes.

Rarer but important cause are **Di George syndrome** and **polyglandular autoimmune syndrome type 1**.

Di George syndrome is due to failure of the development of the third and fourth pharyngeal pouches. It results in hypoplasia or absence of thymus including hypoplasia or absence of the parathyroid, cleft lip and palate, and congenital heart defects.

Polyglandular autoimmune syndrome type 1 comprises hypoparathyroidism and Addison's disease plus any two or three of:

- insulin-dependent diabetes mellitus
- primary ovarian failure
- vitiligo
- alopecia
- malabsorption
- pernicious anaemia
- chronic active hepatitis
- autoimmune thyroid disease.

Pseudohypoparathyroidism is due to resistance to parathyroid hormone (PTH) causing hypoparathyroidism. It is characterized by severe hypomagnesaemia (<0.40 mmol/l) and is due to Crohn's disease or a disorder of the renal tubules.

The main **clinical features** of hypoparathyroidism are due to the hypocalcaemia. Other features depend on the cause. There are a number of signs associated with Di George syndrome and other genetic causes of hypoparathyroidism:

- mental subnormality
- dry, coarse skin
- delayed tooth development
- nail dystrophy
- papilloedema
- calcified basal ganglia
- signs of other autoimmune disorders.

BOX 14.2 Dental relevance of hypoparathyroidism

- Candidosis of the mouth and hands in polyglandular autoimmune syndrome type 1 Treatment of candidosis is extremely difficult and recurs.
- Other problems such as hypertension, hypocalcaemia, and hypoglycaemia all influence appropriate dental treatment.
- Neuromuscular instability.
- Circumoral paraesthesia.
- Chvostek sign—circumoral twitching secondary to gentle tapping of the facial nerve arterial to the ear.
- Trousseau's sign—carpal spasm when blood pressure cuff is >20 mmHg higher than systolic pressure.
- Seizures and fits.
- Laryngospasm and bronchospasm.
- Associated organ-specific autoimmune disease may impact on oral care.

Table 14.3 Causes of hyperparathyroidism

Cause	Per cent of cases
Adenoma	80
Hyperplasia	15–20
Carcinoma	0.5
Multiple endocrine neoplasia types I and II	0.5–5

Hyperparathyroidism

Patients with hyperparathyroidism are usually asymptomatic and present any age. It is more common in females (female : male ratio 3 : 1). Incidence is 1 per 1000 and the worldwide prevalence is 4–5 million. Age presentation is usually between 50 and 53 years.

The causes of hyperparathyroidism are shown in Table 14.3. Patients with an adenoma or hyperplasia are usually asymptomatic whereas those with carcinoma have severe hypercalcaemia and are symptomatic.

Clinical features
- Most patients are asymptomatic with no clinical signs.
- Ten per cent of patients have 'bones, stones, groans, and abdominal pain'.
- Non-specific features are weakness, malaise, and depression.
- Patients may have hypertension and peptic ulceration.
- Renal problems include nephrocalcinosis and nephrolithiasis.
- Skeletal problems include salt-and-pepper skull, bone cysts, brain tremors, and subperiosteal resorption of the distal phalanges.
- Neuromuscular problems are very rare.

Investigations and treatment
Investigations include:

- serum calcium
- serum PTH
- localization of the lesion by ultrasonography or using sestamibi parathyroid scan and MRI.
- renal function
- bone mass using dual-energy X-ray densitometry (bone loss is usually due to cortical not cancellous bone).

Treatment is conservative.

- check serum and urinary calcium every 6 months;
- bone scan and density measured yearly;
- if the patient is a post-menopausal woman HRT and oestrogen help reduce serum calcium.

Surgery may be done if the tumour is large and the patient symptomatic.

> **BOX 14.3 Causes of hypercalcaemia**
>
> - Primary hyperparathyroidism
> - Carcinoma: primary disease or metastatic disease.
> - Abnormal vitamin D metabolism: vitamin D toxicity or granulomatous disease (e.g. sarcoid, TB, histoplasmosis).
> - Immobilization.
> - Other endocrine disorders: thyrotoxicosis, phaeochromocytoma, VIPoma (vaso-intestinal polypetide hormone), acute adrenal insufficiency.
> - Drugs and medication: thiazide diuretics, milk-alkali syndrome, vitamin A toxicity, lithium, aluminium excess, parenteral nutrition.
> - Renal disease: acute and chronic.

> **BOX 14.4 Dental relevance of hyperparathyroidism**
>
> - Brown tumours of the mandible or maxilla.
> - Loss of lamina dura around teeth is pathognomonic.
> - Ostopenia, and patients are prone to pathological fractures.
> - May be associated autoimmune disorders which have oral implications: consider hyperparathyroidism in patients with recurrent epulides.

THE THYROID GLAND AND ITS DISORDERS

The thyroid gland is the most vascular organ in the body. It is a large bi-lobed gland in the shape of a butterfly, situated in the neck above the manubrium sternii and in front of the trachea. The butterfly wings represent the left and right thyroid lobes. It enlarges to extend below the level of the manubrium sternii in the neck.

The thyroid produces thyroxine, the thyroid hormone, which is under pituitary and hypothalamic control, by TSH secreted by the pituitary and TRH secreted by the hypothalamus. A negative feedback loop for hormone secretion occurs.

The main function of the gland is to regulate the metabolism of the body. The gland is subject to abnormalities of growth and enlargement, hormone secretion, the occurrence of nodules and cancerous growths.

Iodine is an essential requirement for development of the thyroid gland. It is used in synthesis of thyroxine (T4) and triiodothyronine (T3). Deficiency leads to cretinism, mental retardation, decreased fertility and the development of a goitre. The minimum daily requirement of iodine for different groups of people is shown in Table 14.4. Prevention of iodine deficiency is by fortification of food, it is added to table salt, bread, and cheese, or by intramuscular injection or oral administration in oil.

Table 14.4 Daily requirement of iodine

Group	Age (years)	Iodine requirement (μg/day)
Children	0–6	90
	7–10	120
Adults		150
Pregnant and lactating women		200

Thyroid imaging techniques

A number of different techniques are used for imaging the thyroid for the purpose of diagnosis of thyroid disease:

- Ultrasound is mandatory in any patient with suspicion of thyroid disease.
- Radionuclide scanning and iodine-131: technetium-99m is preferred for thyroid scanning because it visualizes functioning thyroid parenchyma, it localizes ectopic thyroid and assesses the functional state of the gland ('cold' or non-functioning nodules are sometimes found in thyroid carcinoma and 'hot' nodules are associated with toxic adenomas).
- Computed tomography (CT) gives a good definition of masses in the neck, mediastinum, and lungs.
- Magnetic resonance imaging (MRI) gives good anatomical images of the head, neck, and chest.

Cretinism

Cretinism is a condition which results from a lack of maternal and fetal iodine and thyroxine during fetal development. Lack of iodine during neurological development has serious consequences. Once neurological damage occurs it is irreversible. In congenital hypothyroidism neurological damage may be limited by administering thyroxine immediately after birth.

BOX 14.5 Dental implications of cretinism

- Late development of teeth.
- Teeth erupt in a haphazard order and are irregular in size and shape.
- Hypocalcification of teeth.
- High incidence of caries.
- Crowding at puberty very common.
- Canines may be missing.
- Teeth may appear in anomalous positions.
- Deficient jaw development.

The **clinical features** of cretinism are:

- typical cretinoid facies noted soon after birth
- defects in the skeleton—skull deformity
- dry skin, scanty hair
- pot belly
- failure to thrive.

Goitre

Goitre is a swelling arising from the thyroid. It is the most common cause of midline swelling in the neck. There are many causes:

- Nodular: adenoma (may be with 'hot nodule'), carcinoma.
- Multinodular: toxic multinodular goitre of elderly, Hashimoto's disease, carcinoma.
- Diffuse: Graves' disease, Hashimoto's disease.
- Simple: goitrogen induced, e.g. excess iodine, lithium, antithyroid drugs; painless thyroiditis; subacute thyroiditis; painful enlargement caused by haemorrhage or infection.

BOX 14.6 General clinical signs of thyrotoxicosis

- Patient looks anxious with lid retraction and lid lag.
- Difficulty of upward gaze is an early sign.
- The patient is thin with fatigue and apathy.
- Warm sweaty peripheries.
- Glucose intolerance.
- If goitre is present it may be diffuse with or without a bruit.
- Thinning hair or hair loss.
- Oligomenorrhoea or amenorrhoea.
- Infertility.
- Tremor of the hands.
- Palpitations; pulse shows resting tachycardia.
- ECG may indicate that tachycardia is atrial fibrillation.
- May find signs of high-output cardiac failure.
- Proximal myopathy affecting the upper and lower limbs.

BOX 14.7 Ocular signs in hyperthyroidism

- Lid lag, lid retraction.
- Periorbital puffiness.
- Increased lachrymation/grittiness of eyes.
- Chemosis.
- Proptosis.
- Ophthalmoplegia.
- Diplopia.
- Papilloedema.
- Loss of visual acuity.

Thyrotoxicosis (hyperthyroidism)

Thyrotoxicosis is due to excess free thyroxine or free triiodothyronine. It affects 10 times as many women as men (about 2% of women may be affected). About 80% of cases of thyrotoxicosis are due to **Graves' disease** (see below). Other causes include:

- toxic adenoma
- toxic multinodular goitre
- metastatic thyroid cancer
- pituitary adenoma secreting TSH
- post-partum thyrotoxicosis
- De Quervain's thyroiditis
- excessive thyroxine administration for hypothyroidism or for cosmetic reasons, e.g. induction of weight loss
- exogenous iodide.

Graves' disease

Graves' disease accounts for about 80% of all cases of thyrotoxicosis. It is an organ-specific autoimmune disease.

Graves' disease has the following **clinical features** (note that thyrotoxicosis may be very difficult to recognize in the elderly):

- There is diffuse swelling of the thyroid in 95% of cases.
- The patient is nervous and agitated.
- There is a heightened state of anxiety (e.g. the patient feels as if they are 'running a marathon and never finishing').
- Inappropriate emotions and emotional lability.
- Heat intolerance.
- Weight loss despite an increased appetite.
- Diarrhoea.
- Amenorrhoea or oligomenorrhoea.
- Muscle weakness.
- Palpitations.

There are a number of clinical signs of thyrotoxicosis specific to Graves' disease:

- One to 5% of patients have pretibial myxoedema. The thickened skin appears as plaque like dusky lesions over the shins or feet.
- One per cent of patients have thyroid acropachy—pseudo clubbing (swelling of the end of fingers).
- Seventy to 90% of patients have ophthalmopathy. This is due to infiltration of the extraocular muscles by lymphocytes, with oedema and fibrosis. This is also seen in other forms of autoimmune thyroid disease (e.g. Hashimoto's disease).

Investigations in thyrotoxicosis

- Thyroid-stimulating hormone (TSH) assay: TSH is reduced in hyperthyroidism.

- Thyroxine (T4): T4 is raised in thyrotoxicosis. Care must be exercised with women on HRT, drugs, e.g. the Pill, protein losing states, and autoantibodies (T3) as all interfere with assay: therefore always measure free T4.
- Triiodothyronine (T3): in T3 toxicosis TSH is low and T4 normal.

Treatment of thyrotoxicosis

Medical treatment consists of combination therapy with the antithyroid drugs carbimazole and propylthiouracil. Both are effective treatments but carbimazole is more widely used in the UK. Both drugs can cause agranulocytosis, but this is rare. Beta-blockers are used at the initiation of treatment to damp down systemic symptoms but should be stopped once the antithyroid drugs begin to work. Treatment last 6–24 months depending on the dosing schedule; if patients relapse after treatment ^{131}I therapy is instituted.

Radioiodine, ^{131}I, is concentrated in the thyroid gland and causes the death of rapidly dividing cells. Treatment either causes ablation or leaves a minimal amount of thyroid tissue. There are a number of problems associated with radioiodine use:

- In the short term: avoid contact with young children; thyroiditis may occur; sialoadenitis; transient hypothyroidism in the first 3 months of treatment.
- In the long term: permanent hypothyroidism (10% in first year, 3–5% later); worsens ophthalmopathy.

Surgical treatment is also used. A subtotal thyroidectomy leaves some functioning glandular tissue and aims to achieve euthyroidism. There are also a number of problems associated with surgery:

- post-surgical haemorrhage;
- hypothyroidism;
- recurrent laryngeal nerve damage;
- thyroid crisis (or storm) may occur post-operatively, characterized by loss of appetite, nausea, vomiting, and tachycardia with thready pulse and fever. The patient becomes semiconscious and very restless. Thyroid crisis can be prevented by rendering the patient euthyroid before surgery;
- hypocalcaemia in 20% of cases—it is transient but in 2% the hypocalcaemia becomes permanent;
- relapse occurs in 10% of cases over a period of 10 years.

BOX 14.8 Dental relevance of thyrotoxicosis
- The patient may have high blood sugar.
- The patient may have hypercalcaemia.
- Patients usually have a resting tachycardia; therefore take care with adrenaline.
- Inadvertent intravascular injection may precipitate a critical arrhythmia.
- Patients are emotionally labile.
- Take care to use protective glasses for patients, who may have proptosis.

Hypothyroidism

Hypothyroidism results from a deficiency of thyroid hormones. More than 85% of patients are females. Hypothyroidism usually occurs between the ages of 40 and 70 years and is commonly underdiagnosed.

The causes of hypothyroidism include:

- iodine deficiency (this is the major cause worldwide)
- thyroid surgery
- thyroiditis, which may be autoimmune or infectious
- previous treatment with radioiodine or thyroidectomy
- antithyroid drugs
- other drugs, e.g. lithium and amiodarone
- cretinism, which is due to severe maternal iodine deficiency
- dyshormonogenesis
- disease of the hypothalamus or pituitary.

Clinical features of hypothyroidism

The clinical signs may be subtle, making condition difficult to diagnose. Patients may or may not have a goitre. The goitre when present is a non-tender, firm, moderately enlarged midline mass.

- **General features**: tiredness, weight gain, cold intolerance, myxoedema 'facies', pallor, coarse features, loss of outer third of eyebrows.
- **Haematological features**: iron deficiency anaemia, macrocytic anaemia, pernicious anaemia, normochromic, normocytic anaemia.
- **Cardiovascular system**: bradycardia, angina, hypertension/hypotension, cardiac failure, pericardial effusion.
- **Cutaneous area**: dry/coarse skin, pale yellow skin colour (hypercarotinaemia), myxoedma, erythema abigne, vitiligo, loss of body hair.
- **Nervous system**: poor memory, depression, auditory hallucinations, slow-relaxing tendon reflexes, cerebellar ataxia, 'myxoedema madness', perceptive deafness.
- **Metabolism**: low basal metabolic rate, hypercholesterolaemia, hypercarotinaemia, hyperglyceamia, delayed puberty, growth and mental retardation.
- **Musculoskeletal system**: aches and pains, myalgia and muscle stiffness, carpal tunnel syndrome.

BOX 14.9 Dental relevance of hypothyroidism

- Patients are at risk of cardiovascular disease.
- Patients are more prone to oral candidosis.
- Patients may be hypertensive.
- These patients are prone to depression and may present with atypical facial pain.

Table 14.5 Types of thyroid cancer

| | Type of thyroid cancer | | | | |
	Papillary	Follicular	Medullary	Anaplastic	Lymphoma
Frequency	80%		1%		Pts? Thyroiditis
Age on onset	20–30			60–70	>55 yr
Sex	Female		Both with family history		Female
Metastases	No, local invasion	Yes, 20%	Yes, cells	Yes	Yes
Treatment	Surgery	Surgery and radiotherapy (DXT)	DXT	Surgery and DXT chemotherapy	DXT
10-yr mobility	95%	80%	0%	0%	

- **Endocrine system**: menorrhagia, infertility, galactorrhoea and hyperprolactinaemia.
- **Gastrointestinal system**: constipation, ileus, ascites.

Investigations and treatment

Thyroid-stimulating hormone (TSH) assay shows raised TSH. Thyroxine levels are low.

Treatment is by supplementation of the body's thyroxine levels by administering synthetic thyroxin. Thyroxine levels must be monitored regularly.

Thyroid cancer

Thyroid cancer presents as a midline goitrous swelling. Thyroid cancer accounts for 0.5% of all malignancies and 0.5% of all deaths from cancer.

The aetiology of thyroid cancer is mainly unknown, but radiation increases the risk: the Chernobyl explosion in Ukraine in April 1986 released huge quantities of radiation, radioactive iodine, and radioactive xenon and an increase in thyroid cancer was observed in children in the areas affected.

Table 14.5 gives details about the different types of thyroid cancer.

Investigations
- TSH, T3 and T4 assay.
- Calcitonin assay.
- Respiratory flow volume loop is better than X-ray when looking for tracheal compression.
- Ultrasound scan shows if goitre is cystic/solid or multinodular.
- Technetium-99m pertechnetate scan.

- 'Cold' nodule may be carcinoma (the majority are benign).
- 'Hot' nodules do not exclude carcinoma.
- Fine needle aspiration biopsy; care is needed with interpretation.

THE ADRENAL GLAND AND ITS DISORDERS

The adrenal glands are triangular-shaped glands located on top of the kidneys. Adrenal diseases are uncommon. They arise from abnormalities in hormone secretion from the adrenal cortex and medulla. There is functional zonation: these are the zona fascicularis, the zona reticuaris, and the zona glomerulosa where the different steroid hormones from the basic cyclopentenoperhydrophenanthrane nucleus are produced. The adrenal cortex produces glucocorticoids, mineralocorticoids (aldesterone and deoxycorticosterone), and sex steroids (mainly androgens but also some oestrogen).

Glucocorticoids (cortisol and corticosterone) are synthesized in zona fascicularis and zona reticuaris and aldosterone is synthesized in the zona glomerulosa. ACTH controls steroidogenesis in the adrenal gland as well as in the gonads and placenta. Aldosterone biosynthesis is under the control of the renin–angiotension system.

The adrenal medulla produces the catecholamines adrenaline and noradrenaline. Diseases due to adrenal disorders include congenital adrenal hyperplasia, Cushing's syndrome, Addison's disease, and pheochromocytoma.

Congenital adrenal hyperplasia

Congenital adrenal hyperplasia is an inherited defect due to low levels of cortisol and/or aldosterone. Negative feedback results in high levels of adrenocorticotrophic hormone (ACTH). Ninety per cent of cases are due to 21-hydroxylase deficiency.

Clinical features of congenital adrenal hyperplasia include:

- In the newborn: female virilized *in utero* secondary to excess adrenal androgen converted into testosterone; aldosterone deficiency occurs in most cases; large clitoris resembling a penis.
- In children: males show precocious sexual development; tall stature; penis remains prepubertal; females have early onset of pubic hair or later hirsutism and menstrual problems.

Treatment involves giving hydrocortisone to all patients and 9α-fludrocortisone for salt losers. Surgery may be used to refashion the clitoris.

Cushing's syndrome

Cushing's syndrome is due to glucocorticoid excess and is the term used to describe all causes of glucocorticoid excess. Cushing's disease describes pituitary-dependent cases; it is caused by basophil adenoma of the pituitary and was first described by H. G.Turney in 1913. The definitive paper was published by Harvey Cushing in 1922.

ACTH-dependent Cushing's syndrome can be:

- iatrogenic
- caused by Cushing's disease
- ectopic, from tumours secreting ACTH (e.g. prostate, bronchial oat cell).

ACTH-independent Cushing's syndrome can be:

- iatrogenic
- due to adrenal adenoma or carcinoma
- caused by excess alcohol consumption
- due to McCune–Bright syndrome
- due to Carney's syndrome.

Cushing's syndrome has the following **symptoms**:

- weight gain
- fatigue and muscle weakness
- hirsuitism
- red striae
- hair thinning and loss
- emotional lability
- frank psychosis or neurosis
- fractures
- irregular menstruation.

Signs of Cushing's syndrome include:

- truncal obesity
- moonface and plethora
- buffalo hump
- bruising
- striae
- hirsuitism
- pigmentation
- osteoporosis
- proximal myopathy
- hypertension
- hyperglycaemia.

Investigations will show:

- raised plasma cortisol (usually nocturnal)
- raised 24-h urinary free cortisol
- low potassium
- sodium raised or at the upper limit of normal
- insulin tolerance test shows ACTH rising in response to hypoglycaemia
- polycythaemia and leucocytosis.

> **BOX 14.10** Dental relevance of Cushing's syndrome
>
> - Patients are prone to infection.
> - There is poor wound healing.
> - Patients may be diabetic.
> - Patients may be hypertensive.
> - Patients may be emotionally labile.
> - Patients with Cushing's disease may have visual loss.
> - Patients may be immunosuppressed.

In the **low-dose dexamethasone suppression test** (high sensitivity, low specificity) 0.5 mg dexamethasone is given 6-hourly for 48 h. Very little suppression of plasma cortisol is found in Cushing's syndrome. In the **high dose dexamethasone suppression test** (high sensitivity and high specificity) 2 mg dexamethasone is given 6-hourly for 48 h. The results indicates the site of the pathology: plasma cortisol suppression occurs in adrenal hyperplasia but no suppression occurs in adrenal adenoma or carcinoma. MRI or CT scan gives a good localization of the tumour site.

The **treatment** of Cushing's syndomre depends the cause:

- Trans-sphenoidal surgery for selective tumour removal.
- Unilateral adrenalectomy.
- Pituitary irradiation, although long-term results are less favourable than surgery.
- Drugs to block the overproduction of cortisol are also used: metapyrone is usually used before irradiation or surgery; other drugs include amino-glutethimide and ketoconazole. These are all toxic. Both metapyrone and ketoconazole inhibit steroid production. Of the two, metapyrone is the drug of choice.

Hypoadrenalism

Hypoadrenalism is the insufficient production of adrenocortical hormones to meet physiological requirements. Primary hypoadrenalism is called Addison's disease. Secondary hypoadrenalism is due to deficiency of ACTH. Lack of function of the adrenal glands may be acute or chronic.

Acute hypoadrenalism may be induced by:

- scepticaemia
- unintentional surgical removal of the adrenal cortex
- abrupt withdrawal of high-dose systemic steroids
- sudden pituitary necrosis as in Sheehan's syndrome

Hypoadrenalism is most likely to be due to corticosteroids causing pituitary–adrenal suppression.

Addison's disease

Addison's disease (primary hypoadrenalism) was first described by Thomas Addison in 1849. It is caused by the destruction of the adrenal cortex. Addison's disease is more common in males than females. Addison's disease can be caused by:

- autoimmune adrenalitis
- tuberculosis
- bilateral adrenalectomy for malignant disease
- meningococcal septicaemia
- metastatic tumour deposits.

Rare causes include: amyloidosis, haemochromatosis, histoplasmosis, congenital adrenal hypoplasia or hyperplasia, and drugs (e.g. rifampicin, etomidate, ketoconazole).

Addison's disease has the following **clinical features**:

- Oral pigmentation is an early sign and occurs initially along the bite line on the buccal mucosa.
- Skin pigmentation may be the first sign of the disease, preceding other symptoms; it occurs in sun-exposed or trauma-associated areas.
- Lassitude and muscular weakness.
- Anorexia, weight loss, epigastric discomfort, nausea and vomiting.
- Postural hypotension, feeling faint and dizzy.
- Loss of body hair.
- Depression.
- Nocturia.
- Impotence and amenorrhoea.
- Diarrhoea.
- Hypoglycaemia.

The main **investigations** is screening for urea and electrolytes (U&E), ACTH, cortisol, and blood sugar. Specific tests include:

- ACTH stimulation tests: synacthen test (short tetracosactrin test). If the results are equivocal, then proceed to the long synacthen test.
- Biochemistry: raised Ca, raised K and low blood sugar; raised renin, low aldosterone.
- Chest and kidney X-rays-may show calcification, e.g. tuberculosis.
- Ectopic corticotrophin-releasing hormone (CRH): tumours may secrete ACTH and CRH and not CRH alone.

Pheochromocytoma

The adrenal medulla produces adrenaline, noradrenaline, and dopamine, which are responsible for helping to maintain blood pressure. It is also produced in response to stress.

Pheochromocytomas are tumours, which arise from the chromaffin tissue of the adrenal medulla. There are about eight cases per million per year. Ninety per cent arise directly from the adrenal glands and ten per cent from extra-adrenal chromaffin tissue, the organs of Zuckerkandl, which is a collection of tissue around the inferior mesenteric artery. Ten per cent of tumours occur bilaterally.

Most tumours usually arise sporadically, and only a few are familial. Familial tumours are multicentric and bilateral, and sporadic tumours unilateral and unicentric.

Clinical features

These are due to the secretion of catecholamines: adrenaline, noradrenaline, and dopamine.

The triad of episodic headache, sweating, and palpitations accompanied by anxiety and/or panic attacks should arouse suspicions

Familial Pheochromocytomas:

Pheochromocytomas occur in four syndromes:

- Multiple endocrine neoplasia type 2 (MEN 2) occurs in 50% of people with pheochromcytomas.
- Von Hippel-Lindau disease occurs in 20% of those with pheochromocytomas. The RET/ret proto-oncogene mutations are found in this group of patients.
- Neurofibromatosis occurs in only 1% of those with pheochromocytomas.
- Familial carotid body tumours occur in less than 1% patients with pheochromocytomas.

Investigations:

- Serum and 24 hour urinary catecholamines and metanephrines

Remember these are not specific for pheochrmocytomas and may be raised in stressful situations, fever and exercise.

- Plasma free metanephrine, the o-methylated metabolite of catecholamine appears to be more specific.

Table 14.6 Clinical features of pheochromocytoma

Clinical feature	% of total signs or symptoms
• Anxiety (episodic feelings of impending doom)	100
• Headaches	90
• Sweating	60–70
• Pallor	30
• Tremor	10
• Flushing	15
• Weight loss	5

Localization of pheochromocytomas:

- Ct scanning and MRI are used as initial imaging but have poor specificity.
- Scintiscan after labelling with 1311- or 1231- labelled meta-iodobenzyl-guanidine (MIBG) which localizes in catecholamine storage vesicles allowing extramedullary tumours to be visualized.
- Positron emission tomography using an analogue of dopamine enables visualization of chromaffin cells allowing both adrenal and extramedullary tumours to be localized

Treatment:

- Definitive treatment is surgical removal of the tumour.
- Preoperatively, an α blocker phenoxybenzamine and a β blocker propanolol, atenolol, or metoprolol is administered.
- Ninety per cent of tumours are cured by surgery.
- Treatments for tumours that have metastasized are chemotherapy, octreotide, or recently radioactive MIBG.

DIABETES

Diabetes mellitus is a clinical syndrome associated with hyperglycaemia. It is diagnosed if fasting glucose >7.8 mmol/l and non-fasting glucose >11.1 mmol/l. Non-insulin-dependent diabetes mellitus is usually diagnosed late, 5–10 years after symptoms first appear.

The following **classification of diabetes mellitus** was proposed by the WHO Study Group on Diabetes Mellitus (from the WHO Technical Report Series No. 727, 1988):

- Insulin-dependent diabetes mellitus.
- Non-insulin dependent diabetes mellitus: obese/non-obese.
- Malnutrition related diabetes mellitus.
- Diabetes associated with other conditions and syndromes: pancreatic disease, hormonal disease, drug or chemical induced conditions, abnormalities of insulin or its receptors, genetic syndromes.
- Gestational diabetes mellitus.
- Impaired glucose tolerance.

BOX 14.11 Dental implications of Addison's disease

- Oral pigmentation may be the first sign of this disease.
- Pigmentation varies from light brown to black and occurs on buccal mucosae, usually associated with the 'bite line'.
- There is an increased susceptibility to oral infection.
- Hypotensive or fainting episodes may occur on alighting from the dental chair.
- Patients with Addison's disease must be given steroid cover.

Abnormal glucose tolerance, obesity, family history, and nitrosamines in food appear to increase the risk of diabetes mellitus. Breast feeding appears to have a protective effect.

Insulin-dependent diabetes mellitus (IDDM) and non-insulin-dependent diabete mellitus (NIDDM)

A quarter of all cases of IDDM present in people between 40 and 90 years of age, but most present in the early teens. The incidence of IDDM varies widely with geographical location (see Table 14.6). In the United States more Whites than Blacks or Hispanics are affected. It is estimated that by 2010 220 million people will have diabetes; of these 210 million will have non-insulin-dependent diabetes mellitus (NIDDM).

Aetiology of IDDM
- Genetic factors:
  - IDDM is a polygenic disorder.
  - The HLA class 2 DR and DQ antigens on chromosome 6 (IDDM1) have the strongest association.
  - HLA-DR4, DQA1*0501, DQB1*0201 predispose to diabetes.
  - HLA-DR2, DQA1*0102, DQB1*0602 confer protection.
  - Polymorphisms in the region of the insulin gene on chromosome 11 are also associated with IDDM.
- Environmental factors: no specific agent has been identified.
- Micro-organisms:
  - Coxsackie virus antibodies (ISM) are found in 30% of new cases, with Coxsackie B virus mRNA in 65% of newly diagnosed diabetic children.
  - Other viruses including rubella, enteroviruses, and cytomegalovirus have all been implicated in an aetiological role.
- Diet
- Associated with other organ specific autoimmune diseases presence of autoantibodies: ICA (islet cell antibodies), IAA (insulin autoantibodies), GAD (glutamic acid decarboxylase), IA2 (protein tyrosine phosphatase).

Table 14.7 Incidence of IDDM (childhood diabetes)

Country	Incidence per 100 000 population
Japan	1.7
UK	15
Finland	29.5
USA	9.4–20.8

Patients with ICA plus two or more antibodies have a greater than 80% risk of developing diabetes mellitus.

Aetiology of NIDDM

NIDDM is a heterogeneous disorder with both genetic and environmental factors playing a part.

- Genetic factors include:
  - Pancreatic insulin secreting cell defect. The loss of β cells may be important in the development of diabetes. Three genes implicated are *MODY1*, *MODY2*, and *MODY3*.
  - Other associated genes are insulin, amylin, and sulphonylurea receptors.
  - Insulin resistance—mutations in insulin receptor gene and post-receptor signalling pathway.
- Environmental: hyperglycaemia impairs β cell function.
- Diet: obesity is the major risk factor for NIDDM. Excessive consumption of large amounts of high-calorie foods causes high plasma levels of non-esterified fatty acids (NEFA).
- Stress through illness or trauma affects glucose tolerance.
- Diabetogenic drugs: e.g. steroids, thiazides, beta-blockers, phenytoin, oral contraceptives.

Clinical features of IDDM

- Thirst, polyuria, and nocturia.
- Weight loss may be first symptom.
- Blurred vision.
- Infection.
- Ketoacidosis.
- A small percentage present with hyperventilation, vomiting, and abdominal pain.

Note that patients may have their initial presentation of IDDM in the 75–90-year age group. The fasting blood sugar may >15 mmol/l.

Clinical features of NIDDM

The clinical features may be non-specific and include:

- obesity
- lethargy
- sore mouth secondary to glossodynia, lichen planus, intraoral candidosis
- loss of concentration and application to the task in hand
- cardiovascular disease
- neuropathy
- retinopathy
- renal disease.

Investigations
- Blood sugar estimation, both random and fasting.
- Check the general health by testing the full blood count, renal and hepatic function, serum lipids, and thyroid function test.
- Test the urine for albuminuria.
- Perform an ECG to check for ischaemic abnormalities.

Treatment
Treatment should aim to control hyperglycaemia, control hypoglycaemic emergencies, improve general health, and prevent long-term complications.

- **Specific treatment for IDDM**: hyperglycaemia is controlled with insulin—the type of insulin and regimes are variable.
- **Specific treatment for NIDDM**:
  - Dietary control: help and encourage patients to lose weight.
  - Oral drug treatment: sulphonylureas stimulate insulin secretion of β cells.
  - Care of long-lasting hypoglycaemia.

In both cases the patient should make regular visits to the diabetic clinic for monitoring of diabetic control. Any infection should be treated aggressively. All patients should be encouraged to eat a healthy diet.

Treatment of diabetic emergencies
Diabetic emergencies include diabetic collapse and coma (hypoglycaemic coma and ketoacidotic coma).

Hypoglycaemic coma
All diabetics are predisposed to hypoglycaemic coma. Onset is usually over a few minutes and can be secondary to a missed meal or starvation, vigorous exercise, or infection.
  Clinical signs of hypoglycaemic coma are:

- Sympathetic stimulation results in sweating, dilated pupils, and tachycardia.
- Rapid shallow breathing may supervene.
- There are marked changes in higher cerebral function.

BOX 14.12 Emergency treatment of hypoglycaemia

If the patient is not unconscious:
- Administer glucose in any form, e.g. glucose drink of 50 g dextrose in 200 ml water.

If the patient is unconscious:
- In a child rub glucose syrup paste on the floor of the mouth.
- In all patients give 1 mg glucagon by intramuscular injection (remember glucagon is lyophilized and needs to be diluted) or 20 ml of 20% dextrose by the intravenous route, or 50 ml of 50% dextrose by the intravenous route. NOTE: very isotonic patients may vomit. It is very difficult to inject and may cause thrombophlebitis.

BOX 14.13 Emergency treatment of ketoacidotic coma

- Insulin needs to be given urgently.
- Intravenous insulin 5–6 U/h until the blood sugar drops below 15 mmol/l then administer 2–3 U/h until levels fall into the normal range.
- Rehydration is also very important, the deficit may be between 5 and 10 l. Start with saline until the blood sugar falls to normal then give 5% dextrose.
- The electrolytes may be deranged and potassium, which may initially be high, usually falls as the patient becomes rehydrated. Patients may become hypokalaemic.
- Hypokalaemia needs urgent treatment with 20–40 mmol potassium.
- Several protocols include bicarbonate supplementation to treat the acidosis, although there is no evidence that it is beneficial.

BOX 14.14 Dental relevance of diabetes mellitus

- There is an increased incidence of caries and other dental infections. These should be treated as a dental emergency as patients are susceptible to the development of ketoacidosis.
- Patients are predisposed to oral candidosis.
- Periodontal disease, which is slightly worse in even in well-controlled diabetics.
- Xerostomia occurs as a result of dehydration or drugs.
- Sialosis (salivary gland swelling) may also occur.
- Oral hypoglycaemia may be associated with the development of lichenoid reactions.
- Peripheral mononeuropathy may present in the facial and oropharyngeal area.
- The timing of appointments is important to minimize the risk of a hypoglycaemic event occurring.
- The dental procedure may also be complicated by the long-term medical problems of diabetes including ischaemic heart disease, chronic renal failure, and autonomic and peripheral neuropathy.
- Avoid appointment times at the end of the day. Remember, if a complication occurs medical assistance may not be available.
- Routine treatment under local anaesthesia should be undertaken so that completion of the dental procedure and recovery occurs before a meal is due.
- For general anaesthesia appropriate referral to a specialist centre is recommended.

Ketoacidotic coma
- Onset of ketoacidotic coma is slow, over hours or days.
- It may be the initial presentation in young adults.
- Ketoacidosis may be preceded by infection.
- Patients are hot but not sweating and dehydrated.
- Deep rapid breathing (Kussmaul breathing) occurs.
- The breath smells 'mousy'.
- The urine is positive for sugar and ketones.

Long-term complications of diabetes

Long-term complications are directly related to the patient's diabetic control. Patients with IDDM are prone to ocular, renal, vascular and neurological complications 10–20 years after diagnosis:

- **Ocular complications.** Diabetes mellitus causes 10% of all blindness. Visual disturbances occur frequently due to fluctuation in blood sugar. Also: cataracts, glaucoma, retinopathy, and new vessel formation over the iris (rubeosis iridis).
- **Renal complications.** Pyelonephritis. Glomerulonephritis (proliferative form or Kimmelstein–Wilson with oesinophilic granules deposited in glomerulosus). Glomerular sclerosis secondary to atherosclerosis and hypertension.
- **Vascular complications.** Both large, medium, and small vessel disease are a major cause of morbidity. Patients are prone to myocardial, kidney, and cerebral infarction as well as endarteritis. Vascular problems and neuropathy cause gangrene of feet which may result in amputation.
- **Neurological complications.** Mononeuritis multiplex results from neuropathy from several individual peripheral or cranial nerves. Peripheral neuropathy: this is sensory and results in a glove and stocking distribution. Autonomic neuropathy: this may present with impotence, diarrhoea, sweating, postural hypotension, and dependent oedema.

DISORDERS OF BONE METABOLISM

Rickets (childhood) and osteomalacia (adult)

Rickets and osteomalacia are due to a deficiency of vitamin D (dietary deficiency or lack of sunlight or both) or an abnormality of vitamin D metabolism. The main causes are:

- **Lack of vitamin D.** Asian women, those who are housebound and on special diets. The elderly (a combination of nutrition and being housebound or in long-term care homes). Malabsorption from the small intestine. Calcium deficiency. Primary hyperparathyroidism. Epileptic patients taking phenytoin, primidone, or carbamazepine.
- **Abnormality in vitamin D metabolism due to renal disease:** vitamin D-dependent rickets; chronic renal failure; Fanconi's syndrome; renal tubular acidosis; hypophosphataemia.

The pathology of rickets and osteomalacia is charactized by abnormal production of unmineralized osteoid bone plus an abnormal cartilaginous growth plate with abnormal arrangement of chondrocytes and reduced vascularity.

Clinical features of rickets and osteomalacia

The bones ache and are tender to the touch. Children have swollen epiphyses and tender costochondral joints; babies have a 'ping-pong' consistency of the skull. Adults have groin pain or pain in the pelvis, spine, or ribs.

Table 14.8 Biochemical investigations in rickets and osteomalacia

Test	Result
Serum calcium (corrected for albumin)	Decreased
Serum phosphate	Decreased
Alkaline phosphatase	Very high
Plasma creatinine	Usually high in patients with renal disease
Plasma parathyroid hormone	High in patients with secondary hyperparathyroidism

BOX 14.15 Dental implications of rickets and osteomalacia

- In rickets tooth eruption is delayed.
- Bones are less radio-opaque than normal (in rickets and osteomalacia).
- Craniotabes due to late closure of the fontanelles.
- Increased risk of fractures.

- Skeletal abnormalities. Children have bow-legs and knock knees. Adults may suffer from vertebral compression.
- There is muscle weakness with the patient unable to stand from the squatting position.
- Hypocalcaemia results in positive Chvostek and Trousseau signs: the Chvostek sign is perioral spasms and twitching secondary to light tapping of the facial nerve anterior to the tragus of the ear. The Trousseau sign is carpal spasm resulting from inflating the blood pressure cuff to 20 mmHg above the patient's normal systolic pressure.
- In severe hypocalcaemia (serum calcium <1.90 mmol/l) tetany develops.

Investigations

The results of biochemical investigations in rickets and osteomalacia are shown in Table 14.8. The haematological picture of macrocytosis and/or microcytic blood may be a result of malabsorption. Radiography shows characteristic changes:

- In children: epiphyses are cupped; metaphyses may show areas of resorption as the result of secondary hyperparathyroidism.
- In adults: Looser's zone or pseduofracture is seen the long bones such as the femur and pubic and ischial rami. They are sometimes also seen in the ribs and scapula.

Bone biopsy from the iliac crest, shows reduced calcification with increased osteoid thickness.

Treatment

- In children the vitamin D required is 10 μg or 400 IU and in adults 2.5 μg or 100 IU per day.

- In adults or children with disease secondary to socioeconomic factors exposure to the sun for 30 min five to six times a week is beneficial.
- Vitamin D supplements.
- Other supplements such as calcium, bicarbonate, and potassium may be needed depending on the underlying abnormality.
- Surgery may be required for deformities.

Osteoporosis

Osteoporosis is the commonest metabolic bone disease. It results from a reduction in the unit volume of bone with a change in its composition. It is characterized by low bone mass, resulting in a loss of the microarchitecture of the bone. Patients present with a mean bone density of more than 2.5 standard deviations below the mean. The WHO estimate that 20 million women worldwide have osteoporosis. The incidence of osteoporosis increases with age: in the UK osteoporosis affects 15% of women aged 50, 30% of women aged 70, and 40% of 80-year-old women.

Peak bone mass occurs between the ages of 24 and 35 years, and is greater in males. Bone consists of both trabecular and cancellous bone which is constantly being turned over and remodelled by a continual process of resorption and deposition, trabecular bone being the more actively remodelled. Eight to 10% of an individual's skeletal bone mass is remodelled each year. Regulation of bone remodelling is dependent on many factors:

- Osteocytes in the Haversian system sense skeletal mechanical load.
- Sex hormones affect remodelling, which is increased by thyroid hormone and growth hormone and suppressed by oestrogen, androgens, and calcitonin.
- Other factors include inflammation by local cytokines, IL-1 and IL-6, calcitropic factors vitamin D and PTH and the effect of the RANK/RANKL/OPG pathway on osteoclast function.

Causes and clinical features of osteoporosis

Osteoporosis has many **causes** of which aging is important. Others are:

- Arthritis: rheumatoid arthritis (steroid usage and immobility).
- Drugs: steroids, heparin sulphate, thyroxine, diuretics, cytotoxic therapy.
- Endocrine: hypogonadism, lack of oestrogen, testosterone deficiency in young men, Cushing's syndrome/disease, hyperthyroidism, primary hyperparathyroidism, diabetes mellitus, Addison's disease.
- Genetic predisposition: positive family history, Black races.
- Females: oestrogen withdrawal menopause or removal of ovaries.
- Osteogenesis imperfecta.
- Gastrointestinal: low protein intake, starvation/fasting, coeliac disease, primary biliary cirrhosis, partial gastrectomy.

Table 14.9 Classification of osteoporosis

Primary	Type I (post-menopausal)
	Type II (senile)
	Idiopathic (<50 years of age)
Secondary	Endocrine
	Gastrointestinal
	Rheumatological
	Medication
	Malignant disease

- Lifestyle: sedentary, alcohol, cigarette smoking, low body weight (slimming/starvation/anorexia nervosa).
- Malignant disease: metastatic carcinoma, multiple myeloma.

Osteoporosis can be classified as primary or secondary (see Table 14.9). Osteoporosis is characterized by the following **clinical features**:

- May be asymptomatic.
- Pain, which usually lasts for 3–4 months.
- Loss of height results in deformity: abdominal protrusion, kyphosis, scoliosis.
- Fractures which result in both pain and deformity. Main sites of fracture are vertebrae, neck of the femur, forearm.

Investigations

Bone densitometry: X-rays of the spine and long bones.

- Biochemistry: serum calcium, phosphate, alkaline phosphatase, 24-h urinary calcium and creatinine, Bence-Jones protein, FBC and ESR, oestrogen and testosterone.
- Bone biopsy should be done only when the differential diagnosis includes metabolic disease. (Differential diagnoses for osteoporosis can be multiple myeloma, osteogenesis imperfecta, metastatic carcinoma, osteomalacia, or hyperparathyridism.)

Treatment

Symptomatic relief of pain.

- Prevent further bone loss, e.g. with hormone replacement therapy (HRT), testosterone and biphosphonates, etidronate, alendronate, calcium, calcitonin, calcitriol.
- Stimulate new bone formation by low-impact weight-bearing exercise.
- Try and prevent fractures.
- Treat secondary causes.

Treatment should be monitored by measuring bone mass at regular intervals.

> **BOX 14.16** Dental implications of osteoporosis
>
> - May affect the mandible and maxilla. Fractures may occur with minimal trauma, e.g. tooth extraction.
> - Patients on corticosteroids for oral mucosal disease may develop osteoporosis. Bone loss may occur soon after starting medication.
> - Care in differential diagnosis with other metabolic bone diseases affecting the mandible and maxilla.

Paget's disease of bone

Paget's disease of bone is a disorder of bone metabolism due to increased but abnormal osteoclast activity resulting in bone resorption with abnormal bone deposition and remodelling. It was described by Sir James Paget in 1876. It affects slightly more men than women: in the UK about 1–3% of men over the age of 55 may be affected.

The aetiology of Paget's disease of the bone is unknown. There is a familial tendency in 40–50% of cases and it is inherited as an autosomal dominant trait. There is a causal relationship with paramyxovirus.

Clinical features of Paget's disease of the bone
Most patients are asymptomatic. Symptomatic patients have:

- Pain—this may be due to primary pathology as well as due to secondary arthritis. It is present in 85% of symptomatic patients.
- Deformity which affects the weight-bearing bones and may result in bowing.
- Skin over the affected bone feels warm.
- Neurological damage due to spinal cord compression.
- Hypervascularity results in steal syndrome and causes ischaemia of adjacent structures.
- Pathological fractures of the long bones occur.
- Osteosarcoma occurs in less than 1% of cases but is the most serious complication.
- Irreversible hearing loss.
- Visual loss resulting in tunnel vision.
- High-output cardiac failure is very rare.

The main bones affected are the pelvis (involvement indicated by pain), the spine (which is shortened), the femur (unilateral bowing), and the skull (increase in the size of the vault).

Investigations
Biochemistry investigations:

- Serum calcium is usually normal, but may be raised if the patient is immobilized.

- Serum phosphate is usually normal.
- Serum alkaline phosphate is raised, and may be very high.
- Urinary hydroxyproline is raised.

Radiography shows a decreased density of affected bone giving a mottled appearance with radiolucent areas scattered throughout the affected area. The bone is deformed with a thickened cortex. The skull has a fluffy outline resembling cotton wool.

Treatment

Calcitonin, the previous mainstay of treatment, is no longer used: bisphosphonates are now the drugs of choice. They work by exploiting their affinity for calcium. They inhibit the action of mature osteoclasts with consequent

---

BOX 14.17 Dental relevance of Paget's disease of the bone

- The maxilla and other facial bones are frequently affected.
- The mandible is rarely involved.
- Development of osteogenic sarcoma.
- Teeth show hypercementosis or root resorption.
- Visual impairment—patients have tunnel vision.
- Bone pain may present as a diagnostic difficulty.
- Hearing loss may affect management.

Table 14.10 Classification of osteogenesis imperfecta

Type	Inheritance	Clinical features affecting bone	Other tissues
I	Autosomal dominant	Few features; minor or no deformity; normal height. Accounts for 60% of all patients	Blue sclera; arcus (juvenile); aortic incompetence; mitral valve prolapse; joint hypermobility; dentinogenesis imperfecta; deafness
II	New dominant mutations	Lethal perinatal period; multiple fractures	
III	New mutations (recessive)	Progressive deformity; short limbs; very short stature; kyphoscoliosis	Dentinogenesis imperfecta; deep blue sclera; early death due to respiratory infections
IV	Autosomal dominant	Shortened stature; moderate bone deformity	Sclera normal colour; hyperplastic callus over long bones

suppression of osteoclastic bone resorption. Examples of biphosphonates include: alendronate, clodronate, risedronate, and tiludronate. Pamidronate can only be used as an intravenous preparation.

Pain is treated with non-steroid anti-inflammatory drugs. Specific therapy may be needed for hearing loss, visual problems, and for decompression of the spinal cord.

Osteogenesis imperfecta

Osteogenesis imperfecta occurs due to defects and mutations in the collagen genes. This results in the faulty conversion of normal mineralized cartilage to defective bone matrix. It occurs in 1–2 per 20 000 births. Clinically the disease is heterogeneous resulting from different molecular defects (see Table 14.10).

Investigations
Prenatal diagnosis and genetic screening can be offered to families at risk. However, most cases arise from new mutations.

- Serum biochemistry is usually normal. However, raised alkaline phosphatase and urinary hydroxyproline as well as hypercalciuria may occur.
- Renal function is normal
- Histology: polarized light microscopy of bone reveals abnormal woven bone.
- Radiology shows: osteopenic changes; cortical thinning; deformity of the spine and long bones; increased callus formation at the site of fractures; osteoarthritis; increase of wormian bones in skull; platybasia; large frontal and maxillary air sinuses.
- Teeth may have dentinogenesis imperfecta.

Treatment
Treatment is mainly supportive. There should be joint management by dental, orthopaedic, and rehabilitation medicine teams. Bisphosphonates are used for medication. Families should be advised about national support groups, e.g. the Children's Brittle Bone Foundation UK.

Marfan's syndrome

Marfan's syndrome is caused by a mutation in the epidermal growth factor regions of the fibrillin gene on chromosome 15. It is inherited as an autosomal dominant trait.

Clinical features
Marfan's syndrome affects a number of body systems:

- **Ocular features**. Dislocation of the lens is the main feature as fibrillin is the major component of the microfibrillar system and lens suspensory ligament.

> **BOX 14.18** Dental relevance of osteogenesis imperfecta
>
> • Patients need extensive rehabilitation.
> • Fluoride given for bones may benefit teeth.
> • Dentinogenesis imperfecta needs careful treatment planning with a paedodontist.
> • Patients may require antibiotic cover if they have associated cardiac defects.
> • Deafness may require referral to a special needs clinic.

> **BOX 14.19** Dental relevance of Marfan's syndrome
>
> • Patients need antibiotic cover.
> • Ehlers–Danlos syndrome may be associated.
> • Marfan's is a heterogeneous disease both genetically and clinically, with nine clinical subtypes identified.

Dislocations occur upwards and/or sideways (in comparison to homocystinuria with downward dislocation). Myopia and retinal detachment also occur.

• **Cardiovascular system**. Cardiovascular complications reduce life expectancy by 40–50%. There is dilation of the aorta resulting in aortic incompetence and dissection.
• **Other features**: hernias, spontaneous pneumothorax, cutaneous striae.
• **Anatomical problems**. The height is increased with heel to pubis length being greater than crown to pubis height. Fingers display arachnodactyly (long and thin fingers). The joints are hypermobile.

Differentation diagnosis is homocystinunia or Stickler's syndrome (severe myopia).

Multiple endocrine neoplasia (MEN)

In multiple endocrine neoplasia patients usually present with two or more tumours, which have arisen from the endocrine organs. MEN is uncommon and is inherited as an autosomal dominant trait, with 1 in 2 of first-degree relatives being affected.

Multiple endocrine neoplasia type I

The *MEN1* gene is located on chromosome 11q13. This gives rise to tumours of the anterior pituitary, parathyroid glands, and pancreatic islets cells:

• Anterior pituitary tumours occur in 30% of patients: of these 30% are prolactinomas, 40% are somatotrophinomas (secrete growth hormone), and 20% are corticotrophinomas.
• Parathyroid tumours occur in 95% of patients giving rise to primary hyperparathyroidism (giving hypercalcaemia).

BOX 14.20 Dental relevance of multiple endocrine neoplasia

- Underlying metabolic/endocrine abnormalities that may affect treatment.
- Parathyroid tumours may cause loss of lamina dura and brown tumours in the facial bones.
- Phaeochromocytomas may be associated with von Recklinghausen's disease, and hypertension.
- MEN IIB associated with Marfenoid habitus.

Table 14.11 Clinical variants of MEN type II

MEN type	Clinical features
MEN IIA	Most common: medullary thyroid carcinoma; phaeochromocytoma; parathyroid tumours
MEN IIB	5% of all cases: medullary thyroid tumour; phaeochromocytoma; mucosal neuroma; intestinalautonomic dysfunction; Marfanoid habitus
Medullary thyroid carcinoma (MTC)	Sole clinical feature

- Pancreatic islet cell tumours occur in 40% of patients giving rise to gastrinomas (lead to Zollinger–Ellison syndrome) and insulinomas.
- Other associated tumours are carcinoid, adrenal cortical tumours, and lipoma.

Multiple endocrine neoplasia type II

The gene for MEN type II (*RET*) is located on chromosome 10cen–10q11.2. MEN type II is the association of medullary thyroid carcinoma (MTC) and phaeochromocytoma. Three clinical variants exist: MEN type IIA, MEN type IIB, and MTC (see Table 14.11).

Management of MEN type II is coordinated by team including geneticists, endocrinologists, and surgeons. Genetic testing will identify a patients genetic background and 50–60% of the family at risk. If a genetic mutation is identified the thyroid should be removed: total thyroidectomy is the best approach as this helps prevent micrometastases.

15 Disability

People with disabilities are very disadvantaged in many societies. They are frequently treated with prejudice and discrimination. The British Social Attitudes Survey 1998 looked at predjudice against disabled people in employment which showed these attitudes still prevail.

The **Disability Discrimination Act 1995** (DDA 1995) gives a definition of disability: an adult or child is disabled if he or she has a physical or mental impairment that has a substantial adverse and long-term effect on his/her ability to carry out 'normal' day-to-day activities. The Act has introduced new procedures aimed at combating discrimination as well as protecting disabled people in the areas of education, employment, the provision of goods, facilities, and services and the selling, letting, or managing of land or premises.

The following terms are used within the Act:

- **Physical impairment** is not defined by the act. Examples of impairments are usually restricted mobility, sight, or hearing.
- **Mental impairment** means a clinically recognized mental illness which covers a wide range of impairments relating to mental functioning, including learning disabilities. An impairment has to be a well-recognized illness, i.e. 'recognized' by a respected body of medical opinion.
- **Substantial** means more than 'minor' or 'trivial'. It takes into account the time taken and difficulty experienced to perform an activity or task compared with someone without the impairment.
- **Adverse** means the combined effects of the disability on tasks or activities.
- **Normal day-to-day activities** means that the impairment will be taken to have an impact on normal day-to-day activities only if it affects one or more specified activities as shown in Table 15.1.
- **Severe disfigurement** means that there is severe physical apparent disfigurement and includes skin diseases and birthmarks. These must have a substantial effect but tattoos or non-medical body piercings are not included.
- **Progressive conditions** that hinder the exercise of normal day-to-day activities, e.g. cancer, multiple sclerosis, or muscular dystrophy.
- An **impairment** which is controlled or corrected by medication, e.g. myasthenia gravis, epilepsy.
- The effect of a disability is considered **long term** if it has lasted at least 12 months, or the total period for which it lasts is likely to be at least 12 months, or it is likely to last for the rest of a person's life. The legislation also covers intermittent disabilities, such as multiple sclerosis and epilepsy, where they are

Table 15.1 Examples of the impact of disability on normal day-to-day activities

Normal day to day activity	Examples
Mobility	Unable to walk, or have difficulty with stairs or walking to toilet
Manual dexterity	Getting dressed unaided or pressing phone buttons
Physical coordination	Placing food into one's own mouth or brushing one's teeth without unusual concentration or help
Continence	Loss of bladder or bowel control whilst asleep
Ability to lift, carry, or move everyday objects	Unable to pick up objects of moderate weight with one hand, or carry a moderately loaded tray steadily
Speech, hearing, or eyesight	Talks much more slowly, unable to hear telephone conversations clearly, unable to differentiate colours, unable to walk safely without colliding with objects
Poor memory, unable to concentrate, learn, or understand	Intermittent loss of consciousness and associated confused behaviour, unable to adapt to change of work or new environments
Poor perception of the risk of physical danger	Persistent inability to cross a road safely

likely to continue for prolonged periods following episodes of symptom remission.

Disabilities not currently covered by the DDA include:

- HIV status where no AIDS related symptoms have developed;
- alcohol or drug dependency;
- wearers of ordinary spectacles or contact lenses;
- seasonal allergic rhinitis;
- genetic disorders.

There are a number of recommmendations for the DDA 2004 (adapted from DDA Report and White Paper). The recommendations of the report give guidance on disability matters and cover a wide range of disablities, including all age groups and impairments.

The DDA 2004 recommendations do not include genetic predispositions but do include:

- HIV infection;
- those with or who have had cancer;
- those who are certified as blind or partially sighted;

Table 15.2 Disability Office guidelines for language use in the field of disability

Language to avoid	Preferred language
The disabled	Disabled person/people
Handicapped person/invalid	Disabled person
Special needs students	Disabled students
Able bodied	Non-disabled person
The blind	Blind person/person with a visual impairment
The deaf	Deaf person/person who is hard of hearing
Suffers from/is a victim of/is crippled by	Person who has/person with
Spastic	Person with cerebral palsy
Epileptic	Person with epilepsy
Wheelchair bound	Wheelchair user

- comprehensive inclusion of mental health conditions;
- dysphasia;
- severe short-term conditions, such as some heart attacks, strokes, or depression.

The recommendations provide guidance to tribunals and courts to:

- Remove 'long-term' from the definition and use the concept of 'substantial' to cover both duration and severity of adverse effects.
- Consider the concept of covering only 'clinically well-recognized' mental illnesses and to identify the advantages and disadvantages of removing the limitation.
- Clarify the legislation on what constitutes normal day-to-day activities in relation to work.
- Consider the true effects of a disability on individuals.
- Consider the issue of the effects on normal day-to-day activities of disability.
- Constantly review exclusion of particular conditions.

The Disability Office has issued guidelines for acceptable use:of language; these are summarized in Table 15.2. It is important for dentists to be aware of current terminology as using improper language or addressing a prospective or current patient inappropriately may cause offence.

EPIDEMIOLOGY

The Health Survey for England 2001 indicated that 18% of all men and women over 16 years of age are affected by a disability. In the 10–15 year age group 1% had a severe disability and 4% of boys and 3% of girls had a disability. The risk factors for disability were found to be:

- age
- male sex

- living in the north of England
- having a musculoskeletal disorder
- having been involved in an accident
- having a circulatory disorder.

The main types of physical disability are locomotor (mobility), sight, hearing, and speech difficulties.

The Health Survey for England 2001 used the WHO International Classification of Functioning, Disability and Health (ICF). This is a dynamic assessment of the interaction between functioning and disability and individual contextual terms (personal and environment). The components it considers are:

- **Body functions**—physiological functions of body systems (including psychological functions).
- **Body structures**—anatomical parts of the body such as organs, limbs and their components.
- **Impairments**—problems in bodily function or structure such as a significant deviation or loss.
- **Activity**—the execution of a task or action by an individual.
- **Participation**—involvement in a life situation.
- **Activity limitations**—difficulties an individual may have in executing activities.
- **Participation restrictions**—problems an individual may experience in involvement in life situations.
- **Environmental factors**—make up the physical, social, and attitudinal environment in which people live and conduct their lives.

This list is taken from the WHO's 'Towards a common language for functioning, disability and health' published in 2002.

PHYSICAL IMPAIRMENT

The term 'physical impairment' refers to a person who has difficulty in moving or using all or part of their body.

Locomotor disability

'Locomotor disability' refers to a person who is unable to achieve distinctive activities associated with moving, both him/herself and objects, from place to place.

Epidemiology
Locomotor disability is found in 10% of men and 12% of women. Locomotor disability accounts for 34% of all disabilities. In care homes locomotor disability accounts for 65% of the causes of all disability whereas fewer than 10% of the elderly in private households have a locomotor disability.

The major causes of locomotor disability are:

- cardiovascular disease (severe angina, myocardial infarct, stroke)
- cerebral palsy
- trauma (falls, road traffic accidents, landmines)
- infection (poliomyelitis)
- musculoskeletal disorders (all types of arthritis, mainly osteoarthritis)
- myasthenia gravis
- multiple sclerosis
- osteogenesis imperfecta
- spinal injury (quadriplegia, paraplegia)
- spina bifida and hydrocephalus.

Hearing impairment

'Hearing impairment' is a term used which includes persons who are both deaf and hard of hearing. The term 'profound hearing impairment' covers those persons with a hearing loss of more than 70–90 decibels in the better ear; 'moderate impairment' covers those with a loss of more than 45 but less than 60 decibels in better ear; 'mild impairment' covers those with a loss of more than 30 but not more than 45 decibels in better ear. The term 'deaf' is used to describe people with profound hearing loss who do not benefit from amplification. 'Hard of hearing' is used for those with mild to severe hearing loss who can benefit from amplification. The preferred termiology is 'persons with hearing problems'.

Epidemiology
Fifty-five per cent of people over 60 years of age are deaf or hard of hearing. In the UK, 690 000 people are severely or profoundly deaf and 509 000 people have hearing loss secondary to noise exposure at work. Ten per cent of persons with hearing loss (70 000) use British Sign Language as their first language.

Aetiology
The main causes of loss of hearing are:

- genetic
- infections, e.g. mumps, meningitis
- exposure to loud noise
- trauma, e.g. head injuries
- drugs, e.g. streptomycin
- recurrent middle ear infection, e.g. recurrent otitis media with effusion
- tumours, e.g. acoustic neuroma
- Ménière's disease

Visual impairment

The World Health Organization define 'profound blindness' as the inability to distinguish fingers at a distance of 3 m or less. 'Partial sight' is the inability to

> **BOX 15.1 Dental implications of hearing impairment**
>
> • Communication may be a major problem between the patient and dentist.
>
> Improve patient-dentist communication by:
>
> • Removing your mask and keeping your face visible.
> • Face the patient when explaining treatment.
> • Be seated at the same level as the patient.
> • Use facial gestures and expressive body language.
> • Do not put your hands near or over your face.
> • Do not talk to the patient from behind the dental seat.
> • Repeat your sentences or phrases if the hard of hearing person finds it difficult to follow.
> • Try different ways of communicating, e.g. written information and patient questionnaires may be helpful.

> **BOX 15.2 Dental implications of visual impairment**
>
> • Patients have a right to good oral health.
> • Always give precise details if you need a blind person to follow instructions.
> • Speak directly to them and not to a companion.
> • Always ask their opinion as you would a normally sighted person.
> • A white cane means the patient has sight problems, but this may not be total loss of sight. Always ask if the patient wants help with direction in the dental surgery.
> • A white cane with a red band means the person has both sight and hearing problems.
> • A guide dog with a white and red harness means the person has both sight and hearing problems.

distinguish fingers at a distance of 6 m. The preferred terminology is 'people with sight problems'.

In the UK more than 2 million people have sight problems. Of these only 25% are blind. Braille is now used by only 10% of persons who are blind.

Causes of sight problems include:

• genetic causes (e.g. retinitis pigmentosa)
• cataract
• glaucoma
• diabetic retinopathy
• infection during pregnancy (e.g. toxoplasmosis, rubella)
• trauma or injury.

MENTAL IMPAIRMENT

The **Mental Health Act 1998** gives the following definition of mental disorder: 'Mental disorder means mental illness, arrested or incomplete development of mind, psychopathic disorder and any other disorder or disability of mind.'

There are four types of mental disorder:

- **Severe mental impairment.** A state of arrested or incomplete development of mind which includes severe impairment of intelligence and social functioning and is associated with abnormally aggressive or seriously irresponsible conduct on the part of the person concerned.
- **Mental impairment.** A state of arrested or incomplete development of mind (not amounting to severe mental impairment) which includes significant impairment of intelligence and social functioning and is associated with abnormally aggressive or seriously irresponsible conduct on the part of the person concerned.
- **Psychopathic disorder.** A persistent disorder or disability of mind (whether or not including significant impairment of intelligence) which results in abnormally aggressive or seriously irresponsible conduct on the part of the person concerned.
- **Mental illness** is **not** defined; however, it is the most common form of mental disorder for which people are dealt with under the Act.

The definition includes psychopathic disorders or learning difficulties, which are associated with abnormally aggressive or seriously irresponsible conduct, personality disorders, behavioural disorders, and head injury disorders. Promiscuity, immoral conduct, sexual deviancy, alcohol, and drug abuse are excluded from this definition of mental disorder.

A new proposed definition states that **mental disorder means** 'any disability or disorder of mind or brain which results in an impairment or disturbance of mental functioning'. This is a much broader definition without exclusions, to be included in the Mental Health Equitable Treatment Act 2003, which aims to address treatment issues and assessments of persons with mental impairment.

In the UK 91 million working days a year are lost due to mental health problems. Fifty per cent of work-related absence is due to stress, depression, and anxiety and nearly three in every 10 employees will have a mental health problem in any one year, mainly due to anxiety and depressive disorders. One in four people have a mental health problem in any one year. Below the age of 40 years suicide is the second most common cause of death.

The WHO Guide to Mental Care lists a large number of mental disorders (the most common disorders are given in bold type):

- Acute psychotic disorders which includes acute schizophrenia-like psychosis.
- Acute delusional psychosis and other acute and transient psychotic disorders.
- Adjustment disorders which including acute stress reaction.
- **Alcohol misuse**.
- Bereavement.
- Bipolar disorder.
- Chronic fatigue syndrome, fatigue syndrome, and neurasthenia.

- **Chronic mixed anxiety and depression**.
- Chronic psychotic disorders which include schizophrenia, schizotypal disorder, persistent delusional disorders, induced delusional disorder, and other non-organic psychotic disorder.
- Delirium.
- Dementia.
- **Depression**.
- Dissociative (conversion) disorder.
- Drug induced disorders.
- Eating disorders.
- **Generalized anxiety**.
- Learning disability which may be known internationally as mental retardation.
- Panic disorder.
- Phobic disorder which includes agoraphobia and social phobia.
- Post-traumatic stress disorder.
- Sexual disorders (male and female).
- **Sleep problems** (insomnia).
- **Unexplained somatic complaints**.

Learning disability

The WHO definition of learning disability is 'a state of arrested or incomplete development of mind'. Somebody with a learning disability is said also to have 'significant impairment of intellectual functioning' and 'significant impairment of adaptive/social functioning' which is present from birth.

The Special Educational Needs and Disability Bill 2001 defines a special educational need (SEN) as follows: 'A child [under the age of 19] has SEN if he has a learning difficulty which calls for special educational provision to be made for him'.

The Warnock Report (Special Educational Needs Report of the Committee of Enquiry into the Education of Handicapped Children and Young People, May 1978) recognized that: '. . . those who work with children with special educational needs should regard themselves as having a crucial and developing role in a society now committed, not merely to tending and caring for its handicapped members, as a matter of charity, but to educating them, as a matter of

---

BOX 15.3 Dental implications of mental impairment
- Persons with a mental impairment have a right to good oral health.
- They are least likely to present for treatment.
- Don't be quick to judge or make assumptions.
- Some patients may have erratic behaviour: maintain a calm aspect and be patient throughout the dental appointment.
- Give the person plenty of time to express themself and come to a decision.

right and to develop their potential to the full.' The report suggested the term 'learning difficulties' to cover specific problems with learning in children which may be related to medical, physical, or emotional impairments and language and communication problems.

Epidemiology

In the UK there are approximately 1.5 million people with a learning disability. Learning disability is one of the most common forms of disability in the UK. Every year about 600 children are born with Down's syndrome.

The final report of the Disability Rights Task Force 'From exclusion to inclusion' found that:

- About 20% all school children have special educational needs (SEN) at some time.
- About 3% (248 000) of all school pupils with statements have severe or complex needs.
- Sixty per cent of all children with SEN can be taught in mainstream education.

Causes of learning disability

Causes of learning disability are varied and include:

- Genetic factors, including abnormal genes or chromosomal abnormalities resulting in metabolic abnormalities: proteins—phenylketonuria, Lesch–Nyhan syndrome; lipids—Tay–Sachs disease; carbohydrates—galactosaemia.
- Infections during pregnancy—syphilis, toxoplasmosis, rubella.
- Environmental insults—irradiation, alcohol abuse, smoking, drugs, and starvation.
- Maternal disease—diabetes, hypothyroidism, toxaemia.
- Hypoxia at birth.
- Infections in the neonatal or childhood period, e.g. meningitis.
- Trauma—road traffic accidents with head injury.
- Non-accidental injuries.
- Emotional, social, and mental deprivation.

Conditions associated with learning disability are:

- Autism: 50% of autistic patients have a severe learning disability.
- Asperger's syndrome.
- Communication difficulties.
- Epilepsy.
- Down's syndrome.
- Attention deficit disorder (ADD)/attention deficit hyperactivity disorder (ADHD).
- Cerebral palsy (CP) which is a physical disability due to a central motor deficit centrally. CP may or may not have an associated learning disability.

> **BOX 15.4** Terminology for specific learning disabilities
> - **Dyscalcula**: difficulty in understanding and using symbols or functions needed for success in mathematics.
> - **Dysgraphia**: difficulty in producing handwriting that is legible and written at an age-appropriate speed.
> - **Dyslexia**: difficulty in understanding or using one or more areas of language, including listening, speaking, reading, writing, and spelling.
> - **Dysnomia**: difficulty in remembering names or recalling words needed for oral or written language.
> - **Dyspraxia**: difficulty in performing drawing, writing, buttoning, and other tasks requiring fine motor skill, or in sequencing the necessary movements.

- Figures quoted for superimposed mental illness in people with learning disabilities are between 10 and 60%. The wide discrepancy is due to the difficulty in assessing mental illness because of communication difficulties.

Assessment of learning disability is by the use of psychometric testing: three levels of disability are noted—moderate, severe, and profound.

Management of learning disabilities

Management aims to break pattern of normalization, i.e. how society deals with individuals within their cultural, religious, and social beliefs. These change with time and cultural norms.

Previously, people with learning disabilities were viewed within those norms as being possessed, subhuman, or diseased. They were subject to constant ridicule, isolation, and punishment and treated as children whatever their age. A recent example is the death of a child from suffocation in a church ceremony to 'drive out the devil' in an autistic child. Normalization means treating people with disabilties as having the same value and importance as oneself. The issues to be addressed are:

- Age appropriateness—the environment for education, living, and socializing should be age appropriate. The service provider should deal with disabled persons on an age-appropriate basis.
- Integration and participation—teach children in mainstream schools supported by special teachers. Integration with other children and members of the public.
- Dignity and respect—people should have their own possessions and live where there is respect for privacy, not in large communal dwellings.

The Diability Rights Task Force recommended that: 'Educating disabled and non-disabled children together should lead to a greater understanding of disabled people's needs and lessen stereotypes. We hope this would increase disabled people's opportunities to participate in the labour market and society more generally.'

> **BOX 15.5** Dental implications of learning disability
> - Patients have a right to good oral health.
> - Some patients do not understand, or find it difficult to follow, conversation.
> - Talk directly to the patient and not the accompanying person.
> - Make sure you interact with clear gestures and use plain English.
> - Some patients cannot read or write: adopt an amicable manner and be patient when communicating.
> - Explanatory leaflets about dental procedures may be helpful: use pictures and large print with clear simple language.
> - Audio or videotapes may improve communication and understanding of different dental procedures and orodental problems.
> - Most patients have other skills and should be made to feel valued in the dental surgery.

COMMUNICATION IMPAIRMENT

Communication impairment refers to both speech and language problems. 'Speech and language impairment' means that a person has significant limitation in language ability in the absence of other problems in intelligence, hearing, oral motor function, and neurology. 'Speech disability' is referred to as a person's inability to speak properly. This may be that the speech is not understood or the manner in which it is spoken is disagreeable. People with speech disability may have problems with articulation, i.e. difficulty in forming sounds, or fluency, i.e. stuttering or stammering.

In the UK 7% of the population (more than 2.5 million people) have a communication impairment. Two hundred and fifty thousand people have aphasia (are unable to use speech to communicate). One in 10 children experience language difficulties.

Causes of speech impairment include:

- cerebrovascular accident
- head trauma or injury
- oral or nasal carcinoma
- cleft lip and palate
- learning disability
- neurological disorders, e.g. multiple sclerosis, Parkinson's disease
- hearing loss
- physical disability, e.g. cerebral palsy
- dementia
- psychiatric disorders
- laryngeal disorders, e.g. polyps and carcinoma
- dysphagia.

> ### BOX 15.6 Dental implications of communication impairment
>
> - People with speech impairment have a right to good oral hygiene.
> - Remember the impairment is not apparent until speech is needed.
> - Lack of speech does not equate with lack of intelligence.
> - Do not shout when talking to the patient.
> - Use other methods to communicate, such as pen and paper.
> - Before you proceed with any treatment make sure that you and the patient have understood each other.
> - Do not hurry the patient: their speech may be present but slow, slurred, or difficult to understand. Do not be tempted to finish their sentences for them.

> ### BOX 15.7 Dental implications of facial disfigurement
>
> - People with facial disfigurement have the right to good oral health.
> - Facial disfigurement is very distressing and causes psychosocial problems.
> - Do not make assumptions because of a person's appearance.
> - Social isolation may mean infrequent visits to dentist.
> - Look directly at the patient and make eye contact.
> - Ask open questions and give patients time to discuss problems.
> - Oral and facial prosthesis may play a major part in improving quality of life. No plastic procedure should be attempted without a multiprofessional assessment with the patient being able to express concerns.
> - Important point to remember: reaction to disfigurement and looking different is not related to the cause, site, or the effect on normal function but on the amount of self-esteem, social skills, and social support experienced by the particular person.

FACIAL DISFIGUREMENT

Facial disfigurement is particularly pertinent to the practice of dentistry.

In the UK almost half a million people are disfigured: 1 in 100 children suffer facial disfigurement and 1 in 500 children are seriously affected by disfigurement.

Causes of disfigurement include:

- dermatological conditions such as severe acne, eczema, vitiligo, and psoriasis
- trauma or injury
- burns
- cancer of the orofacial structures.

Congenital causes of disfigurement include:

- cleft lip and palate
- birth marks
- Sturge–Weber syndrome with a facial haemangioma
- Goldenhar syndrome with hemifacial microsomia
- cri du chat syndrome with facial asymmetry and poorly formed ears
- Treacher–Collins syndrome with malformed or absent ears and facial bones
- fibro-osseous dysplasia (cherubism) affects one or more facial bones.

16 Dermatology

The skin is the largest organ in the body and makes up 15–16% of body weight. It plays an important role in maintaining the body's homeostasis.

Skin lesions are common. The prevalence of self-reported work-related skin disease in the UK is 66 000 cases per year, of which approximately two-thirds were dermatitis or eczema (Self-Reported Work Related Illness Survey, 1995).

The functions of the skin are:

- Temperature regulation.
- Acts as two-way barrier function preventing fluid loss, preventing entry of toxins and allergens, and preventing infection.
- Protection from ultraviolet and other radiation.
- Immunological barrier.
- Mechanical support.
- Contains sweat glands to excrete waste and toxic substances.
- Vitamin D_3 is produced in the skin
- Sensory organ: touch, pressure, temperature, chemosensory, proprioception.

The skin is a layered structure made up of the epidermis, the dermis, and the subcutis:

- The epidermis: consists mainly of epithelial cells. The surface stratum corneum consists of keratin covered by a lipid layer. The spinous layer is separated by a granular layer of differentiated keratin-containing cells. There is a basal layer containing rapidly dividing and differentiating cells, including melanocytes. Langerhans cells are distributed are scattered throughout the epidermis.
- The dermis: the dermis is relatively acellular. It contains blood vessels, connective tissue, nerve endings, hair follicles, sweat and sebaceous glands. The intervening connective tissue consists of dermal proteins, glycosaminoglycans, collagen, and elastin.
- The subcutis contains fatty tissue and muscle, including the erector pili.

PIGMENTED LESIONS OF THE SKIN

Pigmented lesions of the skin are common and almost all are benign. However, the incidence of malignant melanoma has been increased in the last 20 years.

- Benign pigmented lesions include: lentigines, freckles, moles, senile warts (seborrhoeic keratosis), and dermatosis papulosa nigra.

- Malignant pigmented lesions include: Hutchinson's melanotic freckle, amelanotic melanoma, acral lentiginous melanoma, and lentigo maligna melanoma.

Benign pigmented lesions

Lentigines

Lentigines are the result of an increased number of melanocytes arranged evenly along the basal layer. They can occur in areas not exposed to the sun. Examples of lentigines are:

- actinic lentigines
- senile, occur on the hands and face in the elderly
- Peutz–Jeghers syndrome (lesions in Peutz–Jeghers are associated with polyposis coli, a pre-malignant lesion)
- leopard syndrome (with associated ocular, CNS, cardiovascular, and genital abnormalities)
- Mongolian spots (grey blue lesions in the lumbosacral region); the colour decreases and fades during childhood.

Freckles

Freckles contain a normal number of melanocytes. Exposure to the increases the melanin production of the melanocytes.

Moles (melanocytic naevi)

These are induced by sunlight. They are common in children and adults. Three forms occur, which are divided according to histology:

- Intradermal naevus: the melanocyte like cells accumulate in the dermis. As they mature they lose their colour as they migrate deeper into the dermis.
- Junctional naevus: the epidermal naevus cells accumulate at the base of the dermis.
- Compound naevus: the epidermal naevus cells accumulate at the base of the dermis with some cells migrating into the uppermost layer of the dermis.

Senile warts (seborrhoeic keratosis)

These are common lesions which have a warty grey to brown appearance. They occur at any site and first appear towards the end of the fourth decade of life.

Dermatosis papulosa nigra

These are not melanocytic proliferations but small pigmented raised lesions. They commonly occur in negroid races.

Malignant pigmented skin lesions

Malignant pigmented skin lesions are malignant tumours of melanocytes (melanomas). The incidence has increased 30-fold over the past 30 years. Incidence is 9.5 per 100 000 in the UK, with more women than men affected.

The causative agents are sunlight (this is the greatest risk factor), viral, or genetic (*CDKN2A* germline mutations). Most melanomas do not arise from moles.

Malignant pigmented skin lesions can be classified into nodular, superficial spreading, acral lentiginous melanoma, and lentigo maligna melanoma. The first two types are the most common.

Nodular and superficial spreading lesions

These arise as a superficial spreading lesion with lateral extension in the dermis. They later enter a nodular phase. Rarely the nodular phase may appear first. Patients affected in their third to sixth decade. The affected site may be the back or lower legs.

The history may vary from asymptomatic to an unusual mole. There may be history of itching, bleeding, or change in shape or colour. On examination of the lesion look for:

- asymmetrical shape and size
- colour variation
- irregular border
- an intradermal component which spreads laterally.

Some **clinical types** of melanoma are:

- **Hutchinson's melanotic freckle**. This is found in areas exposed to the sun. Patients are older than 6 years. It is a flat lesion which spreads superficially. It may remain in a preinvasive phase for a long time before becoming rapidly invasive.
- **Amelanotic melanoma**. This is an erythematous papule or nodule with no pigmentation. Diagnosis usually late and it is often misdiagnosed as another lesion. Prognosis is poor.
- **Acral lentiginous melanoma**. These lesions are coloured and are found on the palms or soles of the feet. The prognosis is poor.

Treatment is by surgical excision, initially with a 4 mm margin. If the subsequent diagnosis is positive then a 0.5 to 2 cm margin of clearance is required for intradermal lesions and larger lesions respectively. Local nodes should be removed followed by radiotherapy or chemotherapy. Monoclonal antibodies and cytokines, e.g. TNFα and IFNγ are sometimes used; however, none of the above are of any proven benefit except surgical excision.

If the depth of invasion is less than 1 mm, with adequate surgical excision the melanoma may be cured.

CONTACT DERMATITIS

In 1999–2000 4300 new cases of work-related skin disease were diagnosed in the UK: 80% of these were contact dermatitis. The Reporting of Injuries,

Diseases and Dangerous Occurrences Regulations 1985 (RIDDOR 85) were introduced in April 1986 and later replaced by RIDDOR 95. Occupational contact dermatitis (e.g. caused by rubber, latex, and X-ray chemicals) is a reportable condition. This is particularly pertinent to dentists and their staff who must report all cases after a doctor's written diagnosis. Health workers reported 15 new cases per 100 000 per year.

Contact dermatitis is a skin eruption which may be irritant induced or allergic in nature. Irritant contact dermatitis is caused by direct contact, whereas allergic contact dermatitis is caused by a type IV hypersensitivity reaction. Atopic dermatitis is an IgE-induced reaction which causes urticaria, which may predispose to development of irritant contact dermatitis.

Irritant contact dermatitis

Irritant contact dermatitis can be caused by domestic irritants such as detergents, cosmetics, or soaps or by occupational irritants such as those encountered by those involved in 'wet work', e.g. nurses, dentists, cleaners, and engineers.

Clinical features
- In the acute phase inflammation occurs; later dryness, skin itching, and scaling may appear.
- The lesions are caused by the irritant penetrating the surface layer of the skin, the stratum corneum.
- The irritant disrupts the cell membranes, causing the release of histamines, prostaglandins, and kinins.
- Mononuclear cells migrate to the area and both cytokines and chemokines are released.
- The resultant lesion is inflammation with the histological appearance of oedema with mononuclear cell infiltrate.
- If there is persistent irritation, the stratum corneum becomes permanently disrupted and the intercellular lipids are damaged.
- The stimulation also increases the production of epidermal cells, which increases skin thickening with scaling.
- The skin is also dry. This is caused by loss of lipids, which contain both ceramides and glycoceramides which are responsible for the water retention properties of the skin.
- There is usually lack of evidence of contact allergy.

Treatment
Treatment is by removal of the irritant. Emollients may help dry skin. Protective clothing should be worn to try and prevent irritant contact dermatitis from developing. However, once chronic dermatitis is established it needs very minimal contact with soap or detergent to maintain it. Even if lesions are cleared it can be easily reactivated. If patients do not respond to exclusion of the irritant, make sure there is no allergic contact dermatitis. This can be done by patch testing.

Allergic contact dermatitis

Any substance may cause sensitization of the skin. Contact may be direct to the skin or by inhalation or ingestion. Dental materials are becoming increasingly common in causing allergic contact dermatitis, e.g. chromates, mercuric formaldehyde, epoxy, resin, nickel sulphate. Medication used for the management of orodental conditions, including topical local anaesthetics, and topical corticostreriods, may also cause problems.

Mechanism and features of allergic contact dermatitis
- A hypersensitivity reaction occurs when low-molecular-weight molecules called haptens penetrate the skin.
- They bind to receptors on antigen-presenting Langerhans cells which in turn sensitize T cells in the regional lymph nodes.
- In sensitized individuals further contact with the hapten causes skin inflammation and dermatitis. This may occur within 48 h.

Clinical features are sharply demarcated lesions on areas of the skin in contact with the allergen, erythema, and rhinitis. A definitive diagnosis is made by patch testing.

Treatment
The main aim should be to prevent allergic contact dermatitis from developing in the first place by means of health education and the identification of workplace hazards using risk assessment procedures:

- There are strict guidelines covering workplace hazards (Control of Substances Hazardous to Health (COSHH)).
- Protective clothing, e.g. gloves, should be non-irritant.
- Barrier creams offer some protection.
- Topical steroids are the main specific treatment.
- Systemic immunosuppressants may be needed for resistant cases.
- Specialist referral may be necessary.

Seborrhoeic dermatitis

Seborrhoeic dermatitis is caused by *Malassezia furfur* a dimorphic fungus which colonizes most individuals in early life. It is usually a harmless symbiont. Under some circumstances, in some people it can induce the process of seborrhoeic dermatitis, but the mechanism for this is unclear. There are other unknown aetiological factors besides the fungus.

Clinical features
Clinical features of seborrhoeic dermatitis include:

- Dandruff, itchy scalp, inflamed scaly scalp.
- Red scaly areas in the naso-labial folds and inside and behind the ears.

- The centre of the chest or upper back may have dry erythematous areas in a petaloid shape.
- The skin lesions can also involve the flexures (axillae, groin, and antecubital fossae).

Treatment

Treatment is with antifungals of the 'azole' type, e.g. ketaconazole, clotrimazole, itraconazole, or fluconazole. These may be in the form of shampoo or cream. Terbinafine should not be used. Occasionally steroids may be needed to reduce the inflammation and irritation.

ALLERGY IN THE DENTAL SURGERY

Hypersensitivity reactions

Hypersensitivity reactions result from an excessive immune response to antigens, which might cause harm clinically. They may be manifest within minutes to 48 h after encounter with the allergen and are secondary responses, in previously sensitized individuals. There are four major types of hypersensitivity: types I, II, III, and IV.

Type I hypersensitivity (anaphylaxis)

Type I hypersensitivity is started by interaction of an allergen with a specific antibody to immunoglobulin (IgE), which is bound to mast cells (and basophils) and which in turn activates an inflammatory response by degranulation of the mast cells (see Figure).

There is a second phase to type I hypersensitivity which is mediated by cytokines: IL10 and IL13 which promote the continued degranulation of mast

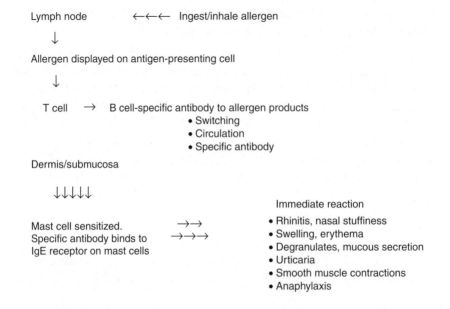

cells and IL15 which enhances the survival and activity of the oesinophils which cause local tissue damage.

Type II hypersensitivity reaction (antibody-dependent cytotoxicity)
This reaction is initiated by the interaction of cell- or connective tissue-bound antigen with specific IgG or IgM antibodies and causes:

- Agglutination of host red blood cells by IgM antibodies.
- Opsonization by IgG antibodies.
- Activation of classical complement antibodies by IgM antibodies.

The classic example of type II hypersensitivity is the transfusion reaction.

Type III hypersensitivity reactions (immune complex hypersensitivity reaction)
This reaction may be either local (i.e. localized to the site of antigen entry, e.g. Arthusas reaction) or systemic. In systemic reactions multiple organs may be involved, e.g. accumulation of antibody–antigen complexes which accumulate on the basement membrane of capillaries and larger blood vessels to give local inflammation such as vasculitis.

Type IV hypersensitivity (delayed type hypersensitivity)
Type IV hypersensitivity is initiated by the interaction of T cells with processed antigen in association with the major histocompatibility complex. Clinical examples of delayed type hypersensitivity are tuberculosis, leprosy, chicken pox, measles, and contact dermatitis. Contact dermatitis is especially important in the dental setting, as dental materials such as nickel chromates and palladium mercuric chloride resins as well as cosmetics all cause clinical signs in the head and neck area, including intraorally.

Latex allergy

The possibility of latex-based allergic reaction within the dental surgery is high. Risk management is an important factor to reduce the number of dental staff developing contact dermatitis and in some cases a type I hypersensitivity reaction.

Latex allergy has markedly increased in the past 10 years. It may affect dental surgeons, hygienist, nurses, and also patients. According to the US Food and Drug Administration the incidence of latex sensitivity in spina bifida patients is 18–40%.

The reactions to latex seen in a clinical setting may vary from contact dermatitis to fatal anaphylactic reaction. It is salutary to remember that latex allergy can occur at any time during exposure to latex even after years of problem-free wear.

Aetiology
- Latex proteins may lead to a type I reaction, initiated by the interaction of antigen (latex) with IgE-specific latex antibodies. Latex proteins also have sequence homology with bananas and avocados and sensitization may lead to problems.

> **BOX 16.1** Factors predisposing to the development of latex allergy
>
> - Atopy: atopic individuals have high IgE antibody levels and quickly develop high specific IgE antibodies to latex. Patients with a history of asthma or other allergic reaction indicate an increased susceptibility to latex allergy.
> - Concurrent infection: infection, either bacterial or viral, can increase the immune response to chemical allergens.
> - Time or length of exposure to the allergen.
> - Quality of the antigen.
> - Allergy to other proteins with homologous sequences: these include common foodstuffs such as chestnuts, bananas and avocados. In the dental surgery, rubber dams and gutta percha points may also have homologous sequences which cross-react with latex allergens.

- Residual chemical accelerators used in the manufacture of latex, including thiurams and mercaptobenzothiazoles, can lead to a type IV reaction.
- The starch powder used in the gloves can cause problems by acting as a hapten binding to the free latex proteins, thus exacerbating the allergic reaction.

Practical problems associated with latex gloves
Skin contact
Free latex proteins are absorbed through the pores of the skin, especially after body heat causes sweating. These act as antigens and cause an antibody response by production of specific IgEs. If powered is bound to the latex the IgE response is even bigger. Repeated exposure to the latex allergen results in repeatedly more severe type I allergic reactions. Examples of this are:

- A female dental surgeon who became increasingly sensitized on exposure to latex gloves. She experienced an anaphylactic reaction during sexual intercourse; her partner used a condom.
- A female patient in a stable relationship using barrier contraceptive methods became increasingly sensitized to latex. She experienced a type I allergic reaction on the second occasion the dentist applied a rubber dam.

Oral or genital mucosal contact
Use of latex within a patient's mouth may result in a gradual leeching of chemical accelerators used in the manufacture. This together with latex covered powder may result in a type IV reaction in the mouth. Clinically this may present as lichenoid reaction, burning erythematous plaque-like lesions, or more commonly as white slough like lesions surrounded by an erythematous halo.
Genital type IV lesions are frequently misdiagnosed as candidiases.

Respiratory contact—nasal or bronchial
Latex powder from gloves remains airborne in surgical areas for hours, and constant use over the clinic opening hours results in aspiration into the respiratory

epithelium resulting in an immune reaction, with both type I and type IV reactions.

Clinically patients complain of nasal stuffiness, rhinorrhoea, and wheezing. In predisposed individuals repeated exposure may result in wheezing, asthma, or even fatal anaphylaxis.

Investigations

The following methods may be used in diagnosis: the skin prick test, the patch test, or *in vitro* tests.

The **skin prick test** is the method of choice, and has a high sensitivity and specificity:

- A solution is made of the extract of rubber latex protein.
- Ten microlitres of solution is introduced into the epidermis.
- In a positive test the diameter of the erythema at the test site is compared with a histamine positive control and a saline negative control.

The **patch test** is used to identify specific contact antigens involved in type IV delayed hypersensitivity reactions causing dermatitis. The test material is applied to the intact skin, usually the back, and read 48–72 h later.

***In vitro* tests** are expensive and have only moderate sensitivity. They are:

- the radioallergosorbent (RAST) test and
- enzyme-linked immunosorbent assay (ELISA).
- Latex-specific IgE distinguishes the positive serum from the control.
- False negatives are may occur.

Management of latex allergy within the work environment

- The COSHH Regulations (1994) impose a statutory obligation on employers (read dentist) to carry out risk assessments for hazardous substances, implement suitable control measures, and carry out any necessary health surveillance.
- All staff must be informed about latex sensitivity on starting employment in a dental surgery.
- Staff must be aware that dental patients may be atopic or have latex sensitivity.
- Staff who are atopic with allergies to banana, avocado, and chestnuts should be advised that should any local reaction occur when wearing latex gloves their use should be stopped and alternative gloves used.
- If an allergy develops, the advice of a specialist physician should be sought. Once a definite diagnosis of contact sensitivity is made the employing dentist should report the matter under the Reporting of Injuries, Diseases and Dangerous Occurrences Regulations 1995 (RIDDOR).
- Allergic reactions should also be reported to the Adverse Incident Centre (AIC) at the Medical Device Agency where national monitoring takes place.
- Dentists must only use gloves which carry the CE marking which indicates that the product complies with the European standards of 'essential requirements'

> **BOX 16.2** Prevention of latex allergy
>
> - Take a careful history regarding allergy in patients.
> - The dental surgeon must know if staff are atopic or suffer from hay fever, asthma, or any known allergy.
> - Choose gloves carefully—powder-free, latex-free gloves or latex gloves with low levels of extractable proteins.
> - Do not wear the same gloves for prolonged periods.
> - Gloves should only be worn when examining or working within a patient's mouth. Forty to 60% of gloves have holes in them before they are used, increasing mucosal contact of patients with latex protein. At the end of a patient's appointment up to 80% of gloves have developed holes.

of safety and performance to ensure minimal risk to both themselves and their staff.

Peanut allergy

In the UK and Europe peanut oil was previously used in infant formulas as well as in cream applied to nipples to prevent cracking. In the UK over 20 000 children are sensitized to peanuts, but peanut allergy is uncommon in Africa, even though peanuts are a major dietary component.

Peanuts are a strong sensitizer in atopic babies, and the sensitizing agent(s) may cross the placenta as well as be excreted in breast milk. The exact incidence of peanut allergy is not known; however, the number of cases are increasing markedly. In an attempt to reduce this trend the Committee on Toxicity of Chemicals in Food, Consumer Products and the Environment (COT) made the recommendations in their Report on Peanut Allergy (Department of Health, June 1998):

- In those families with a history of allergic diseases, pregnant and lactating women and infants may wish to avoid peanuts and peanut products in order to reduce the risk of the development of peanut allergy in later life.
- In common with the advice given for all children, those infants with a parent or sibling with an atopic disease should, if possible, be breast-fed exclusively for 4 to 6 months.
- During weaning of such infants, and until they are at least 3 years of age, they should not be exposed to peanuts or peanut products.
- Irrespective of family history no child under 5 years of age should eat whole peanuts because of the risk of choking.
- A number of recommendations for research have been made to address some of the scientific uncertainties.

Components of peanuts

Peanuts contain 45% oil, 25% protein, and 8% carbohydrate. Peanut oil contain 3.3 μg/ml of peanut protein. Peanut proteins are globulins, which are composed of arachin and conarachin fractions, and albumins, which consist of agglutins, lectin-reactive glycoprotein inhibitors, alpha amylase inhibitors and phospholipases. The major peanut allergens are Ara hI and Ara hII.

Peanut allergy is like other food allergies which are IgE mediated and dependent on type I hypersensitivity reactions. It is the commonest food allergy, and is more common in children than adults.

Peanuts are found in peanut butter, breakfast cereals, and numerous sweets and sauces, especially Indian, Thai, and Chinese foods. Peanut-derived ingredients are also contained in cosmetics, including zinc and castor oil cream. Many medical products state that arachis oil is one of the ingredients—many lay people and professionals fail to recognize this as peanut oil.

Epidemiology

Peanut allergy affects males and females equally. Seventy per cent of cases manifest before 5 years of age. Peanut allergy accounts for 60% of all nut allergies. Other nuts including brazil nuts, cashew nuts, and walnuts can all cause severe type I reactions. Cross-reaction with soya protein is very common and sometimes airborne allergens can be inhaled.

Clinical features

Symptoms begin up to 1 h after ingestion or contact with the allergen. Severe reactions resulting in anaphylaxis may occur from 30–90 min after ingestion or as early as just a few minutes after inhalation of allergens. Touching or kissing someone who has been handling or eating peanuts may also cause symptoms.

Common symptoms of peanut allergy are:

- perioral tingling
- nausea
- facial oedema with a variable amount of airway obstruction
- feeling of throat constriction
- colicky abdominal pain.

Treatment involves the avoidance of offending foods. For mild sensitivity with minimal swelling of the face and lips, itching of mucous membranes, and rhinitis or nasal stuffiness, antihistamine syrup, e.g. chlorphenaremine, or tablets, e.g. piriton, should be given. Remember that absorption may take up to 30 min. The above features plus vomiting will prevent absorption of oral antihistamines and adrenaline is then the drug of choice.

Dental material allergy

Allergy to dental materials is probably under-reported. Clinical signs of type IV hypersensitivity reactions in the mouth are frequently not recognized. They are:

- tingling sensation or itching of the mucosa next to the restoration
- erythematous attached gingivae and buccal mucosae opposing the restoration

> **BOX 16.3** Signs and treatment of anaphylaxis
>
> **Signs of anaphylaxis**
> - urticaria, rhinitis, nasal stuffiness
> - nausea
> - vomiting
> - wheezing
> - hypotension
> - airway obstruction
>
> **Treatment of anaphylaxis**
> - Adrenaline is the mainstay of treatment.
> - In children administer adrenaline spray (e.g. Medispray), 5 or 10 puffs repeated every 5 min up to 15–20 puffs in a child (20 puffs in an adult).
> - This is not as effective as subcutaneous or intramuscular adrenaline.
> - Patients should be taught to self-administer adrenaline 1 : 1000 up to 1 ml via an Epi-pen, which gives 0.3 ml at each injection up to 1 ml, or a Minijet containing adrenaline 1 : 1000 0.3 ml and repeat if necessary in adult up to 1 ml.

- frank lichenoid reaction
- lesions mimicking vesiculobullous disease.

Commonly known allergens in dental materials are nickel sulphate, potassium dichromate, cobalt chloride, palladium chloride, and gold sodium thiosulphate. Gold positivity is seen in up to 25% of repeated symptomatic patients. This material is still thought of as being inert when used in the oral cavity. In the dental surgery, rubber dams and gutta percha points may also have homologous sequences which cross-react with latex allergens (see section on latex allergy).

In a testing of 1730 children and adults nickel and thimerosal were the most frequent dental material allergens in females, ethylmercuric chloride and thimerosal in boys, and Balsam of Peru in the elderly. Resins used in composites constantly leach resulting in type IV hypersensitivity reactions in the mouth.

PSORIASIS

Psoriasis is a common skin disease: in the UK it affects 1.4–1.6% of the population. It is clinically characterized by inflammation of the skin with plaque formation resulting from hyperproliferation of keratinocytes. A seronegative arthropathy develops in approximately 7–10% of patients.

Psoriasis has a well documented genetic component to its **aetiology**, with twin studies revealing a concordance rate of up to 70%. Patients with skin disease may be HLA-B13, -B17 or -B27 as well as HLA-Cwb and -DR7. Both HLA-B27 and -DR7 are associated with joint disease.

Environmental factors also play a part in the aetiology. Episodes of trauma, drug reactions, infection, pregnancy and stress may all precipitate an attack of psoriasis. Although sunlight may be a relieving factor in most patients, exacerbations may be caused in approximately 10%.

The **pathogenesis** of psoriasis involves antigenic stimulation, e.g. by streptococcal superantigens. These activate T cells and cause dilatation of dermal vessels. The activated T cells and neutrophils migrate into the dermis and epidermis where they release cytokines which stimulate proliferation of keratinocytes.

The **clinical features** are typically are multiple, well defined erythematous plaques with a silvery scale. The silvery scale can be removed leaving pin-point capillary bleeding (Auspitz's sign). Koebner's phenomenon occurs in sites of trauma, such as operation scars, where localized areas of psoriasis are seen. (Koebner's phenomenon is also seen in lichen planus but was first described in psoriasis.)

The clinical variants of psoriasis are:

- erythrodermic psoriasis
- generalized pustular psoriasis
- guttate psoriasis
- palmoplantar pustulosis
- psoriatic arthritis
- nail psoriasis
- napkin psoriasis
- unstable psoriasis
- psoriasis vulgaris

Erythrodermic psoriasis

Erythrodermic psoriasis is a severe disease which may be life threatening. It usually arises in patients with long-standing disease and almost all of the body surface may be affected. The skin becomes uniformly erythrodermic and scaly. A rise in body temperature results in problems with thermoregulation and loss of surface water results in dehydration. The hyperdynamic metabolism results in high-output cardiac failure. This constitutes a medical emergency and requires hospital admittance and circulatory support.

Generalized pustular psoriasis

This form of psoriasis is also potentially lethal. It may arise *de novo* or in patients with long-standing disease on cessation of therapy. Almost all surfaces may be affected. The skin becomes acutely inflamed and sore and large

BOX 16.4 Dermatological psoriatic emergencies
- Erythrodermic and generalized pustular psoriasis.
- Treatment is by supportive care as an inpatient.
- Rehydration and thermoregulation are essential.
- Systemic therapy includes acitretin or ciclosporin.

sheets of small, sterile pustules appear and become confluent. Like erythrodermic psoriasis this condition is a medical emergency.

Guttate psoriasis

Guttate psoriasis occurs in children and young adults. Patients usually have a genetic predisposition. Lesions arise 14–21 days after an acute attack of streptococcal tonsillitis. The lesions are usually less than 1 cm in size and the morphology is drop-like. They are numerous and occur as non-itchy lesions on the limbs and trunk. The lesions resolve spontaneously after about 3 months.

The underlying tonsillitis should be treated with antibiotics and PUVA (psoralen and UVA radiation) phototherapy applied. Topical treatments are not used as they irritate the skin.

Palmoplantar pustulosis

Palmoplantar pustulosis is much more common in patients who smoke (or have smoked) cigarettes. The lesions are yellow pustules which later turn brown. They occur on the palmar and plantar surfaces of the hands and feet.

Treatment is difficult. UVA therapy may be helpful and topical corticosteroids are used. Resistant cases may need acitretin.

Nail psoriasis

Nail psoriasis occurs in almost all patients with psoriatic arthritis and about half of patients who have skin lesions. The lesions occur on any or all of the nails of the hands and feet. These are:

- **Onycholysis**—the occurrence of small pin-head pits causing separation of the nail plate from the distal nail bed. Onycholysis also occurs in fungal nail infections, hypothyroidism, and thyrotoxicosis.
- **Psoriatic nail dystrophy**—the occurrence of the appearance of longitudinal ridges and areas of discoloration of the nail.
- **Superinfection** may occur with *Candida* or *Pseudomonas*.

If superinfection is present it should be treated; however, treatment is usually not successful.

Napkin psoriasis

Napkin psoriasis usually develops in infants. The lesions, which are erythrodermic plaques typical of psoriasis, appear in the nappy area. The lesions are self-limiting but topical emollients may be helpful.

Psoriasis vulgaris

The lesions may occur on the extensor surfaces of the limbs, the back, the hairline and scalp, body flexures as well as the vulva and penis. The lesions are characteristically well demarcated with erythematous plaques. The plaque size

Table 16.1 Clinical subtypes of psoriatic arthritis

Clinical features	% of cases
Oligo- or monoarthritis which is asymmetrical	70
Rheumatoid arthritis with a symmetrical distribution	15
Ankylosing spondylopathy in HLA-B27 patients	5
Arthritis mutilans, a destructive arthritis which involves the small joints of the hands and feet. This usually affects patients with severe disease	5

varies from very small to larger plaque areas where smaller lesions have become confluent.

The treatment of choice is topical applications:

- Dithranol and coal tar both stain clothing and have a pungent smell.
- Vitamin D analogues can be applied as either an ointment or cream.
- Calcipotriol is a common first-line treatment and can be used for long-term treatment. It should not be used in the face or in flexors.
- Tazarotene, a retinoid, is effective but limited experience is available with this drug
- Steroids only should be used in the short term on the face and scalp.
- Second-line treatment includes PUVA phototherapy.
- Rarely methotrexate, ciclosporin, and acitretin.

Psoriatic arthritis

Psoriatic arthritis is a seronegative arthropathy. It may occur in 10% of patients with skin disease or in some patients with no apparent skin disease. There are several distinct clinical subtypes of psoriatic arthritis (Table 16.1).

The diagnosis is usually clinical and is confirmed by biopsy.

ATOPIC ECZEMA

Atopic eczema has increased markedly in the past 30 years. In UK over all age groups 5% of the population are affected by eczema. There is a distinct age profile to atopic eczema:

- In the UK 75% of cases occur in children less than 6 months old.
- Ninety per cent of cases occur in the under 5s.
- A few cases begin later, even in the elderly.
- Between the ages of 10 and 20 years 50–90% of atopic eczema disappears.
- Ten per cent of cases recur.
- Most atopic conditions clear by the age of 30.

Apart from eczema, other atopic clinical disorders are asthma and hayfever. All three conditions occur in 30–50% of cases.

Aetiology

Genetic background and environmental factors both play a part.

Genetic background

There is a positive family history of atopy in approximately 60–70% of cases. Linkage studies indicate a likage to three loci:

- chromosomes 2, 5, 6, 9, 11, 12, 13 in asthma
- high-affinity IgE receptor on chromosome 11q13 in asthma but not eczema
- mast cell chymase, chromosome 14q11.2, in eczema.

There are also mutation polymorphisms/variants:

- IL-4 receptor alpha variants in atopy or eczema.
- IL-4 and IL-13 induce IgE synthesis in B cells and T helper 2 (Th2) type differentiation in T cells.
- Both bind to heterodimer receptors with the IL-4R alpha chain as a component.

Environmental factors

Known environmental precipitating factors are:

- House dust mite (*Dermatophagoides pteronyssinus*) in dust, beds, cuddly toys, and especially damp inadequately heated houses.
- Animal/pet danders and pollens.
- Food proteins, e.g. milk, fish, flour (very rare).

Known environmental exacerbating factors are:

- Infections.
- Temperature/humidity (skin drying/house dust mite numbers).
- Woollen clothing.
- Stress.

Pathogenesis

The basic defect is unknown. Most patients (80%) have an increase in total IgE but 20–40% have normal total or specific IgE levels. IgE is unlikely to be a primary defect in eczema. The higher the IgE level the greater chance the patient has of developing concomitant asthma/hayfever; they also have a more severe dermatitis and a poorer prognosis in any eczematous disorder.

Congenital defects such as: transient IgA deficiency, a Th2 defect in the foetus, and a Th1 defect in the neonate.

Clinical features

Clinical features are variable with a fluctuating course. The rash found in eczema has characteristic features:

- it is symmetrical
- it is very itchy

- there are erythematous patches/papules/vesicles
- skin is scaling and dry
- there are excoriations/fissures
- weeping/crusting are present
- lichenification.

The distribution of rash depends on the age of the patient:

- In infants aged 0–18 months rash is found on the face and extensors (elbows/knees, especially when crawling). The napkin area is usually spared.
- In childhood (18–24 months onward) rash is found on the flexures (antecubital/popliteal fossae, sides of the neck, wrists, and ankles) and nail pits and ridges. Rash on the hands is usually limited.
- In adults the picture is similar to childhood but the face and hands are often affected.

Investigations

There is no diagnostic test. Investigations are mainly carried out in adult patients. These are:

- Total serum IgE (remember 20% of patients have normal IgE and 15% of apparently normal individuals have raised IgE).
- Radioallergosorbent test (RAST).
- Specific serum IgE—house dust mite/danders/pollens/foodstuffs: negative result suggests allergy is unlikely.
- Skin prick tests—a test solution is put on the skin and a prick made with a sharp needle.
- Patch test to allergens thought to cause contact allergic dermatitis.
- 'Atopy patch test' with aeroallergens is still under investigation.
- Skin biopsy stained with haematoxylin and eosin (H&E). These may show: hyper/parakeratosis, acanthosis, spongiosis, dermal lymphocytic infiltrate, exocytosis.
- Skin swab should be sent for bacterial culture and sensitivity testing.

Complications

Superinfection of lesions is a common problem in patients with eczema. Bacterial infections (*Staphylococcus aureus*) cause impetigo. Viral infections with Herpes simplex can cause eczema herpeticum or Kaposi's varicelliform eruption. Papulovesicles such as warts and molluscum contagiosum may be secondary to eczema.

BACTERIAL INFECTIONS OF THE SKIN

Normal skin is colonized by huge numbers of bacteria, which live harmlessly as commensals on its surface and within its follicles. At times overgrowth of some of these resident organisms may cause minor disease of the skin. On other occasions bacteria not normally found there may colonize the epidermis and rapidly lead to disease.

Some of the normal flora found on the skin and their locations are as follows:

- The hair follicles are inhabited by anaerobes (e.g. *Propionibacterium* spp.) in their deeper parts and nearer the surface by aerobic cocci in addition to yeast of the *Pityrosporum* spp.
- There are no bacterial inhabitants of sweat ducts or glands.
- Resident aerobic flora are: Gram-positive cocci, e.g. *Staphylococcus*, *Micrococcus*, a variety of Gram-positive rods, e.g. the coryneforms or diphtheroids, and gram-negative *Acinetobacter*.

Staphylococcus aureus

Staphylococcus aureus is one of the most important causes of skin infections and of serious systemic disease. *Staphylococcus aureus* is part of the normal skin flora and is carried by all patients with *Staphylococcus*-induced skin infection. It can be distinguished from other staphylococci by its positive test for coagulase. Testing for carriage of staphylococcus gives the results shown in Table 16.2.

Staphylococcal-induced diseases include impetigo, ecthyma, folliculitis, furunculosis, carbuncle, and occasionally cellulitis. Staphyloccoci also cause secondary infections when lesions are already present, for example in eczema, ulcers, and skin infestations. Stapylococci can also cause staphylococcal scalded skin syndrome, toxic shock syndrome, and staphylococcal scarlatina.

Other bacteria infecting the skin

Coagulase-negative staphylococci

Staphylococcus epidermidis is the main pathogen in this group. It causes minor skin infections including folliculitis.

Streptococci

Streptococci are Gram-positive chains. Nearly all streptococci are facultative anaerobes. *Streptococcus pyogenes* is carried in the throat by about 10% of the population. Streptococcal-induced diseases include: impetigo, ecthyma,

Table 16.2 Sites of carriage of *Staphylococcus aureus*

Site	% positive
Anterior nares	35
Perineum	20
Axillae	5–10
Toe webs	5–10

erysipelas, cellulitis, vulvovaginitis, perianal infections, streptococcal ulcers, blistering distal dactylitis, and necrotizing fasciitis. Streptococci also cause secondary infection:

Toxins from the streptococci may be a major problem in scarlet fever and toxic shock-like syndrome. Hypersensitivity to streptococcal antigens can cause erythema nodosum, with vasculitic like lesions. Streptococci may also provoke guttate psoriasis.

Cellulitis and erysipelas

Cellulitis is an acute, subacute, or chronic inflammation of loose connective tissue. Erysipelas is a bacterial infection of the dermis and upper subcutaneous tissue. Erysipelas is classically a facial infection (that is not to say it is cellulitis of the face).

Bacteria are present in small numbers and are often very difficult to culture. Cellulitis and erysipelas are predominantly streptococcal diseases, usually group A streptococci. Staphylococci are sometimes also found in cellulitis and less frequently *Streptococcus pneumoniae* and *Haemophilus influenzae* (especially on children's faces). Fungi may be involved in immunocompromised patients.

Clinical features
- A wound or ulcer is usually the portal of entry.
- Constitutional upset may occur with fever and malaise.
- Local features include erythema, heat, swelling, pain, or tenderness.
- Lymphadenopathy and lymphangitis are common.
- The leg is the commonest site for infection, but erysipelas occurs on the face.
- Erysipelas has a raised edge; blistering is common and there may be superficial haemorrhage.
- Severe cellulitis may show bullae and can progress to dermal necrosis; it uncommonly proceeds to fasciitis or myositis.

Complications are common without effective treatment: fasciitis, myositis, subcutaneous abscesses, septicaemia and in some streptococcal cases, nephritis. Also, staphylococcal scalded skin syndrome.

Investigations and treatment
Swabs can be taken from eroded or ulcerated surfaces. Vesicle fluid can be cultured. Also blood cultures and serology.

Treatment is with appropriate antibiotics in adequate dosages. In severe cases intravenous antibiotics may be needed.

Impetigo

Impetigo is a contagious superficial pyogenic infection of the skin. Causal organisms are staphylococci and streptococci or both together. In impetigo the epidermis splits just below the stratum granulosum forming large blisters. There are many neutrophils.

Epidemiology

Cases of impetigo peak in the summer. It affects all ages but mostly pre-school and young school-age children. Impetigo can be very widespread in neonates. Factors leading to infection include:

- Poor hygiene and overcrowded conditions (however, it is also commonly found in clean and healthy individuals).
- Existing skin disease.
- Minor abrasions in those with chronic carriage.

Clinical features

- There may or may not be systemic upset.
- Impetigo is highly contagious.
- There is a well localized area of erythema with either vesicles or bullae at center, the bursting to leave.
- The exudate is honey crusted.

Complications and treatment

Complications include deeper infections, e.g. celulitis, post-streptococcal acute glomerulonephritis, scarlet fever, urticaria, and erythema multiforme (but NOT rheumatic fever).

Treatment is with topical antibiotic or oral antibiotic if infection is severe or if there is systemic upset.

Superficial folliculitis

Superficial folliculitis is very common. It is caused by infection of a physical or chemical injury by *Staphylococcus aureus*. It can be acute or chronic and heals without scarring.

Furuncle (boil)

A furuncle is an acute, usually necrotic, infection of a hair follicle with *Staphylococcus aureus*. It is common in adolescence and early adulthood. In the UK furuncles are most common in the winter.

The furuncle starts as a small, follicular, inflammatory nodule and soon becomes pustular then necrotic. The necrotic core discharges to leave a violaceous macule which ultimately heals leaving a permanent scar. Lesions are either single or multiple and appear on the face, neck, arms, wrists, fingers, buttocks, and anogenital region. Attacks consist of single crops, or multiple crops at irregular intervals, with or without periods of freedom.

Treatment is with a systemic antibiotic, e.g. flucloxacillin.

Carbuncle

A carbuncle is a deep infection of a group of follicles with *Staphylococcus aureus*. It occurs in middle aged and old men.

The sites affected are the neck, shoulders, hips, or thighs. The lesion appears as a painful, hard, red lump, which suppurates with an area of central necrosis.

Cutaneous larva migrans

Cutaneous larva migrans is a 'creeping eruption' due to moving parasites in the skin. It can be caused by many different hookworm varieties, the dog hookworm *Ancylostoma braziliense* being the commonest cause in humans.

The adult hookworm lives in the intestines of dogs and cats. The ova are shed in the faeces, and only in the right climate (i.e. humid, warm, moist sandy areas) will the infective larvae be able to hatch. These larvae penetrate human skin that is in contact with them, i.e. through the web spaces of feet when walking barefoot on the beach, or through the buttocks or other parts of the body in contact with the sand, when lying on the beach. The patient complains of a localized area of itching, and an erythematous serpiginous (worm-like) eruption is observed in the affected area. These are the tracks left behind by the moving larvae.

Treatment is with oral albendazole 400 mg/day for 3 days (this may cause gastric upset) and topical thiobendazole 10%.

Scabies

Scabies is caused by the scabies mite *Sarcoptes scabei var. hominis*. This mite is around 0.4 mm long and travels 2 mm/day laying two or three eggs a day.

The scabies mite is spread by direct physical transfer, including sexual contact. The fertilized female mite burrows through the stratum corneum where she lays her eggs. The eggs hatch after 3 days into larvae which form shallow pockets in the stratum corneum where they mature within 2 weeks. Mites mate in these pockets. The male dies but the fertilized female continues to burrow and continues the cycle.

The first signs of itching (pruritus) occurs approximately 4–6 weeks after infection. The pruritus is caused by a hypersensitivity reaction to the mites. Patients develop a secondary eczematous rash and nodules—no mites are present here unless burrows are seen.

The commonest sites include finger web spaces, palms, wrist, arch of feet, and the penis. Scabies rarely infects the face and scalp, except in babies.

Treatment is by one application of permethrin (Lyclear). If infestation is severe the process should be repeated the following week. All close contacts must have the same treatment at the same time.

DERMATOLOGICAL EMERGENCIES

Classification of urticaria and angioedema

- **Chronic**. Idiopathic.
- **Acute**. Food: in childhood milk, eggs, tomatoes, fish, wheat; in adults strawberries, shellfish.
- **Drugs**. Aspirin, opiates, NSAIDs, antibiotics, e.g. penicillins.

- **Hereditary**. C1 esterase inhibitor deficiency.
- **Physical**. Dermographism, cholinergic, cold, sun, heat, pressure.
- **Systemic**. Systemic lupus erythematosus, lymphoma, infestations.

Acute anaphylaxis

Acute anaphylaxis is an exaggerated response to a substance to which an individual has become sensitized. Histamine, serotonin, and other vasoactive substances are released from basophils and mast cells in response to an IgE-mediated reaction.

Clinical features

Symptoms vary; it usually starts with pruritus and rhinitis and may end in death:

- pruritus and rhinitis
- urticaria
- nausea
- vomiting
- diarrhoea
- erythema
- flushing
- angioedema
- laryngeal oedema
- bronchospasm
- hypotension
- cardiovascular collapse and death.

Treatment

Immediate therapy:

- Stop the offending agent.
- Maintain airway with 100% oxygen.
- Lay the patient flat with his or her feet elevated.
- Give adrenaline: intramuscular 0.5 mg to 1 mg (0.5 to 1.0 ml of 1:1000). Repeat every 10 min until blood pressure and pulse are stable.
- Intravenous therapy (colloid).

Secondary therapy:

- Intravenous (IV) antihistamines, e.g. piriton 10 mg IV. This will stop mast cell degranulation.
- Intravenous corticosteroids (100–300 mg hydrocortisone IV). This will deal with the late phase of anaphylaxis.

Long term:

- Patient should have an Epi-pen and Medicalert bracelet.

Erythroderma

Erythroderma is any inflammatory dermatosis which involves all or nearly all of the skin surface (usually more than 90% of the surface area is involved).

Differential diagnosis
- 40% eczema: contact allergic dermatitis, atopic (endogenous), seborrhoeic, unclassified
- 25% psoriasis: pustule psoriasis
- 15% lymphoma: Sezary's syndrome
- 10% drug eruptions
- 1% pityriasis rubra pilaris
- 1% other skin disease
- 8% unknown

Complications
- Dehydration: increased transepidermal water loss; increased capillary permeability.
- Impaired temperature regulation: excess heat loss; failure to sweat.
- Hypoalbuminaemia: increased plasma volume; protein loss in exfoliated scale; protein-losing enteropathy.
- Cutaneous oedema: increased capillary permeability; increased plasma volume; hypoalbuminemia.
- Cardiac failure: increased cardiac output; increased plasma volume.
- Secondary infections: staphylococcal, streptococcal.

Clinical features
- Widespread erythema
- lymphadenopathy related to primary pathology and secondary to widespread inflammation (dermopathic)
- fever
- rigors
- light-headedness
- clinical dehydrated
- widespread oedema
- collapse.

Investigations
Patients must be admitted within 24 h and all cases treated seriously. The following tests should be done:

- swab skin and pustules if present
- perform a septic screen: blood cultures and mid-stream urine
- chest X-ray (if indicated).

Measure vital observations blood pressure, pulserate and temperature at least 4-hourly. Make a fluid balance chart to monitor fluid intake and urine output (insert a urinary catheter if necessary) and measure daily electrolytes.

Treatment
- All patients should receive bland greasy emollients to prevent fluid loss.
- Maintain normal haemodynamics, i.e. intravenous fluids to maintain blood pressure.
- Nutritional support.
- If skin infection is suspected or secondary infection likely, give intravenous antibiotics to cover staphylococci and streptococci.
- If patient is haemodynamically unstable, admit to acute care unit.

The following treatments are specific to the cause and in addition to the above:

- Eczema: treat additionally with systemic prednisolone orally and topical steroids.
- Psoriasis: intramuscular or oral methotrexate.
- Lymphoma: as for eczema.
- Drug induced: stop the offending drug if known.

CARE OF THE ELDERLY

The ageing process is complicated and not completely understood. The body becomes mature around the age of 18 years after which ageing begins. The body replaces and repairs tissue constantly but with ageing this slows down and become less consistent as well as less precise. The process is progressive and irreversible. The ageing mechanism is dependent on several factors including genetic background and environment (including lifestyle):

- hereditary factors
- environment and lifestyle factors:
  - cellular damage from heat, radiation, and metabolism producing free radicals.
  - smoking, which accelerates changes associated with ageing.
  - exercise may improve functional capacity later in life.
  - stress.
  - diet.

The affects of ageing can be seen in every system of the body. Age-related diseases are called degenerative diseases.

Problems associated with ageing

General changes

The presence of **multiple diseases** is very common in the elderly, with multidrug therapy resulting in an ever-increasing list of complications.

Clinical features may be non-specific or present in an uncharacteristic way, e.g. clinical signs of thyroid disease in the elderly may be masked or present atypically with depression (hypothyroidism) or falls. Difficulty and delay in the ability of the body to respond quickly to pathological insults results in sudden and rapid deterioration of major systems, e.g. cardiac and renal failure and life-threatening pneumonia.

Fractures, falls, and mobility problems

Common causes of **fractures** in the elderly are:

- age—there is an increase in falls after the age of 65 years;
- osteoporosis due to loss of bone mass;
- hormonal—perimenopausal vertebral fractures;
- osteoarthritis—increases in incidence with age.

Causes of **falls** in the elderly can be systemic or environmental. Systemic causes ionclude:

- episodic confusion or disorientation due to alcohol, drugs, or hypoglycaemia
- hypotension due to autonomic or drug induced
- arrhythmias
- faints
- dementia
- visual impairment
- Parkinsonism
- cerebrovascular accidents or transient ischaemic attacks (TIAs)
- epilepsy.

Environmental causes of falls include:

- unfamiliar surroundings
- poor lighting
- uneven surfaces
- shoes undone or poorly fitting.

Bone disease is a problem in the elderly which has an impact on the occurrence of fractures and falls:

- Osteoporosis and Paget's disease of the bone are seen increasingly in elderly.
- Vitamin D deficiency causing osteomalacia is not uncommon in elderly people who are sedentary with a poor diet. It can cause problems of diffuse bone pain and lumbar pain. Together with proximal muscle weakness this can lead to falls.
- Age-induced muscle weakness and osteoporosis may cause fractures of the neck of the femur.

Mobility disorders increase with age. The reasons for this are not clear but changes in nerve conduction and loss of muscle mass may be important.

Nervous system

Changes in the **central nervous system** with age are very important because of their impact on intellectual function and communication. However, the reasons for these changes are not well understood. The responses of neurons are variable, with decreases in some areas while other areas maintain the status quo. The changes are also very individualized.

In the **peripheral nervous system** there is a reduction in the conduction of nerve impulses and a number of changes occur in the **autonomic nervous system**:

- modification in the control of heart rate
- baroreceptor responses are decreased, resulting in a reduced postural response with increased hypotensive episodes
- abnormalities of temperature regulation.

Dementia

Half a million people in the UK suffer from dementia, of these 250 000 live in residential care and 250 000 with informal carers. With the increasingly ageing population this number is likely to rise to a million in 20 years' time placing a huge drain on resources.

Dementia in the elderly has a number of **causes**:

- **Alzheimer's disease** is the commonest cause. It affects half a million people in the UK. Early stages may include memory lapses, confusion, especially about recent actions, and emotional lability. Initially sufferers have insight into their problems of intermittent confusion, and become depressed and scared by their increasing loss of memory and control of their environment, eventually becoming withdrawn and unable to cope with daily living.
- Vascular disease causes 25% of cases of dementia, e.g. after a stroke or multiple small infarcts in the brain due to cerebrovascular disease.
- Lewy bodies causes 10–16% cases of dementia: Lewy bodies are structures found within the cytoplasm of nerve cells, leading to degeneration of brain tissue. Memory, language. and concentration are all affected.
- Fronto-temporal dementia, e.g. Pick's disease, causes fewer than 5% of cases of dementia. The frontal area of the brain is affected. Patients lack insight and lose their ability to empathize with others—they may appear selfish and unfeeling. Behavioural changes occur such as loss of inhibitions, becoming very withdrawn or very aggressive, exhibitionism. Sufferers cannot concentrate and may show obsessive-compulsive behaviour. Personality and behaviour are affected more than memory.
- Alcoholic Korsakoff's syndrome causes fewer than 3% of cases of dementia.
- Creutzfeldt–Jacob disease (CJD) causes fewer than 3% of cases of dementia.

Headache and facial pain

Headache and facial pain are a constant source of morbidity in the elderly. Cause of headache and facial pain in the elderly include:

- dental problems including ill fitting dentures
- depression and social isolation
- temporal arteritis
- herpes zoster of the 5th cranial nerve
- atypical facial pain
- trigeminal neuralgia
- oral dysaesthesia
- temporomandibular joint dysfunction.

Endocrine changes

The **menopause** in women is the most evident endocrine change associated with ageing.

With ageing there are decreases in thyroid hormone levels resulting in hypothyroidism, the amount and rate of secretion of insulin secretion, and glucose tolerance with a rise in age-associated diabetes mellitus. There is no change in the secretion and rate of response of the pituitary glands, the response of the adrenals, or the activity of the parathyroid.

Diabetes in elderly may present atypically. The development of complications, e.g. cataract or peripheral vascular disease, may be the first presentation. Visual disturbances secondary to retinopathy and cataracts are common.

Thyroid disease in the elderly is insidious in onset and has atypical clinical features. Both hyper- and hypothyroidism occur but hypothyroidism is more common.

Vision, hearing, taste and smell

- **Presbycusis** or high-tone deafness occurs due to background environmental noise as well as physiological age related loss.
- **Presbyopia** or long sightedness results from a decrease in elasticity of the lens and begins early in life causing symptoms in the late fourth and fifth decades.
- **Hypogeusia** results from loss of taste buds and decline in the sense of smell over the age of 60 years.

Cardiovascular changes and cardiovascular disease

Cardiac output remains unchanged with age. There are decreases in the muscle mass, which is replaced by fibrous tissue, and an increase in myocardial stiffness. The heart rate is increased in the response to physiological change. This results in increases in blood pressure and arrhythmias, such as atrial fibrillation.

The **clinical features of heart disease** in old age are often absent or modified. Cardiac pain may be trivial or absent. Symptoms of breathlessness or hypotension and dizziness may occur during episodes of angina or myocardial infarction. In heart failure fatigue may be the dominant symptom.

Postural hypotension is common in the elderly (a fall of greater than 20 mmHg in the systolic BP may occur on standing). In the dental surgery there may be a drop in blood pressure on rising from dental chair or seating in the reception area. This may give rise to dizziness or syncope.

Gastrointestinal system and liver

- Xerostomia or dry mouth is a major problem resulting commonly from drugs and more rarely from systemic disease.
- Neuroleptic drugs, antidepressants and other antimuscarinic drugs may worsen xerostomia.
- Atrophy of the stomach and small intestine results in impairment of absorption of nutrients.
- There is reduced motility of the large bowel with increased diverticular disease.
- Faecal incontinence affects around 1% of people over the age of 65 years. This results from dementia and anorectal and neurological disorders as well as previous and current laxative abuse. The resultant faecal impaction of the lower bowel can lead to overflow incontinence from liquid faeces.

- The liver decreases in size by 25–30% but its cellular structure and function is unchanged resulting in very little change in liver function except for the metabolism of some drugs.

Genitourinary system

There is a decline in the glomerular filtration rate which falls by 1–2% per year over the age of 45, with consequent problems in excretion of metabolic and drug by products. There is also an increased risk of dehydration because of the decline in response to antidiuretic hormone.

Urinary incontinence affects 10–16% of those aged over 70. Twenty per cent of women over the age of 65 are affected by incontinence. Urinary incontinence in elderly has a number of causes both non-urological:

- generalized systemic illness,
- stroke causing CNS damage,
- behavioural problems,

and urological:

- infection of the bladder or kidneys,
- stress incontinence resulting in loss of urine on coughing or straining,
- urge incontinence due to instability of the bladder detrusor muscle,
- overflow incontinence due to obstruction of the bladder outflow tract by the prostate, constipation, or tumour,
- tumour causing a fistula between the bladder and vagina.

Drug therapy in the elderly

The elderly make up 20% of the population but receive 43% of all prescribed drugs. The main problem with prescribing in the elderly is polypharmacy. The reasons for this are multiple pathology and frequent visits to GPs: this often results in inappropriate prescribing, which occurs in up to 80% of patients.

Drugs	Percentage of total drugs prescribed
• diuretics	25%
• analgesics	20%
• antirheumatic drugs	15–20%
• hypnotics, sedatives, and anxiolytics	15%
• beta-blockers	11%
• digoxin	6%

The complication of drugs commonly used in elderly are shown in Table 17.1.

Pharmacokinetics

Pharmacokinetics is the effect of the body on drug metabolism:

- **Absorption** is relatively unchanged with age
- **Bioavailability**. Reduced first-pass metabolism results in increased circulating levels of drugs. Low albumin levels lead to increased competition for binding sites, e.g. warfarin, sulphonylureas.

Table 17.1 Complications of drugs commonly used in the elderly

Drug	Complications
NSAIDs	Gastric erosion, renal failure
Tricyclic antidepressants	Confusion, dry mouth, postural hypotension, constipation
Warfarin	Bleeding especially post-extraction
ACE inhibitors	Angioedema, renal failure, postural hypotension
Neuroleptics	Athetoid movements, xerostomia or hyperptylism, Parkinsonism, confusion, hypothermia, postural hypotension
Diuretics	Postural hypotension, xerostomia, hypokalaemia, urinary incontinence

- **Volume of distribution**. Changes in the volume of distribution result in the modification of the plasma half-life making it difficult to use as a measure of drug elimination. The reduction in total body water and lean body mass reduce the volume of distribution of water-soluble drugs. Lipid-soluble drugs are increasingly stored in fat, prolonging the half-life of these drugs, e.g. the half-life of diazepam is increased.
- **Metabolism and elimination**. The glomerular filtration rate decreases with age, resulting in reduced elimination of drugs which are normally excreted by the kidney, e. g. penicillin, digoxin, and aminoglycosides. Endogenous production of serum creatinine decreases with age and is not a good indicator of renal function in the elderly. Age-related reduction in hepatic blood flow will reduce clearance of drugs which largely undergo first-pass metabolism (e.g. propranolol, warfarin, and verapamil).

Pharmacodynamics

Pharmacodynamics is the effect of the drug metabolism on the body. These are changes in target organ and sensitivity, receptor responsiveness, and homeostatic responses:

- **Target organ sensitivity**. Responses to beta-adrenoreceptor drugs, both beta blockers and agonists, reduces with age. Synthesis of clotting factors is increased in the elderly.
- Increased brain **receptor sensitivity** results in psychomotor impairment with psychosedative drugs, e.g. benzodiazepines, anticholinergics, opiates. Thiazide diuretics in elderly patients cause of potassium depletion.
- **Homeostatic responses**. Response to drugs may be enhanced or decreased by changes in homeostatic mechanisms. These are:
  - Thermoregulation: phenothiazines, many other centrally sedating drugs, alcohol, postural control sedative drugs.

- Orthostatic circulatory responses: antihypertensives, diuretics, ACE inhibitors, nitrates, phenothiazines, tricyclic antidepressants, levodopa.
- Visceral muscle function (bowel, bladder and eye): anticholinergic drugs, diuretics.
- Cognitive function: cholinergic transmission, digoxin, cimetidine, NSAIDs.

Compliance

Compliance is a common problem. It is estimated that between 30 and 50% of patients are non compliant. This may be due to:

- Poor motivation—especially if the person is asymptomatic.
- Elderly people become confused with the numbers and different treatment protocols for different drugs.
- Elderly people may find labelling confusing and may have poor vision.
- Practical problems—taste, size, and 'sticking', and inability to open bottle tops or use inhalers.
- Patients find it difficult to follow instructions and frequently forget to take medication.

Common dental problems in the general elderly population

- General dental problems: patients may be edentulous, suffer from periodontal disease or xerostomia, and have poor alveolar bone to support dentures.
- Headache and facial pain: temporal arteritis, atypical facial pain, herpes zoster, trigeminal neuralgia.
- Specific tooth problems: root caries, teeth are brittle and chip easily, soft tissue is atrophic.
- Mucosal lesions: ulcers, keratosis, squamous cell carcinoma.

Elderly patients in residential and nursing homes

Elderly patients in residential and nursing homes are not given adequate access to proper basic dental care (see Table 17.2). Residents have increased rates of dental pathology because of:

- Lack of perceived need by the patient.
- Lack of perceived need by carers. Help is usually only sought when either the resident or a relative complains of a broken denture or an acute problems such as pain.
- Lack of knowledge by carers or patients about accessing dental care.
- The elderly may be unable to express their needs, e.g. following a stroke.

There are a number of specific problems concerning dental treatment of the elderly in the dental surgery. These are discussed below.

Anaesthesia

- Local anaesthesia is preferred.
- Avoid intravenous sedation in the dental chair in patients with cerebrovascular disease, hypertension, or cardiovascular disease.

Table 17.2 Dental problems in the elderly in residential care

Dental problem	% of dentulous residents[†]
Caries	20
Periodontal disease	75
Poor oral hygiene	80
Difficulty eating	25
Problems with taste perception	22
Practical difficulty in maintaining oral hygiene either cleaning their dentures or brushing their teeth	30

[†]Forty per cent of the elderly in residential care are edentulous.

BOX 17.1 Dental relevance of ageing

- Only 37% of those aged 65–75 years and 27% of those over 75 years are registered with a dentist.
- In the elderly poor dental health together with a diminished ability to communicate results in increased morbidity including problems with speech, eating and chewing, weight loss, dehydration, and incapacity.
- Patients have who are edentulous or have ill-fitting dentures suffer pain, discomfort and functional limitation, which may lead to social embarrassment and isolation.

- Benzodiazepines are preferred to opioids for sedation.
- The risks of general anaesthesia are increased because of the altered pharmacodynamics.
- General anaesthesia predisposes patients to diverse complications, e.g. pneumonia, pulmonary embolism, deep vein thrombosis.

Mobility
- Domiciliary visits may be necessary because of a reduction in mobility and increasing frailty.
- People using wheelchairs and walking frames may have difficulty with access into the dental surgery and chair.
- The elderly are prone to falls.

Positioning
- Elderly patients dislike been treated in the supine position.
- The supine position may provoke breathlessness, e.g. congestive cardiac failure, be uncomfortable due to arthritis or kyphosis, or be life-threatening in patients with rheumatoid arthritis of the cervical spine.
- The supine position can worsen postural hypotension.

CARE OF CHILDREN

Childhood is a time of rapid physical, mental, intellectual, and emotional growth. Children are not mini-adults and their experience of pathology and responses to environmental stress and medication is unique. They are prone to acute illnesses, especially infections. The average child in the UK experiences 10–12 infective episodes in the first year of life.

Fever

Fever is a common symptom in children. Normal body temperature fluctuates between 36.1 °C (97 °F) and 37.4 °C (99.3 °F), being lower in the morning and higher in the evening. Temperatures are considered raised when the temperatue is >37.8 °C (100.0 °F) orally or in the ear, >37.2 °C (99.0 °F) in the axilla, or >38 °C (100.4 °F) measured rectally.

Causes of fever in children include:

- Viral infections: childhood exanthems, e.g. mumps, rubella, measles; rhinoviruses and coronaviruses (common cold); influenza; encephalitis.
- Bacterial infections: ear infections; streptococcal sore throat; urinary tract infections; topical dermatological infections; bacterial meningitis; pneumonia.
- Other causes include: teething; recent vaccination; crises in sickle cell disease; autoimmune disorders; ulcerative colitis flare; malignant disease.

Treatment of fever consists of:

- Immediate management: sponge baths with tepid water (children with very high temperatures may need cooler water); prevent dehydration by watching fluid intake; paracetamol or ibuprofen are suitable anti-pyretics (do not give aspirin because it may precipitate Reye's syndrome).
- Treat the underlying problem.
- Children with persistent high temperature should be referred for special investigations.

Vaccination

Diphtheria, tetanus, pertussis (whooping cough) (DTP)

Diphtheria is caused by *Corynebacterium diphtheriae* which produces a potent toxin and severe respiratory tract inflammation by coating the mucous membrane of the respiratory tract with a thick fibrinous exudate. The toxin causes degeneration of peripheral nerves and cardiac muscle. The disease results in 20–30% of patients dying.

Tetanus is caused by *Clostridium tetani* found in animal faeces and as spores in soil. It causes infection by contamination of an open wound or cut. The organism produces a powerful neurotoxin which attaches to the motor neurons causing painful rigid muscle spasms (tetany). These are particularly severe in the neck and jaw (lockjaw) and cause dysphagia. Pain is intense. Twenty per cent of patients who contract tetanus die.

Pertussis (whooping cough) is caused by *Bordetella pertussis* which has two stages: a catarrhal stage similar to a cold and a paroxysmal stage of ferocious 'whooping 'coughing associated with cyanosis and vomiting.

The diphtheria, tetanus, and pertussis vaccines are usually combined and given as a single injection. They can be given separately or in different combinations. The vaccination schedule is:

- First dose at 2 months.
- Second dose at 3–4 months.
- Third dose at 4–6 months.
- Booster of tetanus and low-dose diphtheria vaccines at 15–18 years.

Hib

Haemophilus influenzae type b (Hib) infection can cause serious illness, e.g meningitis, severe croup, septicaemia, pneumonia, and joint and bone infections. A child under the age of 13 months needs a course of three doses given by injection. After the age of 4 years acquired immunity is adequate and Hib becomes unnecessary. No boosters are needed for Hib immunization.

Hib may be offered as a separate injection at the same time as the DTP and polio vaccines, or it may be combined with the DTP.

Polio

Poliomyelitis is caused by poliovirus. The virus affects the anterior horn cells in the spinal cord, causing muscular paralysis. If the muscles of the upper and lower limbs are involved permanent paralysis may ensue. Severe infection may affect the respiratory centre causing life-threatening complications.

A course of three doses of the vaccine is given by mouth at the same time as DTP and Hib vaccines. Single booster doses are given at $3\frac{1}{2}$–5 years (school entry) and at 15–18 years (school leaving).

Measles, mumps, and rubella (MMR)

Measles is highly infectious. It starts like a cold with nasal stuffiness and rhinitis with intra-oral Koplick spots, after which ear infections, bronchitis, and pneumonia develop. Cerebral complications include convulsions, blindness, and brain damage. The morbidity and mortality is high.

Mumps causes painful swelling of the parotid glands. Serious complications include deafness, meningitis, and brain damage. Testicular involvement may result in sterility.

Rubella although rubella is mild in children, it can cause serious complications to the fetus if a pregnant woman who has not had the disease or been immunized comes into contact with the disease during the first 3 to 4 months of her pregnancy. It can result in many severe defects in the fetus, including deafness, blindness, cardiac abnormalities, and brain damage.

The MMR vaccine is offered in a single injection, which gives protection against all three diseases. The vaccination schedule is

- First dose at 15 months (12–24 months).
- Booster dose at 3½–5 years.

The controversy regarding the triple vaccine versus separate vaccines or whether there is an association between the triple vaccine and autism and Crohn's disease led to a public statement in February 2002 by the Royal College of Paediatrics and Child Health, the Public Health Medicine Environmental Group, Community Practitioners and Health Visitors Association, and the Faculty of Public Health Medicine all endorsing the use of the MMR triple vaccine. The debate is ongoing. However, poor uptake of the MMR triple vaccine has lead to sporadic outbreaks of measles.

Tuberculosis (BCG)
The BCG injection is usually offered to children aged 10–14 years after skin tests indicate they have no immunity to TB; however, there is poor uptake. Babies at increased risk of coming into contact with TB are given BCG vaccine within the first 6 weeks of life.

Poisoning in children

More than 40 000 poisoning incidents occur per annum in the UK. The commonest cause of accidental poisoning in children is due to children putting small objects in their mouths or drinking household chemicals, e.g. household cleaners, cosmetics, alcohol, or medication. Forty-five per cent of episodes involve poisoning by two or more toxic agents, e.g. with medication such as analgesics, benzodiazepines, tricyclic antidepressants, cardiac drugs, and ferrous sulphate taken accidentally.

Male teenagers are more likely to unwittingly poison themselves with volatile substances (e.g. solvent abuse). Children aged around 10–15 years under emotional stress sometimes deliberately poison themselves, usually with the drugs of a close adult relative. Deliberate poisoning of children by adults also occurs.

Most deaths from poisoning are from carbon monoxide poisoning, due to faulty gas appliances, and from ingestion of antidepressants.

The **clinical features** of poisoning are variable and depend on the type of poison ingested.

Treatment requires assessment of cardio-respiratory function. Depression of either will need hospital support. Any child thought to have ingested aspirin, paracetamol, ferrous sulphate, or antidepressants should be admitted to hospital and given specific treatment.

> **BOX 17.2** Mechanisms of fluoride toxicity
>
> - If ingested it acts on the intestinal mucosa to form hydrofluoric acid which corrodes the stomach.
> - Absorbed, it binds calcium and magnesium ions leading to hypocalcaemia and hypomagnesaemia disrupting neurotransmission and causing seizures.
> - Metabolically, it blocks glycolytic degradation of glucose.
> - Direct cytotoxicity causing disruption of coagulation, oxidative phosphorylation, and glycolysis. Inhibits Na^+/K^+-ATPase leading to extracellular potassium accumulation.
> - Direct cardiotoxicity caused by vasomotor depression occurs.
> - Direct neurotoxicity caused by calcium binding to enzymes to prevent neurotransmission.
> - Inhibits acetylcholinesterase, which is partly responsible for the cholinergic symptoms of hypersalivation, vomiting, and diarrhoea.
> - Severe toxicity results in multiorgan failure.
> - Death usually results from respiratory paralysis, dysrhythmia, or cardiac failure.

Fluoride poisoning

The estimated toxic dose of fluoride is 5–10 mg/kg body weight, with death occurring at 12–16 mg/kg in children. In children the lethal dose is 500 mg.

Fluoride poisoning is usually accidental in young children. In teenagers it may be either accidental or intentional. Fluoride may be available to children from any of the folowing sources:

- sodium monofluorophosphate in toothpaste (toothpastes contain 1 mg/g of fluoride with low solubility and low risk),
- sodium fluoride in dietary supplements,
- sodium fluoride in insecticides and rodent poisons,
- ammonium bifluoride in chrome cleaning agents.

Clinical features of fluoride poisoning are diverse and widespread:

- Gastrointestinal effects: nausea, vomiting, hypersalivation, mucositis, erosion, dysphagia, diarrhoea, abdominal pain.
- Electrolyte abnormalities: hypocalcaemia, hypomagnesaemia, hypoglycaemia, hyperkalaemia.
- Neurological effects: headache, seizures and faints, tremor, decreased muscle power, muscular spasm, tetany, hyperreflexia.
- Cardiovascular effects: widening of the QRS complex, arrhythmias, cardiogenic shock, cardiac arrest.

After the acute phase jaundice and oliguria develop.

The mainstay of **treatment** is calcium. This competes with the action of fluoride at the cellular level: milk, calcium chloride, calcium gluconate or calcium lactate should be immediately administration to precipitate calcium fluoride.

Calcium chloride is used in preference to calcium gluconate or lactate as it provides more free calcium on an equal volume basis.

Child abuse

Trauma to the head is the main cause of morbidity and mortality in abused children. Skeletal and non-skeletal injuries and fractures are highly suggestive of abuse. Non-skeletal injuries include seizures, unexplained bruises, and retinal haemorrhages due to shaking (the most common cerebral abnormality is a subdural hematoma). Skeletal injuries include fractures inconsistent with the clinical history. These are usually multiple fractures and of different ages, with the extremities being most commonly affected: 55% of children less than 1 year old and 73% of children less than 2 years old present with fractures.

Differential diagnosis—these are all rare but should be considered:

- metabolic bone disease, e.g. rickets, renal osteodystrophy
- osteogenesis imperfecta
- congenital syphilis
- multifocal osteomyelitis
- congenital insensitivity to pain
- Menke's syndrome
- metaphyseal dysostosis
- infantile cortical hyperostosis (Caffey's disease).

Gastrointestinal system

Diarrhoea

Diarrhoea is defined as a stool volume of more than 200 ml/m^2/day or a stool weight of more than 150–200 g watery stool/m^2/day. In infancy and early childhood diarrhoea it is defined as an increase in stool frequency with the development of loose or watery stools.

Characteristics of diarrhoea are a sudden increase in number of stools, lessening of stool consistency, watery stools, and a propensity for the stools to change colour and become yellow or green. Acute diarrhoea lasts less than 2 weeks after which it becomes chronic.

Causes diarrhoea in childhood include:

- acute gastroenteritis—this is the commonest cause of acute diarrhoea;
- infection due to viruses, bacteria, or parasites—an important cause of diarrhoea in developing countries;
- ear infection;
- urinary tract infection;
- contaminated food and water;
- person to person contact in cases of diarrhoea caused by infection.
- Other causes include antibiotic therapy, food allergy, malabsorption, and introduction of new foods into an infant's diet.

Gastroenteritis

Gastroenteritis is diarrhoea accompanied by vomiting. Differential diagnosis of gastroenteritis are:

- infections, including upper respiratory infections, meningitis, septicaemia, and urinary tract infection;
- acute appendicitis;
- food intolerance, e.g. to cows' milk protein;
- pyloric stenosis or tumour;
- intussusception.
- coeliac disease.

Gastroenteritis has the following **clinical features**:

- Abdominal cramps which occur before the onset of diarrhoea.
- Fever.
- Dehydration secondary to excessive water loss. This is the most important clinical feature in childhood gastroenteritis. Signs of dehydration include listlessness, dry lips and tongue, skin that is pale and dry, reduced tissue turgor, and sunken eyes.

The following **investigations** need to be performed:

- Examine the stool for bacteria, viruses, and parasites.
- Culture bacteria from the stool, urine, ears, throat, blood, and CSF as indicated.
- Estimate the degree of dehydration (see Table 17.3).
- Check the electrolyte balance.

Treatment of diarrhoea/gastroenteritis involves:

- Oral rehydration with replacement fluids and minerals; this is the mainstay of treatment.

Table 17.3 Degree of dehydration: amount of body fluid lost expressed as a percentage of the total body weight

Fluid loss	Classification	Signs
<2–3%	Very mild dehydration	No clinical signs
3–5%	Mild dehydration	Loss of tissue turgor
5%	Moderate dehydration	Loss of skin turgor, depressed fontanelle, sunken eyes, extremities warm
>10%	Severe and often fatal	As above plus tachycardia and cold extremities

- The intake of clear liquids should be increased.
- Intravenous fluids are required only when the child is 10% dehydrated.
- Food that normally gives a child loose bowel movements, as well as milk, should be avoided.
- Symptomatic relief for cramps using muscle relaxant.

Colic

Colic is the occurrence of severe recurrent bouts of crying in an otherwise healthy baby. It is common, usually begins at 2–3 weeks of age, and may last for 3 months. The cause is unknown. Crying usually starts in the early evening and may continue for several hours.

It is important to exclude other causes of abdominal pain. Check for signs of pyrexia, upper respiratory tract, ear, or urinary infection, abdominal swelling, diarrhoea and/or vomiting, and blood in the stool.

There is no specific medication for colic, and the parents should be given reassurance.

Cardiovascular system

Cardiovascular defects occur as common congenital defects. One in every 145 births has a cardiac defect, resulting in 4600 children being born each year with cardiac abnormalities. There are 150 000 people aged 16 years or older who have a cardiac defect, of whom 12 000 have complex abnormalities.

Congenital cardiac defects include:

- **Atrial septal defect**: patent foramen ovale.
- **Ventricular septal defect**: this is the most common congenital heart defect.
- **Atrioventricular septal defect**: there is an opening between the aorta and the ventricles in this defect and only one atrioventricular valve is present.
- **Coarctation of the aorta**: there is a stricture of the descending or thoracic aorta, resulting in a high blood pressure proximal to stricture which is usually in the upper limbs.
- **Patent ductus arteriosus** is more common in girls (female : male ratio 2 : 1). The ductus arteriosus is the connection between the pulmonary artery and the aorta of the normal fetal heart. It does not close but remains patent after birth and allows shunting of oxygenated blood from the aorta back to the pulmonary artery.
- **Tetralogy of Fallot**. This the most serious congenital defect. It is a combination of four defects—pulmonary valve stenosis which is due to a stricture into the pulmonary artery restricting blood flow to the lungs; ventricular septal defect which allows oxygenated blood to flow from the left to the right ventricle; hypertrophy of the right ventricle due to increased workload; and an abnormally placed aorta which opens over the ventricular septal defect allowing blood from both ventricles into the aorta. The consequence of the

combination of defects is central and peripheral cyanosis which increases with age. Other symptoms include dyspnoea, failure to thrive, and frequent upper respiratory tract infection. Toddlers tend to squat to increase venous return and reduce dyspnoea.

• **Transposition of the great arteries**. The aorta originates at the right ventricle in place of the pulmonary artery. The pulmonary artery originates at the left ventricle in place of the aorta. The result is the circulation of deoxygenated blood. The resultant defect is fatal.

The **cause** of congenital heart defects is unknown in most cases:

• Genetic and environmental factors are both contributing factors. Examples of genetic/chromosomal disorders associated with cardiac abnormalities include Down's syndrome (trisomy 21), Turner's syndrome, Marfan's syndrome, Noonan syndrome, and Holt–Oram syndrome.
• Systemic disease in a pregnancy may predispose to congenital defects. Some of these are phenylketonuria, rubella, systemic lupus erythematosus, and diabetes mellitus.
• Drugs such as cocaine, alcohol, thalidomide, phenytoin, isoretinoin, and lithium.

The **clinical features** are usually variable and depend on the severity of the defect. In severe cases there may be:

• malaise
• irritability
• difficulty feeding and failure to thrive
• cyanosis
• dyspnoea (child may squat to improve venous return)
• fainting
• cough and/or wheezing
• tachypnoea and or tachycardia
• weak pulses
• cold peripheries
• clubbing of fingers and toes
• hepatomegaly
• oliguria
• swelling around the eyes and swollen abdomen and/or legs.

Ear, nose, and throat

Middle ear infection
Middle ear infections are acute otitis media (AOM) and otitis media with effusion (OME). AOM is common in children with 70% of cases occurring before the age of 10 years. It is more common in boys. OME is also common, with 80% of episodes occurring in children less than 4 years old.

Streptococcus pneumoniae and *Haemophilus influenzae* are the main causative organisms, and occasionally *Moraxella catarrhalis*.

Clinical features are as follows:

- In AOM: earache, fever, history of upper respiratory tract infection, tugging or rubbing ear, irritability, immobile ear drum which may discharge pus, hearing loss.
- In OME: earache, loss of balance, behavioural problems, speech problems, impaired drum mobility, hearing loss; irritability and fever are usually absent.

The infection usually lasts a few days, but persisting deafness may last a few weeks.

Treatment differs for AOM and OME:

- For AOM: analgesia for pain (paracetamol or ibuprofen not aspirin); decongestants and antihistamines are of no benefit; if indicated, a 5-day course of amoxicillin.
- For OME: for bilateral disease with >25 dB hearing loss surgery may be indicated, with the insertion of grommets. An ENT specialist should screen children older than 3 years who have poor language development or behavioural problems.

Immune and respiratory systems

Allergy

In the UK 1 in 3 people has an allergy-related problem. One to 2% of children have a food allergy. All children may develop allergies, but atopic children are at greater risk. Children commonly show allergies to peanuts, milk, avocado, medication, bee and wasp stings, kiwi fruit, and latex. Common allergic disorders in children are eczema, atopic asthma, food allergies, and hay fever.

Clinical features of allergic reactions in children are:

- coughing, which may be persistent without obvious precipitating cause,
- rhinitis,
- itchy eyes, ears, lips, palate, and throat,
- sneezing,
- wheezing,
- shortness of breath,
- vomiting and diarrhoea,
- nettle rash or hives.

Eczema

Eczema develops in 8–20% of children. The disease is usually mild, but results in a thousand hospital admissions a year. Eczema disappears in 75% of children by around 16–17 years of age. Eczema in infants is usually mild and may be confined to the face, flexures, and scalp.

Acute eczema involves dry skin, with itching weeping and scaling. In chronic eczema the inflamed skin becomes thickened and lichenified and scaling increases with fissuring.

Most children respond well to **treatment** with emollients and topical steroids and pimecrolimus. Resistant cases are treated with tacrolimus in specialist units.

Asthma

Asthma is a common chronic condition in children. Eight to twelve per cent of children in the population are affected. In the 12 months from August 2002 to August 2003, around 4 million asthma attacks occurred in children in the UK. Asthma is an important cause of absenteeism from school. Most children who suffer from asthma have atopic asthma.

Clinical features vary according to age:

- In very young children (0–3 years): wheezing, coughing, which may be worse at night, and recurrent colds.
- In children aged 3–5 years: as above, including early morning coughing, malaise and listlessness.

Symptoms are exacerbated by allergens, upper respiratory tract infections, exercise, tobacco smoke, and pollution and dust.

Treatment for asthma is with:

- Beta agonists such as salbutamol and terbutaline and the longer-acting salmeterol, the effect of which lasts for 12 h; these relax bronchiolar muscles.
- Steroids by inhaler and systemically in pulsed doses in severe cases.
- Cromones such as sodium cromoglicate and nedocromil which act to reduce inflammation are more effective in children than in adults.
- Anti-leucotrienes such as montelukast and zafirlukast which antagonize airway constriction. Montelukast is licensed for children over 2 years and zafirlukast for children over 12 years.

Pneumonia

Infection of the alveoli is common in children. In children between 3 months and 6 years 85–90% of cases are caused by the virus *Haemophilus influenzae* and 10% of cases are caused by bacteria *Streptococcus pneumoniae*. Between 5 and 35 years the most common cause is *Mycoplasma pneumoniae*.

The **clinical features** of bacterial pneumonia are:

- productive cough
- high temperature and fever
- chills
- chest pain
- dyspnoea.

Viral pneumonia has clinical features as above with rhinitis and pleural effusion. If *Haemophilus influenzae* type b is the causative organism children may develop severe epiglottis and/or meningitis.

Mycoplasma pneumonia lasts longer than viral or bacterial pneumonia. Sufferers usually develop a dry non-productive cough, with malaise and rash. Later the cough becomes productive.

Treatment depends on the cause:

- Antibiotics are the mainstay treatment in bacterial or mycoplasma pneumonia.
- For pneumonia resulting from measles or herpes simplex antibiotics should be used as the pneumonia is commonly a secondary bacterial infection.
- Treatment of viral pneumonia is supportive. Pneumonia caused by *Haemophilus influenzae* type b can be prevented by the Hib vaccine.

Central nervous system

Seizures and fits in children

In England about 400 000 people suffer from epilepsy; it is the commonest neurological condition in children. Almost a thousand people die every year during or after a seizure, and teenagers die of epilepsy suddenly in their sleep without any other known cause. Childhood problems of epilepsy are compounded by frequent misdiagnosis.

Triggers for an epileptic seizure in children include:

- hunger
- tiredness
- non-compliance with medication
- flashing lights
- sudden loud noises
- stress and anxiety
- boredom
- extreme heat
- dehydration or excessive liquid intake
- menstruation
- alcohol.

There are a number of seizure types which have different **clinical features**:

- Absence seizures. The child abruptly becomes unaware of their surroundings and stares ahead. The attacks may occur several times a day. Seizures may affect school-work and concentration.
- Tonic–clonic seizures. The clinical features are the same as in adults; however, incontinence and confusion are more common post-ictally.
- Myoclonic seizures. Jerks or contractions of muscles occur suddenly. Associated with brief episodes of loss of consciousness. There is no post-ictal confusion.
- Atonic seizures. The child unexpectedly drops to the ground with the sudden relaxation of the muscles. There is very brief loss of consciousness with almost instantaneous recovery.

Table 17.4 Treatments used in childhood epilepsy

Type of seizure	Treatment
Tonic–clonic seizure	Carbamazepine or sodium valproate
Absence seizure	Sodium valproate or ethoximide
Partial seizures	Carbamazepine, phenytoin or sodium valproate
Poorly controlled seizures	Combination of drugs
Refractive epilepsy	Ketogenic diet may help

- Tonic seizures. The child falls to the ground as the muscles suddenly contract. Breathing may also become difficult.
- Complex partial seizures. The child appears conscious but cannot communicate and does not respond to commands. There may be repetitive behaviour such as tugging or pulling at the clothes or hair.
- Febrile seizures. Occur in 2–5% of all children when running a high temperature. Clinically they are usually simple fits, which may recur.

In the acute phase the **treatment** is supportive and symptomatic. Not all seizures need treatment. The chance of recurrence after an initial episode is only 30%, but this increases to 75% after the third fit. Forty per cent of deaths from seizures are avoidable and it is estimated that about 80% of children receive inadequate treatment for their seizures.

Care should be taken with medication. Drugs used in adults may not work or may be harmful in children. Commonly used drugs are shown in Table 17.4.

Cerebral palsy

Cerebral palsy is characterized by the failure to fully control motor function. Motor function affects mobility, speech, eating, and swallowing. Involuntary movements and problems with muscle tone occur. In severe cases of mental retardation, epilepsy may cause great limitation to the quality of life.

Cerebral palsy is caused by hypoxia affecting the brain of the fetus during pregnancy or delivery or in premature babies. It can also arise from trauma to the head in neonates as a result of accident or child abuse, and from viral infections or lead poisoning.

There are a number of types of cerebral palsy having different **clinical features**:

- Spastic cerebral palsy is the most common type of cerebral palsy. It affects the muscle tone, which is increased causing spastic jerky movements of the limbs.
- Ataxic cerebral palsy affects the muscle tone, which is decreased resulting in poor coordination. People with ataxic cerebral palsy are unsteady on their feet with a pronounced tremor.

- Athetoid cerebral palsy affects the muscle tone, which is intermittently increased or decreased resulting problems with posture and position and involuntary movements affecting both the face and the limbs.
- Quadriplegia affects all four limbs. Children with quadriplegia have general movement disorders affecting the limbs, face, and trunk.
- Hemiplegia affects one side of the child's body only. Mobility is usually normal with one side either limping or dragging during walking or running.
- Diplegia is very rare. It affects only the lower limbs not the upper limbs, causing problems with mobility of the lower body.

Treatment should be by a combined multidisciplinary approach with speech and language therapy, occupational therapy, physiotherapy, medical intervention, family support services, and early education with use of assistive technology.

Autism

Autism is a disability that affects the way in which a person communicates and interacts with the people around them. One in every 2000 people has an autistic spectrum disorder. Autism is more common in boys than girls (male:female ration 4 : 1). The autistic spectrum includes Asperger's syndrome in which children display characteristics of autism but are of average or above average intelligence and have good communication skills.

Clinical features are variable; they include:

- Difficulty with verbal and non-verbal communication: an inability to value social interaction; talking 'at' rather than 'with' people; limited and eccentric use of language with the use of a few repetitive words and phrases.
- Difficulty with developing imagination: inability to interact or play imaginatively with objects, animals or people; limited or no understanding or appreciation of emotions, ideas, and beliefs of their own or others; inability to comprehend gestures, facial expression, or change of vocal tone; inappropriate gesturing.
- Difficulty with social relationships: appearance of being detached and apathetic; interaction when it occurs is usually inappropriate, and repetitive; appearance of being oblivious to the other person's response.
- Other features include poor coordination and difficulties with fine control of movement.

The **causes of autism** are unknown but may be due to problems influencing the development of the brain before, during, or after birth. There is probably a genetic basis, but as yet no genes have been identified. Other factors include maternal rubella, hypoxia at birth, childhood infections, e.g. measles, herpes simplex, pertussis, and tuberous sclerosis.

There is no specific **treatment** for autism. Parental support and structured support for the child, namely specialized education and behaviour therapy, are important.

Attention deficit hyperactivity disorder (ADHD) or
attention deficit disorder (ADD)
ADHD/ADD affects 3–5% of children in the United States. Five per cent of 5–15-year-old children in the UK have significant conduct disorders.

There are three types of disorder with differing clinical features:

- Inattentive (previously known as attention deficit disorder, or ADD): child is easily distracted, unable to pay attention to details, unable or unwilling to following directions, is forgetful and misplaces objects.
- Hyperactive–impulsive (previously known as attention deficit hyperactivity disorder, or ADHD): child fidgets and wriggles, blurts out answers before hearing the full question, is impatient, and shows inappropriate behaviour such as running or jumping around when it is customary to sit quietly.
- Combined: the most common clinical type Signs from both ADHD and ADD with or without hyperactivity.

Diagnosis made if the behaviour is present before the age 7 and lasts for 6 months or more and if the behaviour negatively affects two or more areas of the child's life, e.g. school, home, or social life.

Treatment is by behaviour management using specific validated programmes. The use of specific medication is uncommon in Europe.

Reye's syndrome
Reye's syndrome is an acute encephalopathy which may be precipitated by aspirin in children under age of 12 years. It is characterized by symptoms of lethargy, nausea and vomiting, hepatomegaly, and seizures with resultant coma and often death.

Urinary system

Urinary tract infection (UTI) in children
Urinary tract infections in children are common, with 2–8% of children developing UTIs. During a UTI more than 10 000 organisms are found per ml of voided urine (which is normally sterile).

Young children may have few **signs and symptoms**. The most common feature is pyrexia with or without vomiting. Other symptoms include bedwetting, odorous urine, frequency, urgency (wetting in class or nursery in a toilet-trained child).

Treatment involves teaching children correct toilet hygiene and maintaing good hydration. The antibiotics nitrofurantoin and cephalosporins may be given. In chronic UTIs long-term antibiotics will decrease risk of pyelonephritis. Any anatomical abnormalities of the urinary system can be dealt with surgically.

Nocturnal enuresis (bedwetting)
Nocturnal enuresis is the involuntary passage of urine at night or during sleep. Enuretic incontinence is normal under 2 years of age. The reason for this is that

before this age the sacral spinal reflex arc is solely responsible for control of urination. At 2–2½ years the nervous system has matured enough for cortical control to govern the spinal reflex allowing voluntary control of enuresis. Boys are slower to become dry at night than girls: at 3½ years 75–80% are dry at night, at 5½ years 10% wet the bed once a week, and at 15 years 1% wet the bed.

Causes of nocturnal enuresis are:

- normal variation in development
- organic disease: urinary tract infection, diabetes mellitus, diabetes insipidus
- neurovesical dysfunction
- obstructive overflow.

Treatment of nocturnal enuresis is by behavioural therapy, e.g. reward, or cognitive therapy, e.g. a bedwetting alarm. Any underlying organic problems should be treated.

Other conditions

Phenylketonuria

Phenylketonuria is common in northern Europeans and Asians but not in Africans. It is inherited as a recessive disorder in which a child has low or defective phenylalanine hydroxylase meaning that dietary phenylalanine cannot be properly utilized. Phenylalanine accumulates in the body and brain causing brain damage and severe mental retardation. All babies are tested for phenylkeonuria within 48–72 h of birth after feeding has begun.

Phenylketonuria shows few symptoms in early infancy except listlessness, vomiting, and poor feeding. Typical clinical features develop in early childhood if the condition is untreated:

- child looks fairer than sibs
- microcephaly
- delayed tooth eruption
- misshapen jaws
- mental retardation
- eczema
- seizures
- urine has a characteristic mousy smell
- hyperactivity and attention deficit disorder.

Dietary measures are very important in the **treatment** of phenylketonuria. A low-phenylalanine diet is essential. The diets of affected children and adults can be supplemented with special formulas low in phenylalanine but containing other essential amino acids. People with phenylketonuria should avoid dairy products, including milk, meat, eggs, fish, and aspartame sweetener (which contain phenylalanine).

Table 17.5 Risk of having a Down's syndrome child versus maternal age

Maternal age (years)	Risk
25	1 : 1250
26	1 : 952
35	1 : 378
40	1 : 106

Table 17.6 Features associated with Down's syndrome

Feature	Percentage affected
Cardiac abnormalities, e.g. atrial septal defect	>50
Visual problems: squinting, hyper- or hypometropia, cataracts in 3rd to 4th decade	50
Hearing problems	30–40
Dementia in early 4th decade	25
Endocrine abnormalities, e.g. hypothyroidism	10
Intestinal malformations	10

Down's syndrome

Down's syndrome results from a genetic defect, in most cases trisomy 21. The risk of having a child with Down's syndrome increases with maternal age (Table 17.5).

A number of assiciated problems are found in Down's patients (Table 17.6). **Clinical features** are variable. The facies are characteristic but other features vary depending on severity:

- flat round face
- upward slant to the eyes with prominent epicanthic skin folds
- small flat nose
- small ears of variable profile
- large tongue
- single crease across the centre of the palm
- fifth finger has only one flexion furrow instead of two
- extra space between the big toe and the second toe
- floppy with decreased muscle tone
- hyperflexible joints.

Treatment is symptomatic. Assess the child for speech and language impairments as well as learning disability. Treat any endocrine disorder. If a cardiac defect is present antibiotic cover will be needed for dental treatment.

Table 17.7 Sequence of tooth eruption

Teeth	Age of eruption
Maxillary central incisors	6 months
Mandibular lateral incisors	7–8 months
Upper lateral incisors	8–9 months
First primary molars	1 year
Primary canines	16 months
2nd primary molars	2 years
Lower first permanent molars and central incisors	6 years
Central and lateral incisors	7–8 years
Lateral incisors	8–9 years
2nd premolars and canines	11–12 years
1st premolars	10–11 years

Down's syndrome patients may also need hearing and visual assessments and treatment.

Dental relevance of childhood disorders

The teeth and supporting tissues are developing dynamically during childhood. Congenital and systemic disease, trauma, nutrition, and medication may all have deleterious effects with serious consequences for the dentition.

The **eruption sequence** of the dentition is shown in Table 17.7: there may be some variation. Common causes of abnormal eruption times are Down's syndrome, congenital heart disease, thyroid disorders, and ectodermal dysplasia.

Gingivitis is due to collection of plaque around the teeth. It is nearly always reversible.

Malocclusion has a number of causes:

- Heredity, with variation in the skeletal morphology in relation to tooth size and eruption pattern.
- Variation from the usual eruption sequence.
- Habits, e.g. thumb sucking. Many children derive reassurance from thumb sucking; however, continued sucking after the age of 4–5 years affects the path of eruption and may result in malocclusion.

Both breast-feeding and bottle feeding can cause **tooth decay**. The nipple or teat when used as a pacifier causes milk to persist and collect around the anterior teeth. The lactose in breast and cow's milk is converted to acid. A healthy diet will not protect children from caries and periodontal disease. Important factors are oral hygiene and fluoride daily or in fissure sealants.

Trauma to the teeth is relatively common and frequently involves the front teeth. The most common age at which accidents occur is 9–10 years: twice as many boys as girls damage their teeth in accidents. Trauma usually results from minor accidents and falls and sports injuries. Trauma to the primary dentition does not usually cause damage to the permanent dentition under the age of 3 years, and does not affect growth pattern of teeth or speech.

Avulsion of a tooth from the permanent dentition is common during **trauma to the face**. If the tooth is left outside the mouth for more than 30 min reimplantation has less chance of success. Occasionally, the replanted tooth may begin to resorb, loosen, and fall out after a few months or years. If the tooth is fractured or chipped tooth but not avulsed, restoration of the tooth is usually undertaken.

Tongue piercing is associated with periodontal disease, chipping of the teeth, swelling of the tongue, problems with talking, chewing, and swallowing, metal hypersensitivity, and sialorrhoea.

Children with **congenital cardiac disease** patients need antibiotic cover during dental treatment.

Down's syndrome children have specific problems:

- they may need antibiotic cover if they have a cardiac defect;
- visual and hearing defects may make communication difficult;
- hypothyroidism impedes mental development increasing problems with communication;
- macroglossia makes intraoral access difficult.

Children with **attention deficit disorder** have difficulty sitting in the dental chair and cooperating during treatment; they may need sedation.

Index